ATLAS OF X-LINKED INTELLECTUAL DISABILITY SYNDROMES

ATLAS OF X-LINKED INTELLECTUAL DISABILITY SYNDROMES

SECOND EDITION

Roger E. Stevenson, M.D.

SENIOR CLINICAL GENETICIST

GREENWOOD GENETIC CENTER

GREENWOOD, SOUTH CAROLINA

Charles E. Schwartz, Ph.D.

DIRECTOR OF RESEARCH

GREENWOOD GENETIC CENTER

GREENWOOD, SOUTH CAROLINA

R. Curtis Rogers, M.D.

SENIOR CLINICAL GENETICIST

GREENWOOD GENETIC CENTER

GREENWOOD, SOUTH CAROLINA

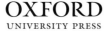

OXFORD
UNIVERSITY PRESS

OXFORD
UNIVERSITY PRESS

Oxford University Press, Inc., publishes works that further
Oxford University's objective of excellence
in research, scholarship, and education.

Oxford   New York
Auckland   Cape Town   Dar es Salaam   Hong Kong   Karachi
Kuala Lumpur   Madrid   Melbourne   Mexico City   Nairobi
New Delhi   Shanghai   Taipei   Toronto

With offices in
Argentina   Austria   Brazil   Chile   Czech Republic   France   Greece
Guatemala   Hungary   Italy   Japan   Poland   Portugal   Singapore
South Korea   Switzerland   Thailand   Turkey   Ukraine   Vietnam

Library of Congress Cataloging-in-Publication Data
Stevenson, Roger E., 1940-
Atlas of X-linked intellectual disability syndromes/Roger E. Stevenson, Charles E. Schwartz, and R. Curtis Rogers.–2nd ed.
p. ; cm.
Rev. ed of: X-linked mental retardation / Roger E. Stevenson, Charles E. Schwartz, Richard J. Schroer. 2000.
Includes bibliographical references and index.
ISBN 978–0–19–981179–3 (alk. paper)
1. X-linked mental retardation–Atlases.   I. Schwartz, Charles E.   II. Rogers, R. Curtis (Richard Curtis), 1953-
III. Stevenson, Roger E., 1940-X-linked mental retardation.   IV. Title.
[DNLM: 1. Mental Retardation, X-Linked–Atlases. QS 17]
RC574.S77 2012
616.85'88042—dc23
2011024318

1 3 5 7 9 8 6 4 2
Printed in the United States of America
on acid-free paper

This Atlas is dedicated to all persons with X-linked intellectual disability, to their families, to the physicians that provide medical care, to the scientists that seek to understand the underlying biology, and to the memory of Ethan Francis Schwartz 1996–1998.

TABLE OF CONTENTS

FOREWORD

The Greenwood Genetic Center in South Carolina was established in 1974 through the efforts of Roger Stevenson and his associates to provide a diagnostic and assessment service for the state for those with intellectual disability (ID). During the eighties and nineties the major contribution of X-linked genes to ID became accepted. This stimulated the Center to publish in 2000 a now classic book entitled *X-Linked Mental Retardation*. The first half gave an account of the history of X-linked ID and the second half was an atlas with pictures and clinical details of the affected males from published families. It included 125 different syndromes. In many, linkage studies had identified the gene location but in only very few had the responsible gene mutation been identified.

This second edition of the *Atlas* is a marvelous 10-year update. It will be essential not only as a reference book for medical geneticists but also for molecular laboratories providing a gene screening service. Over the past ten years since the publication of the previous edition, around 100 genes and their mutations have been identified in those with clinical syndromes and over 33 in 95 families with nonsyndromic XLID. Some clinical diagnoses have now been recognized as different manifestations of the same gene as in the 24 base-pair duplications in the *ARX* gene. There has also been a merging of the syndromic with the non-syndromic, as families have been found in which different affected members may have features of either syndromic or non-syndromic ID but carry the same mutation.

Atlas of X-Linked Intellectual Disability Syndromes will have two main functions. The first is as a help in clinical diagnosis when the facial gestalt or a cluster of clinical features brings a particular diagnosis to mind. A quick look at the atlas will help confirm this suspicion and the clinician know whether the gene has been identified.

The second, more important function is just becoming apparent. In the immediate past if one made a clinical diagnosis of an X-linked ID condition and if the gene had been identified, the next step was to look for a laboratory willing to test for that mutation. Now the scene has been reversed. In investigating a singleton male with ID or someone from a family that might have a mutation in a gene coded on the X, one can order an X gene screen covering most of the a

multigene sequencing panel that includes all genes associated with XLID. This is a service now offered not on by Greenwood Genetic Center but is also available in through other laboratories. A result comes back reporting a mutation in gene *ABC*. This atlas can provide both the information of the clinical features associated with mutations in that gene with some idea of the prognosis and references to more detailed clinical reports. The classical sequence of clinical diagnosis to causal mutation has given way to causal mutation to clinical diagnosis.

This will lead to major changes in clinical practice. There will be far less discussion, in the clinic and at meetings as to whether a particular set of clinical findings fits in with one syndrome as opposed to another. The laboratory will often be able to settle the matter. All undiagnosed males with ID will have a molecular karyotype and, if necessary, will be followed by a screen of the genes on the X chromosome, soon to be followed by looking for de novo mutations. Is this the death knell of the clinical dysmorphologist? Lay and professional support groups will be known more by their mutations than by their eponymous or anatomical syndromes as is happening with chromosomal disorders. The Internet will provide increasingly accurate clinical and molecular data.

Molecular testing is rapidly becoming less expensive. This will allow the introduction of pre-pregnancy testing for carriers of X-linked ID to be added to the routine screenings. This *Atlas of X-Linked Intellectual Disability Syndromes* will be invaluable in interpreting the findings.

The authors are to be congratulated on producing a major new reference similar in importance today as was the publication of Dave Smith's *Recognizable Patterns of Human Malformations* in the sixties. Information in this field continues to accumulate rapidly and we look forward to the next edition in less than 10 year's time. This atlas is one more step in the mission of the Greenwood Genetic Center of having all babies born free of physical and mental disabilities.

Gillian Turner OA Mb.Ch.B MRCPE. D.Sc.
University of Newcastle
New South Wales
Australia

PREFACE

In the early days of human development, the brain dominates the embryological landscape. As other organ systems develop and the fetus grows, the brain becomes less formidable anatomically, but progressively more complex functionally. Soon after postnatal life begins, it engages the environment and issues responses that bind the child to parents and to others. It enables the acquisition of skills that serve as benchmarks of developmental progress. Ultimately, the brain defines the essence of human existence through the control of thought processes, neurological function, and behavior.

A certain fragility of the developing brain is suggested by the high prevalence in the population of significant impairment of cognitive and adaptive performance. Such impairments may be associated with faulty formation or function of the brain, occur in one to three percent of the population, and are considered collectively under the general term intellectual disability. The high frequency with which developmental failure of the brain occurs is found in no other organ system. The developing brain may, thus, be easily damaged or minor damage may be more readily expressed. Alternatively, other organ systems may have structural or functional redundancy that gives greater capacity in reserve.

Intellectual disability – significant impairment of cognitive and adaptive functions – exists as a human phenomenon with numerous dimensions. For the affected individual, it represents a cloak that limits capacity to learn, ability for expression, freedom of movement, and achievement of goals. For society, it represents a disability characterized by reduced productivity, some measure of dependency, and vulnerability to discrimination and exploitation. For public health, it is a common abnormality, one that is distributed throughout all strata of the population, and imposes a costly and lifelong burden. For medicine, intellectual disability represents an aberration in the formation and/or function of the central nervous system that demands evaluation and explanation.

Partition of intellectual disability by cause is informative on several counts. Scientifically, it confirms that the developing brain is susceptible to a wide variety of insults including faulty genetic instructions, environmental influences, and a combination of these two forces. Only with recognition of the causes can specific strategies for treatment and prevention be devised. From a practical clinical standpoint, knowledge of causes gives the clinician a basis to judiciously select diagnostic tests, predict natural history, calculate recurrence risks, direct counseling, and make reasonable medical and educational plans.

A pervasive finding among persons with intellectual disability has been the excess of males. In most populations, the excess is about 20–40%. The biological inequity between males and females conferred by the different number of sex chromosomes has been considered primarily responsible for the excess. Accepting a male excess of 30%, one would estimate that XLID constitutes one of the most common causal categories of intellectual disability, equaling that of chromosome aberrations. However, the current ability to identify intellectual disability due to X-linked genes in clinical populations accounts for only a fraction of this number.

X-linked intellectual disability has been divided into two broad categories, syndromal and nonsyndromal (or nonspecific). In syndromal X-linked intellectual disability, somatic, neurologic, behavioral, or metabolic abnormalities accompany the intellectual disability and often constitute a recognizable pattern. In nonsyndromal X-linked intellectual disability, males have no somatic, neurologic, behavioral, or metabolic findings that distinguish them from nonaffected brothers or from other males with intellectual disability.

A large number of families with syndromal and nonsyndromal forms of XLID have been reported, primarily during the past 50 years. Although there have been recent advances to confirm diagnoses with biochemical or molecular testing, the clues to identification of most XLID syndromes come from the family history and phenotype. This *Atlas of X-Linked Intellectual Disability* is intended to provide the clinicians, scientists, and students with a resource to differentiate the various types of XLID on the basis of craniofacial or other somatic findings, neurologic signs or symptoms, behavioral manifestations, brain imaging, and laboratory testing. Separate genes exist for many, but not all, of the 150 syndromal forms of XLID.

Delineation of the various forms of XLID has been possible only through the contributions of affected families and their physicians. To them, we are indebted and to them we dedicate this monograph. Researchers worldwide have followed up the clinical observations with systematic biological investigations, including a wide variety of imaging, histologic, molecular and cytogenetic studies, which have permitted delineation of the phenotype and localization of the majority of the X-linked intellectual disability syndromes. The responsible genes have now been identified in two-thirds of the syndromes.

Prior to publication of *X-Linked Mental Retardation* in 2000, the laboratory approach to gene localization and identification was limited to pursuit of genes where the gene products were known (enzymes in all cases: *HPRT*, *PGK1*, *OTC*, and *PHDA1*), exploration of chromosome rearrangements (predominately X-autosome translocations), and linkage analysis in large families in which XLID appeared to segregate. Since that time, the study of breakpoints in chromosome rearrangements and linkage analysis coupled with candidate gene testing, have continued to be the most productive means of gene identification. Brute force sequencing of the X chromosome and genomic microarrays for copy number variants coupled with candidate gene testing, have been added to these technologies in recent years. Prior to 2000, 30 XLID genes had been identified; since then an additional 72 XLID genes have been identified. Among families suspected to have XLID, 40–50% of the responsible mutations can now be identified with the most commonly affected genes, besides *FMR1*, being *ARX* (5–6%), and *MECP2*, *OPHN1*, *PQBP1*, and *KDM5C* (each 1–4%). Mutations are detected in a much lower percentage of sporadic males with ID.

Segmental duplications involving one or more genes on the X chromosome have been associated with intellectual disability. The most common of the segmental duplications involves the *PLP1* gene at Xq22 and is responsible for the majority of cases of Pelizaeus–Merzbacher disease (Mimault et al. 1999). A second important duplication occurs in Xq28 and includes *MECP2* with or without adjacent genes. The phenotype includes severe intellectual disability (sometimes with co-occurring autism or autistic manifestations), hypotonia, absent or limited speech, absent or limited ambulation, spasticity, seizures, and recurrent respiratory infections (Van Esch et al. 2005, Friez et al. 2006). In some cases of X chromosome segmental duplications, it is unclear whether the whole gene duplication, partial duplication of adjacent gene or other position effect is most important in the causation of ID. In many cases of clinically important segmental duplication of the X chromosome, marked skewing of X-inactivation has been documented in carrier females.

The clinical re-evaluation of families with XLID previously reported, observations in more recently ascertained families, and the incorporation of molecular technologies in diagnosis have resulted in lumping, splitting and reclassification of a number of XLID. With the variability and imprecision with which clinical evaluations are carried out, it is inevitable that some individuals with X-linked intellectual disability will be incorrectly included in existing diagnostic categories while others will be incorrectly excluded. The extent to which individuals/families can be evaluated is dependent on the setting, access to historical information, availability and ages of affected and nonaffected family members, and the experience and expertise of the observers. Differences in phenotype can result from mutations in different domains of a gene and by contributions from the balance of the genome. The identification of many causative XLID genes has provided the opportunity to compensate for some of these variables, resulting in the lumping of entities previously considered to be separate and the splitting of other entities previously considered the same. At the same time, the phenotypic limits of some XLID entities have been established with some degree of objectivity.

Several XLID entities have been most instructive. Discovery that mutations in the *ATRX* gene (Xq21.1) cause Alpha-Thalassemia Intellectual Disability allowed testing of large number of males with hypotonic facies, intellectual disability, and other features (Gibbons et al. 1995a, 1995b; Villard and Fontes 2002). Five named XLID syndromes – Carpenter–Waziri, Holmes–Gang, Chudley–Lowry and XLID–Arch Fingerprints–Hypotonia – have been found to be allelic variants of Alpha-Thalassemia Intellectual Disability as have certain families with spastic paraplegia and nonsyndromal XLID (Abidi et al. 1999, Lossi et al. 1999, Stevenson et al. 2000, Guerrini et al. 2000, Yntema et al. 2002, Abidi et al. 2005). One family clinically diagnosed as Juberg–Marsidi syndrome was found to have an *ATRX* mutation (Villard et al. 1996). This is now known to be based on misdiagnosis of Juberg–Marsidi syndrome since the original family with this syndrome has a mutation in *HUWE1* at Xp11.22 (Friez et al. 2011). One family clinically diagnosed as Smith–Fineman–Myers syndrome was also found to have an *ATRX* mutation, although the gene has not been analyzed in the original family (Villard et al. 2000). A clinically similar condition, Coffin–Lowry syndrome, was found to be separate from Alpha-Thalassemia Intellectual Disability and due to mutations in the serine–threonine kinase gene, *RPS6KA3* (*RSK2*) located at Xp22.13 (Trivier et al. 1996).

Kalscheuer et al. (2003) found mutations in *PQBP1* (Xp11.23) in two named XLID syndromes – Sutherland–Haan syndrome and Hamel Cerebro-Palato-Cardiac syndrome – and in MRX55 and two other families with microcephaly and other findings. Lenski et al. (2004), Stevenson et al. (2005), and Lubs et al. (2006) added Renpenning, Porteous, and Golabi-Ito-Hall syndromes to the list of XLID syndromes caused by mutations in *PQBP1*. As with the *ATRX* phenotypes, a wide variety of phenotypic expressions result from different mutations in *PQBP1* and we remain challenged to better understand the molecular and developmental mechanisms leading to these differences (Germanaud et al. 2011, Sheen et al. 2010, Musante et al. 2010).

ARX (Xp22.11) was also found to be an important XLID gene encompassing multiple phenotypes. Mutations, most commonly a 24 bp expansion of a polyalanine tract, were found in a number of nonsyndromal families (MRX29, 32, 33, 36, 38, 43, 54, and 76), an X-linked dystonia (Partington syndrome), X-linked infantile spasms (West syndrome), X-linked lissencephaly with abnormal genitalia, hydranencephaly and abnormal genitalia, and Proud syndrome (Strømme et al. 2002a, 2002b; Bienvenu et al. 2002, Frints et al. 2002, Kitamura et al. 2002, Uyanik et al. 2003, Kato et al. 2004, Stepp et al. 2005).

Perhaps the most prominent example of syndrome splitting is FG syndrome. This syndrome, initially described in 1974 by Opitz and Kaveggia, is manifest by macrocephaly (or "relative macrocephaly"), downslanting palpebral fissures, imperforate anus or severe constipation, broad and flat thumbs and great toes, hypotonia, and intellectual disability. In the ensuing years, the manifestations attributed to FG syndrome have become protean, but none was pathognomonic or required for the diagnosis (Opitz et al. 1988, Romano et al. 1994, Ozonoff et al. 2000, Battaglia et al. 2006). Clinical heterogeneity was thus introduced and as a result different families were found to have different localizations on the X chromosome (Briault et al. 1997, 2000; Piluso et al. 2003, Dessay et al. 2002, Jehee et al. 2005, Tarpey et al. 2007, Unger et al. 2007).

In 2007, Risheg et al. found a recurring mutation, pR961W, in *MED12* (Xq13.1) in six families with the FG phenotype, including the original family reported by Opitz and Kaveggia. In addition to the above noted manifestations, two other findings, small ears and friendly behavior, were consistently noted.

Although most patients that have carried the FG diagnosis have one or more findings that overlap with those in FG syndrome, they do not have *MED12* mutations (Lyons et al. 2009, Clark et al. 2009). Some have been found to have other X-linked gene mutations (*FMR1, FLNA, ATRX, CASK, MECP2*) and others have had duplications or deletions of the autosomes (Lyons et al. 2009, Clark et al. 2009). So great is the currently existing heterogeneity within FG syndrome, that the vast majority of individuals so designated should best be considered to have intellectual disability of undetermined cause. The designation of multiple loci on the X chromosome for FG syndrome appears to be ill conceived (Opitz et al. 2008) and illustrates the hazards involved in nosology without a laboratory basis.

In a number of instances, certain mutations of genes have been associated with nonsyndromal XLID while other mutations of the same genes have caused syndromal XLID. Seventeen genes that may cause either type of XLID, depending on the mutation, have been identified (www.ggc.org/xlmr.htm, Figure 2). In some cases (e.g., those with

OPHN1 and *ARX* mutations) reexamination has found syndromal manifestations in families previously considered to have nonsyndromal XLID (Turner et al. 2002, Frints et al. 2002, Bergmann et al. 2003, Philip et al. 2003).

The frequency with which the process of lumping and splitting in this limited field of investigation has occurred has been extremely instructive to both clinical and molecular investigators. The underlying mechanisms or pathways by which mutations in different genes result in similar phenotypes and different mutations in a single gene result in disparate phenotypes, however, remain to be fully elucidated.

An exponential increase in the understanding of molecular pathways and neuronal complexes involved in brain function has occurred in the past decade. Many of the genes and their protein products involved in the critical processes of proper brain development and function – neurogenesis, neuronal migration, and synaptic connectivity – have been identified. It has become obvious that the "brain genes" may play multiple roles in these areas of central nervous system development at different critical developmental periods. Neurogenesis is likely affected by many X-linked genes given the finding of microcephaly in over 40 of the syndromes described in this text. Neuronal migration abnormalities are a common pathogenic finding on cranial imaging studies in individuals with mutations of *ARX, DCX,* and *FLNA*. Synaptic connectivity has emerged as the single most important functional deficit in individuals with ID and the synapse is the site of expression for a majority of the associated X-linked genes. Gene products are involved in pre- and post-synaptic processes of synaptic vesicles (*SYN1, SYP*), cellular adhesion (*L1CAM, NLGN3, NLGN4, PCDH19*), neurotransmitter release and receptor function (*GRIA3, IL1RAPL1*), neurite outgrowth and dendritic spine maturation (*FMR1, PAK3, OPHN1*), and cytoskeletal homeostasis (*CASK, FLNA*). Additionally, several X-linked genes function as transporters: *ATP7A, MED12, SLC16A2* (*MCT8*) and *SLC6A8*, and transcription regulation and chromatin remodeling: *ARX, MECP2, KDM5C, RPS6KA3, BRWD3* and *ATRX*. Rho GTPase genes – *ARHGEF6, ARHGEF9, OPHN1, GDI1, FGD1* and *PAK3* – mediate organization of the cytoskeleton, cell shape, and motility. The RAS-MAPK transcription-signaling cascade includes proteins encoded by *ARX, PHF6, ZNF41, PAK3,* and *RPS6KA3*. Some genes are involved in basic cellular processes, including RNA splicing (*PQBP1*), translation (*FTSJ1*), energy metabolism (*SLC6A8*), endocytosis (*DLG3, AP1S2*), ubiquitination (*CUL4B, UBE2A*) and nonsense mediated decay (*UPF3B*). Elucidation of the molecular etiology of Fragile X syndrome has allowed greater understanding of the interplay and balance necessary between both excitatory glutaminergic and inhibitory GABAergic neurons, and provided insight to possible treatments targeted at restoring this balance, an approach that may also be applicable to other types of ID and autism.

We wish to thank our clinical and research colleagues who have taught us about X-linked intellectual disability. In particular, we thank Herbert Lubs (Painter, VA), Fernando Arena (National Cancer Institute, Bethesda, MD), Hunt Willard (Duke University, Durham, NC), Jean-Louis Mandel (Institut de Chimie Biologique, Strasbourg), Grant Sutherland (Women's and Children's Hospital, Adelaide), Gillian Turner, Anna Hackett, and Michael Field (Hunter Genetics, New South Wales), Josef Gecz (Women's and Children's Hospital, Adelaide), Giovanni Neri (Universitá Cattolica del Sacro Cuore, Rome), Patrick Tarpey and Mike Stratton (Wellcome Trust Sanger Institute, Hinxton, Cambridge, UK), Lucy Raymond (Cambridge Institute of Medical Research, Cambridge, UK), and Michel Fontés (INSERM, Marseille). Our current and former colleagues at the Greenwood Genetic Center: William Allen, Ellen Boyd, Sara Cathey, Katie Clarkson, David Everman, Joseph Geer, Michael Lyons, Robert Saul, Laurie Seaver, Richard Simensen, Steven Skinner, Yuri Zarate and our laboratory colleagues: Fatima Monica Basehore Abidi, Lauren Cason, Mike Chandler, Barbara DuPont, Michael Friez, Bernhard Häne, Lynda Holloway, Darci Horne, Julie Jones, John Longshore, Melanie May, Ron Michaelis, Retecher Nelson, Lisbeth Ouzts, Katy Phelan, Laura Pollard Anand Srivastava, Monica Stepp, Jack Tarleton, Harold Taylor, and Tim Wood have made important contributions to the evaluation and understanding of X-linked intellectual disability. They have made suggestions on content of this Atlas, reviewed drafts of the manuscript and have taken on additional responsibilities to give us time to devote to this effort.

Numerous authors and publishers have provided figures to illustrate the XLID syndromes. Individual credits are given in the figure legends. Literature searches, citation verification, and other library resources have been provided by Rachel Collins. Karen Buchanan and Patti Broome have organized the materials used to produce this monograph and have provided invaluable assistance and advice.

The production of *Atlas of X-Linked Intellectual Disability* gave us the opportunity to work with Anne Dellinger and Catherine Barnes at Oxford University Press. Their valuable suggestions from concept through production have enabled us to work with some degree of efficiency and equanimity.

REFERENCES

Abidi F, Hall BD, Cadle RG, et al.: X-linked mental retardation with variable stature, head circumference, and testicular volume linked to Xq12–q21. Am J Med Genet 85:223, 1999.

Abidi FE, Cardoso C, Lossi AM, et al.: Mutation in the 5' alternatively spliced region of the XNP/ATR-X gene causes Chudley–Lowry syndrome. Eur J Hum Genet 13:176, 2005.

Battaglia A, Chines C, Carey JC: The FG syndrome: Report of a large Italian series. Am J Med Genet A 140:2075, 2006.

Bergmann C, Zerres K, Senderek J, et al.: Oligophrenin 1 (OPHN1) gene mutation causes syndromic X-linked mental retardation with epilepsy, rostral ventricular enlargement and cerebellar hypoplasia. Brain 126:1537, 2003.

Bienvenu T, Poirier K, Friocourt G, et al.: ARX, a novel Prd-class-homeobox gene highly expressed in the telencephalon, is mutated in X-linked mental retardation. Hum Mol Genet 11:981, 2002.

Briault S, Hill R, Shrimpton A, et al.: A gene for FG syndrome maps in the Xq12–21.31 region. Am J Med Genet 73:87, 1997.

Briault S, Villard L, Rogner U, et al.: Mapping of X chromosome inversion breakpoints [inv(X)(q11q28)] associated with FG syndrome: a second FG locus [FGS2]? Am J Med Genet 95:178, 2000.

Clark RD, Graham JM, Friez MJ, et al.: FG syndrome, an X-linked multiple congenital anomaly syndrome: the clinical phenotype and an algorithm for diagnostic testing. Genet Med 11:769, 2009.

Dessay S, Moizard MP, Gilardi JL, et al.: FG syndrome: linkage analysis in two families supporting a new gene localization at Xp22.3 [FGS3]. Am J Med Genet 112:6, 2002.

Friez MJ, Jones JR, Clarkson K, et al.: Recurrent infections, hypotonia, and mental retardation caused by duplication of MECP2 and adjacent region in Xq28. Pediatrics 118:e1687, 2006.

Friez MJ, Brooks SS, Stevenson RE, et al.: Juberg–Marsidi syndrome and Brooks syndrome are allelic X-linked intellectual disability syndromes due to a single mutation (p.G4310R) in HUWE1. 15th International Workshop on Fragile X and Early-Onset Cognitive Disorders. September 5, 2011, Berlin, Germany.

Frints SG, Froyen G, Marynen P, et al.: Re-evaluation of MRX36 family after discovery of an ARX gene mutation reveals mild neurological features of Partington syndrome. Am J Med Genet 112:427, 2002.

Germanaud D, Rossi M, Bussy G, et al.: The Renpenning syndrome spectrum: new clinical insights supported by 13 new PQBP1-mutated males. Clin Genet 79:225, 2011.

Gibbons RJ, Brueton L, Buckle VJ, et al.: Clinical and hematologic aspects of the X-linked α-thalassemia/mental retardation syndrome (ATR-X). Am J Med Genet 55:288, 1995.

Gibbons RJ, Picketts DJ, Villard L, et al.: Mutations in a putative global transcriptional regulator cause X-linked mental retardation with α-thalassemia (ATR-X syndrome). Cell 80:837, 1995.

Guerrini R, Shanahan JL, Carrozzo R, et al.: A nonsense mutation of the ATRX gene causing mild mental retardation and epilepsy. Ann Neurol 47:117, 2000.

Jehee FS, Rosenberg C, Krepischi-Santos AC, et al.: An Xq22.3 duplication detected by comparative genomic hybridization microarray (Array-CGH) defines a new locus (FGS5) for FG syndrome. Am J Med Genet A 139:221, 2005.

Kalscheuer VM, Freude K, Musante L, et al.: Mutations in the polyglutamine binding protein 1 gene cause X-linked mental retardation. Nat Genet 35:313, 2003.

Kato M, Das S, Petras K, et al.: Mutations of ARX are associated with striking pleiotropy and consistent genotype-phenotype correlation. Hum Mutat 23:147, 2004.

Kitamura K, Yanazawa M, Sugiyama N, et al.: Mutation of ARX causes abnormal development of forebrain and testes in mice and X-linked lissencephaly with abnormal genitalia in humans. Nat Genet 32:359, 2002.

Lenski C, Abidi F, Meindl A, et al.: Novel truncating mutations in the polyglutamine tract binding protein 1 gene (PQBP1) cause Renpenning syndrome and X-linked mental retardation in another family with microcephaly. Am J Hum Genet 74:777, 2004.

Lossi AM, Millán JM, Villard L, et al.: Mutation of the XNP/ATR-X gene in a family with severe mental retardation, spastic paraplegia and skewed pattern of X inactivation: demonstration that the mutation is involved in the inactivation bias. Am J Hum Genet 65:558, 1999.

Lubs H, Abidi FE, Echeverri R, et al.: Golabi–Ito–Hall syndrome results from a missense mutation in the WW domain of the PQBP1 gene. J Med Genet 43:e30, 2006.

Lyons MJ, Graham JM Jr., Neri G, et al.: Clinical experience in the evaluation of 30 patients with a prior diagnosis of FG syndrome. J Med Genet 46:9, 2009.

Mimault C, Giraud G, Courtois V, et al.: Proteolipoprotein gene analysis in 82 patients with sporadic Pelizaeus–Merzbacher disease: duplications, the major cause of the disease, originate more frequently in male germ cells, but point mutations do not. The Clinical European Network on Brain Dysmyelinating Disease. Am J Hum Genet 65:360, 1999.

Musante L, Kunde SA, Sulistio TO, et al.: Common pathological mutations in PQBP1 include nonsense-mediated mRNA decay and enhance exclusion of the mutant exon. Hum Mutat 31:90, 2010.

Opitz JM, Smith JF, Santoro L: The FG syndrome (Online Mendelian Inheritance in Man 305450): Perspective in 2008. Adv Pediatr 55:123, 2008.

Opitz JM and Kaveggia EG: Studies of malformation syndromes of man XXXIII: The FG syndrome. An X-linked recessive syndrome of multiple congenital anomalies and mental retardation. Z Kinderheilk 117:1, 1974.

Opitz JM, Richieri-da Costa A, Aase JM, et al.: FG syndrome update 1988: note of 5 new patients and bibliography. Am J Med Genet 30:309, 1988.

Ozonoff S, Williams BJ, Rauch AM, Opitz JO: Behavior phenotype of FG syndrome: cognition, personality, and behavior in eleven affected boys. Am J Med Genet 97:112, 2000.

Philip N, Chabrol B, Lossi AM, et al.: Mutations in the oligophrenin-1 gene (OPHN1) cause X linked congenital cerebellar hypoplasia. J Med Genet 40:441, 2003.

Piluso G, Carella M, D'Avanzo M, et al.: Genetic heterogeneity of FG syndrome: a fourth locus (FGS4) maps to Xp11.4-p11.3 in an Italian family. Hum Genet 112:124, 2003.

Risheg H, Graham JM Jr., Clark RD, et al.: A recurrent mutation in MED12 leading to R961W causes Opitz-Kaveggia syndrome. Nat Genet 39:451, 2007.

Romano C, Baraitser M, Thompson E: A clinical follow-up of British patients with FG syndrome. Clin Dysmorphol 3:104, 1994.

Sheen VL, Torres AR, Du X, et al.: Mutation in PQBP1 is associated with periventricular heterotopia. Am J Med Genet A 152A:2888, 2010.

Stepp ML, Cason AL, Finnis M, et al.: XLMR in MRX families 29, 32, 33 and 38 results from the dup24 mutation in the ARX (Aristaless related homeobox) gene. BMC Med Genet 6:16, 2005.

Stevenson RE, Abidi F, Schwartz CE, et al.: Holmes–Gang syndrome is allelic with XLMR-hypotonic face syndrome. Am J Med Genet 94:383, 2000.

Stevenson RE, Bennett CW, Abidi F, et al.: Renpenning syndrome comes into focus. Am J Med Genet A 134:415, 2005.

Strømme P, Mangelsdorf ME, Shaw MA, et al.: Mutations in the human ortholog of Aristaless cause X-linked mental retardation and epilepsy. Nat Genet 30:441, 2002a.

Strømme P, Mangelsdorf ME, Scheffer IE, Gécz J.: Infantile spasms, dystonia, and other X-linked phenotypes caused by mutations in Aristaless related homeobox gene, ARX. Brain Dev 24:266, 2002b.

Tarpey PS, Raymond FL, Nguyen LS, et al.: Mutations in UPF3B, a member of the nonsense-mediated mRNA decay complex, cause syndromic and nonsyndromic mental retardation. Nat Genet 39:1127, 2007.

Trivier E, De Cesare D, Jacquot S, et al.: Mutations in the kinase Rsk-2 associated with Coffin–Lowry syndrome. Nature 384:567, 1996.

Turner G, Partington M, Kerr B, et al.: Variable expression of mental retardation, autism, seizures, and dystonic hand movements in two families with an identical ARX gene mutation. Am J Med Genet 112:405, 2002.

Unger S, Mainberger A, Spitz C, et al.: Filamin A mutation is one cause of FG syndrome. Am J Med Genet 143A:1876, 2007.

Uyanik G, Aigner L, Martin P, et al.: ARX mutations in X-linked lissencephaly with abnormal genitalia. Neurology 61:232, 2003.

Van Esch H, Bauters M, Ignatius J, et al.: Duplication of the MECP2 region is a frequent cause of severe mental retardation and progressive neurological symptoms in males. Am J Hum Genet 77:442, 2005.

Villard L, Fontes M: Alpha-thalassemia/mental retardation syndrome. X-linked (ATR-X, MIM #301040). ATR-X/XNP/XH2 gene MIM #300032). Eur J Hum Genet 10:223, 2002.

Villard L, Fontès M, Adès LC, Gecz J: Identification of a mutation in the XNP/ATR-X gene in a family reported as Smith-Fineman-Myers syndrome. Am J Med Genet 91:83, 2000.

Villard L, Gecz J, Mattei JF, et al.: XNP mutation in a large family with Juberg–Marsidi syndrome. Nat Genet 12:359, 1996.

Yntema HG, Poppelaars FA, Derksen E, et al.: Expanding phenotype of XNP mutations: mild to moderate mental retardation. Am J Med Genet 110:243, 2002.

R.E.S.
C.E.S.
R.C.R.

AARSKOG SYNDROME

(AARSKOG-SCOTT SYNDROME, FACIOGENITAL DYSPLASIA, FACIODIGITOGENITAL SYNDROME)

OMIM 305400

Xp11.22

FGD1

Definition. XLID with short stature, hypertelorism, downslanting palpebral fissures, joint hyperextensibility, and shawl scrotum. The gene (*FGD1*), a guanine nucleotide exchange factor, exerts its influence, at least in part, by activating Rho GTPase. More than 100 mutations, the majority of which lead to truncated proteins, have been identified.

Somatic Features. Prominent forehead, widow's peak, hypertelorism, downslanting palpebral fissures, ptosis, short nose with anteverted nares, cupped ears, wide upper lip, indistinct philtral pillars, and small chin comprise the facial phenotype. In adults, the face elongates and the prominent forehead and hypertelorism may not be apparent. When extended, the fingers are held in flexion at the MP joints, hyperextension at the PIP joints, and flexion at the DIP joints, presumably because of shortening of the flexor tendons. Other musculoskeletal findings include brachydactyly, horizontal palmar crease, varus foot, and generalized joint hyperextensibility. The scrotum tends to surround the penis,

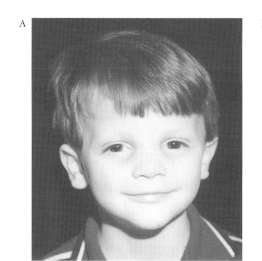
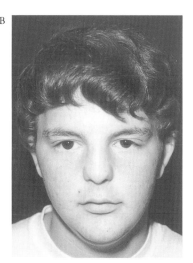
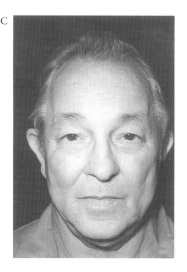

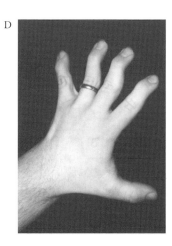
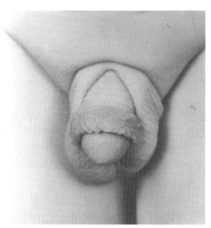

Aarskog Syndrome. Four-year-old with hypertelorism, downslanting palpebral fissures, and prominent forehead (**A**); 17-year-old with prominent forehead, ptosis, and cupped ears (**B**); 60-year-old with balding and cupped ears but less apparent widening of midface (**C**); characteristic posturing of extended fingers (**D**); shawl scrotum (**E**).

giving the "shawl scrotum" appearance. Protruding umbilicus, cryptorchidism, and inguinal hernias may occur.

Growth and Development. From birth, linear growth follows the lower centiles. Head circumference is normal.

Cognitive Function. Intelligence is usually normal but is quite variable from normal into the mildly impaired range. Severe intellectual impairment is the exception.

Neurological Findings. Hypermobility of the cervical spine may lead to cord impingement.

Heterozygote Expression. Carrier females tend to be shorter than noncarriers and may have subtle facial features (hypertelorism, fullness of tip of the nose), brachydactyly, and unusual posturing of the fingers.

Comment. Aarskog syndrome has one of the distinctive recognizable somatic phenotypes with which very few conditions are likely to be mistaken. Noonan syndrome shares ptosis, downslanting palpebral fissures, short stature, and pectus excavatum. However, patients with Noonan syndrome often have broad and webbed neck and a cardiac defect; patients with Aarskog syndrome often have shawl scrotum. These findings serve as distinguishing but not pathognomonic findings. Teebi Hypertelorism syndrome and Robinow syndrome – both autosomal syndromes – should be included in the differential diagnosis.

Only about one-fifth of the individuals suspected on clinical findings to have Aarskog syndrome harbor *FGD1*

mutations. One family with nonsyndromal XLID had a missense mutation.

REFERENCES

Aarskog D: A familial syndrome of short stature associated with facial dysplasia and genital anomalies. J Pediatr 77:856, 1970.

Fryns JP: Aarskog syndrome: The changing phenotype with age. Am J Med Genet 43:240, 1992.

Lebel RR, May M, Pouls S, et al.: Non-syndromic X-linked mental retardation associated with a missense mutation (P312L) in the FGD1 gene. Clin Genet 61:139, 2002.

Logie LJ, Porteous MEM: Intelligence and development in Aarskog syndrome. Arch Dis Child 79:359, 1998.

Orrico A, Galli L, Cavaliere ML, et al.: Phenotypic and molecular characterization of the Aarskog-Scott syndrome: A Survey of the clinical variability in light of FGD1 mutation analysis in 46 patients. Eur J Hum Genet 12:16, 2004.

Pasteris NG, Cadle A, Logie LJ, et al.: Isolated and characterization of the faciogenital dysplasia (Aarskog-Scott syndrome) gene: A putative Rho/Rac guanine nucleotide exchange factor. Cell 79:669, 1994.

Porteous MEM, Curtis A, Lindsay S, et al.: The gene for Aarskog syndrome is located between DXS255 and DXS566 (Xp11.2-Xq13). Genomics 14:298, 1992.

Porteous MEM, Goudie DR: Aarskog syndrome. J Med Genet 28:44, 1991.

Scott CI, Jr.: Unusual facies, joint hypermobility, genital anomaly and short stature: A new dysmorphic syndrome. Birth Defects: Orig Art Ser VII(6):240, 1971.

Stevenson RE, May M, Arena JF, et al.: Aarskog-Scott syndrome: Confirmation of linkage to the pericentromeric region of the X chromosome. Am J Med Genet 52:339, 1994.

DIFFERENTIAL MATRIX

Syndrome	Telecanthus/ Hypertelorism	Brachydactyly	Urogenital Anomaly	Comments
Aarskog	+	+	+	Short stature, downslanting palpebral fissures, ptosis, cupped ears, anteverted nares, horizontal palmar crease, midfoot varus, joint laxity, shawl scrotum, cryptorchidism, inguinal hernias
Atkin-Flaitz	+	+	+	Macrocephaly, short stature, downslanting palpebral fissures, broad nasal tip, thick lower lip, macroorchidism, seizures
ATRX-Associated XLID	+	+	+	Microcephaly, short stature, small triangular nose, tented upper lip, open mouth, wide spacing of teeth, musculoskeletal anomalies, hemoglobin H inclusions in erythrocytes
Simpson-Golabi-Behmel	+	+	+	Somatic overgrowth, supernumerary nipples, polydactyly
Kang	+	+	0	Microcephaly, frontal prominence, downturned angles of mouth
Otopalatodigital I (*FLNA*-Associated XLID)	+	+	0	Cleft palate, hearing impairment, short stature, skeletal dysplasia, mild cognitive impairment
Hall Orofacial	+	0	+	Normal growth, upslanted and short palpebral fissures, prominent nasal tip, high nasal bridge, inguinal hernia
Telecanthus-Hypospadias	+	0	+	High broad nasal root, dysplastic ears, cleft lip/palate, abnormal cranial contour or symmetry
Wittwer	+	0	+	Microcephaly, short stature, microphthalmia, hearing loss, vision loss, hypotonia, seizures
XLID-Psoriasis	+	0	+	Open mouth, large ears, hypotonia, seizures, psoriasis
Hereditary Bullous Dystrophy, X-linked	0	+	+	Microcephaly, short stature, upslanting palpebral fissures, protruding ears, short and tapered digits, cardiac defects, bullous dystrophy, small testes, early death from pulmonary infection

ABIDI SYNDROME

OMIM 300262

Xq12-q21

Definition. XLID with variable manifestations, but usually short stature, small head size, and small testes. The gene maps to Xq12-q21.

Somatic Features. Based on a single family, manifestations tended to be mild and variable. The head circumference was smaller than unaffected brothers but in only one case was less than the 3rd centile. Stature was usually below the 10th centile, again with a single case being below the 3rd centile. Sloping forehead and cupped ears were present in some cases. Two affected males had cleft lip with or without cleft palate, but this was noted in nonaffected family members as well. Testicular volume was below the 10th centile in four of six for whom measurements were available. Large ears, hearing loss, high foot arches, and excessive arch fingerprints were present in some cases.

Growth and Development. Birth weights were in the lower centiles. Adult height and head circumference tended to be at or below the 10th centile. Developmental milestones were globally delayed in most cases.

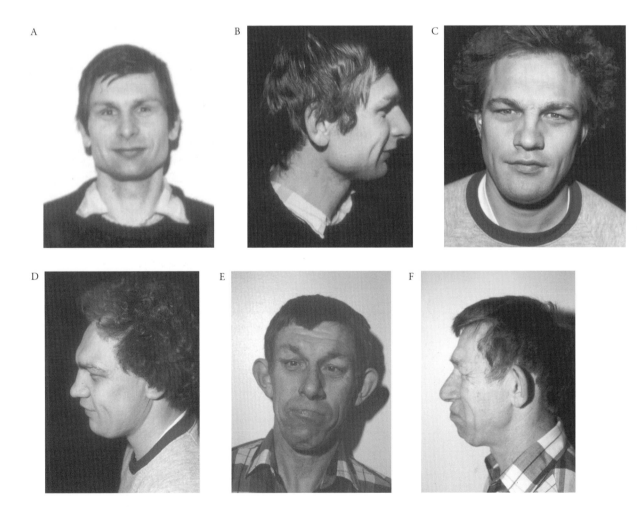

Abidi Syndrome. Facial appearance of three males ages 31, 34, and 37 years, showing sloping forehead and prominent brow (**A-D**) and sloping forehead, cupped ears, and repaired cleft lip (**E-F**).

Cognitive Function. IQ measurement varied between 12 and 61.

Neurological Findings. Muscle tone was normal, and in several cases there was a mild increase in deep tendon reflexes.

Heterozygote Expression. None

Comment. The manifestations were so mild and variable as to limit their usefulness in clinical diagnosis. In many respects, the syndrome resembles Renpenning syndrome, which maps to Xp11.

REFERENCE

Abidi F, Hall BD, Cadle RG, et al.: X-linked mental retardation with variable stature, head circumference, and testicular volume linked to Xq12-q21. Am J Med Genet 85:223, 1999.

DIFFERENTIAL MATRIX

Syndrome	Microcephaly	Short Stature	Small Testes	Comments
Abidi	+	+	+	Sloping forehead, cupped ears
ATRX-Associated XLID	+	+	+	Telecanthus/hypertelorism, small triangular nose, tented upper lip, open mouth, wide spacing of teeth, minor musculoskeletal anomalies, hypotonia, erythrocyte HbH inclusions in some
Börjeson-Forssman-Lehmann	+	+	+	Coarse face, large ears, gynecomastia, narrow sloped shoulders, visual impairment, tapered digits, hypotonia, obesity
Hereditary Bullous Dystrophy, X-linked	+	+	+	Upslanting palpebral fissures, protruding ears, digits short and tapered, bullous dystrophy, early death from pulmonary infection, cutaneous lesions, cardiac defects
Renpenning	+	+	+	Upslanting palpebral fissures
XLID-Microcephaly-Testicular Failure	+	+	+	Prominent supraorbital ridges, high nasal bridge, prominent nose, macrostomia
Cornelia de Lange Syndrome, X-linked	+	+	0	Arched eyebrows, synophrys, long philtrum, thin lips, cutis marmorata, small hands and feet, hirsutism, enlarged cerebral ventricles, proximal thumbs, elbow restriction
Miles-Carpenter	+	+	0	Ptosis, small palpebral fissures, open mouth, pectus excavatum, scoliosis, long hands, camptodactyly, rockerbottom feet, arch fingerprints, unsteady gait, skeletal abnormality, spasticity
Roifman	+	+	0	Spondyloepiphyseal dysplasia, retinal pigmentary deposits, antibody deficiency, eczema, hypotonia
Pettigrew	+	0	+	Dandy-Walker malformation, microcephaly or hydrocephaly, long face with macrostomia, contractures, choreoathetosis, cerebellar hypoplasia, spastic paraplegia, iron deposits or calcification of basal ganglia, seizures
XLID-Hypogonadism-Tremor	0	+	+	Prominent lower lip, muscle wasting of legs, abnormal gait, obesity, seizures, tremor

ADRENOLEUKODYSTROPHY

(ADDISON DISEASE AND CEREBRAL SCLEROSIS, ADRENOMYELONEUROPATHY, SIEMERLING-CREUTZFELDT DISEASE, BRONZE SCHILDER DISEASE, MELANODERMIC LEUKODYSTROPHY)

OMIM 300100

Xq28

ABCD1

Definition. XLID with variable and progressive vision and hearing loss, spasticity, and neurological deterioration associated with demyelination of the CNS and adrenal insufficiency. The gene, *ABCD1*, encodes a peroxisomal membrane ATP-binding cassette (ABC) protein.

Somatic Features. Malformations are not features of this peroxisomal disorder. With elevated melanocyte-stimulating hormone in overt or covert adrenal insufficiency, the skin may become diffusely darkened.

Growth and Development. In childhood-onset adrenoleukodystrophy, normal growth and development for the first several years are followed by developmental stagnation or regression and growth failure.

Cognitive Function. Cerebral demyelination during childhood results in cognitive arrest and in adulthood results in dementia.

Neurological Findings. X-linked adrenoleukodystrophy usually presents with neurological features. The neurological presentation, age of onset, and progression are variable. Cerebral involvement predominates in childhood. Spinal cord presentation is more common in adulthood. At any age, the presence of cerebral demyelination signals a more rapid progression.

Natural History. Cerebral adrenoleukodystrophy usually presents at ages 4 to 8 years but may present in adolescence. Slowing and then arrest of motor, mental, and social development, with behavioral changes, are followed by spasticity, vision and hearing impairments, and, in a matter of years, death in an extremely debilitated state. The adult-onset cerebral presentation includes dementia and psychosis and is also rapidly progressive. More commonly, however, adults present with more slowly progressive spastic paraparesis (adrenomyeloneuropathy). They may develop sphincter incompetence and impotence. About half will develop cerebral involvement.

By the time of neurological manifestations, frank adrenal insufficiency or, more commonly, compromise of adrenal reserve, may be found. About 15% of people who suffer

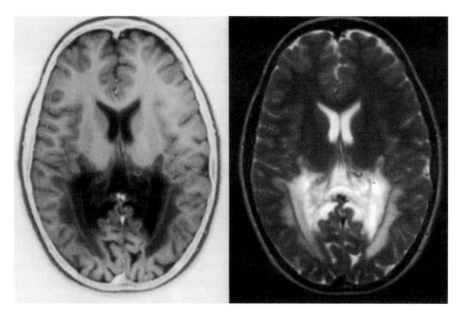

Adrenoleukodystrophy. T-2 axial images of the brain (image on the left is video-inverted) showing bilateral, symmetric abnormal signal in the occipital lobe white matter, and splenium of the corpus callosum caused by dysmyelineation/demyelination.   Courtesy of Dr. G. Shashidhar Pai, Medical University of South Carolina, Charleston.

from childhood-onset adrenoleukodystrophy present with adrenal insufficiency. About 40% of adrenomyeloneuropathy patients have clinical adrenal insufficiency before the onset of neurologic symptoms. Of those with neurological presentation, 85% have compromise of adrenal reserve by ACTH provocative testing. Variable presentations within families is common.

Heterozygote Expression. Heterozygotes may be affected in this condition, most commonly with adrenomyeloneuropathy but sometimes with cerebral involvement. One-half or more of carriers show some mild neurological manifestation, and about 20% have adrenomyeloneuropathy. Adrenal insufficiency is very rare in heterozygotes.

Neuropathology. Brain demyelination commences in the parieto-occipital region and progresses anteriorly in 85% of cerebral cases. The demyelination is accompanied by an inflammatory response. Spinal cord pathology is that of a distal axonopathy fiber loss with minimal or no inflammatory response. Adrenal pathology is characterized initially by cellular edema followed by atrophy.

Laboratory. Very-long-chain fatty acids are increased in blood and other tissues. Cortisol may be low or decreased cortisol reserve may be detected with provocative tests.

Treatment. Cortisol replacement is indicated for adrenal insufficiency. Evaluation of intervention for neurologic features is complicated by the variability of presentation. Dietary therapy with GTO–GTE oils (glyceryl trioleate–glyceryl trierucate) normalizes very-long-chain fatty acid levels but does not alter the progression of pre-existing neurological impairment. The efficacy of the diet in preventing the onset of neurological symptoms is under investigation. Also under study are bone marrow and stem cell transplantation and anti-inflammatory interventions.

Comment. The existence of a modifier gene has been proposed because the severity of the neurological involvement does not correlate with gene mutations, very-long-chain fatty acid levels, or adrenal insufficiency. It is proposed that the modifier gene may affect the cerebral inflammatory response.

X-linked adrenoleukodystrophy accounts for about 5% of the leukodystrophies, is less frequent than Pelizaeus-Merzbacher disease and metachromatic leukodystrophy, but is more common than Krabbe disease and Tay-Sachs disease.

REFERENCES

Berger J, Pujol A, Aubourg P, et al.: Current and future pharmacological treatment strategies in X-linked adrenoleukodystrophy. Brain Pathol 20:845, 2010.

Bonkowsky JL, Nelson C, Kingston JL, et al.: The burden of inherited leukodystrophies in children. Neurology 75:718, 2010.

Cartier N, Aubourg P: Hematopoietic stem cell transplantation and hematopoietic stem cell gene therapy in X-linked adrenoleukodystrophy. Brain Pathol 20:857, 2010.

Dodd A, Rowland SA, Hawkes SLJ, et al.: Mutations in the adrenoleukodystrophy gene. Hum Mutat 9:500, 1997.

Gartner J, Braun A, Holzinger A, et al.: Clinical and genetic aspects of X-linked adrenoleukodystrophy. Neuropediatr 29:3, 1998.

Moser HW: Adrenoleukodystrophy: phenotype, genetics, pathogenesis and therapy. Brain 120:1485, 1997.

Mosser J, Lutz Y, Stoeckel ME, et al.: The gene responsible for adrenoleukodystrophy encodes a peroxisomal membrane protein. Hum Mol Genet 3:265, 1994.

DIFFERENTIAL MATRIX

Syndrome	Spastic Paraplegia	Vision Loss	Hearing Loss	Comments
Adrenoleukodystrophy	+	+	+	Adrenal insufficiency, diffuse skin pigmentation, progressive neurological deterioration and dementia, elevated very-long-chain fatty acids in plasma
Gustavson	+	+	+	Microcephaly, short stature, optic atrophy with blindness, large ears, joint contractures, rockerbottom feet, brain undergrowth, hydrocephaly, cerebellar hypoplasia, seizures
Mohr-Tranebjaerg	+	+	+	Neurological deterioration with childhood onset, dystonia
Schimke	+	+	+	Microcephaly, sunken eyes, downslanting palpebral fissures, narrow nose, wide spacing of teeth, cupped ears, hypotonia, abducens palsy, choreoathetosis, contractures
Paine	+	+	+	Microcephaly, short stature, optic atrophy, seizures
Proud (*ARX*-Associated XLID)	+	+	+	Microcephaly, agenesis of corpus callosum, cryptorchidism, inguinal hernias, ataxia, seizures
Ataxia-Deafness-Dementia, X-linked	+	+	+	Optic atrophy, ataxia, hypotonia, seizures, childhood death
Cerebro-Oculo-Genital	+	+	0	Microcephaly, hydrocephaly, short stature, agenesis of corpus callosum, microphthalmia, ptosis, hypospadias, cryptorchidism, clubfoot
Goldblatt Spastic Paraplegia	+	+	0	Optic atrophy, exotropia, nystagmus, ataxia, dysarthria, muscle hypoplasia, contractures
Pelizaeus-Merzbacher	+	+	0	Optic atrophy, nystagmus, hypotonia, ataxia, dystonia, CNS dysmyelination
XLID-Blindness-Seizures-Spasticity	+	+	0	Poor growth, postnatal microcephaly, clubfoot, seizures, contractures, scoliosis, hypomyelination
XLID-Spastic Parapleglia, type 7	+	+	0	Nystagmus, reduced vision, absent speech and ambulation, bowel and bladder dysfunction, spastic quadriplegia
Wittwer	0	+	+	Microcephaly, short stature, microphthalmia, hypertelorism, genitourinary anomalies, hypotonia, seizures

AGENESIS OF THE CORPUS CALLOSUM, X-LINKED

(MENKES-KAPLAN SYNDROME)

OMIM 304100

Maldevelopment of the corpus callosum may occur as an isolated and perhaps asymptomatic finding or may co-exist with other anomalies. XLID syndromes that may have dysgenesis of the corpus callosum include Aicardi, *ARX*-Associated XLID, Bertini, Cerebro-Oculo-Genital, Hydrocephaly-MASA Spectrum, Juberg-Marsidi-Brooks, Kang, Lujan, MIDAS, Optiz FG, Oral-Facial-Digital I, Pyruvate Dehydrogenase Deficiency, and X-Linked Lissencephaly. Although a number of families with apparently X-linked partial or complete agenesis of the corpus callosum have been reported, it is not clear that they do not represent one of these syndromes.

Boyd et al. (1993) and others have noted that dysgenesis of the corpus callosum may be a frequent finding in some families with X-Linked Hydrocephaly-MASA Spectrum. The families reported by Menkes et al. (1964) and Kaplan (1983) may, in fact, be examples of this spectrum. Menkes et al. (1964) reported five cases with agenesis of the corpus callosum that experienced severe developmental impairment and seizures beginning in the neonatal period. Kaplan (1983) reported a 2-year-old boy with developmental disability, small head size, enlarged ventricles, hypoplasia of the inferior vermis and cerebellum, right ptosis, adducted thumbs, upper limb weakness, and Hirschsprung disease. The child's maternal uncle had intellectual disability, microcephaly, and agenesis of the corpus callosum.

REFERENCES

Boyd E, Schwartz CE, Schroer RJ, et al.: Agenesis of the corpus callosum associated with MASA syndrome. Clin Dysmorphol 2:332, 1993.

Kaplan P: X linked recessive inheritance of agenesis of the corpus callosum. J Med Genet 20:122, 1983.

Menkes JH, Philippart M, Clark DB: Hereditary partial agenesis of corpus callosum. Arch Neurol 11:198, 1964.

Serville F, Lyonnet S, Pelet A, et al.: X-linked hydrocephalus: clinical heterogeneity at a single gene locus. Eur J Pediatr 51:515, 1992.

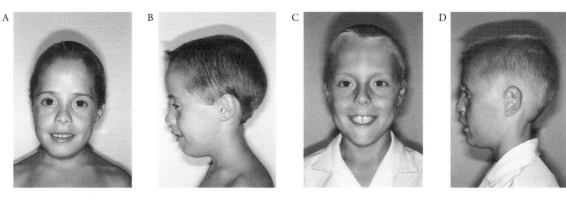

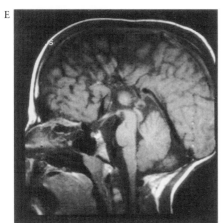

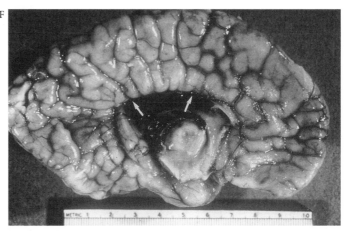

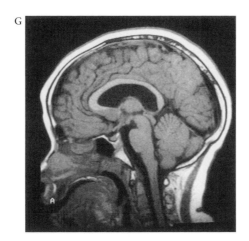

Agenesis of the Corpus Callosum, X-Linked. Seven-year-old male with total agenesis of the corpus callosum (A-B). Brother of patient in A and B at age 9 years with total agenesis of the corpus callosum (C, D); sagittal MRI scan of patient shown in C and D showing absence of the corpus callosum (E). Sagittal brain section showing absence of the corpus callosum [arrows] (F); sagittal MRI scan of a child with macrocephaly and normal-appearing corpus callosum (G).   Illustrations A-E courtesy of Dr. E.M. Honey, University of Pretoria, Republic of South Africa.

AHMAD SYNDROME

OMIM 300218

Xp11.3-q23

MRXS7

Definition. XLID with short stature, obesity, and hypogonadism.

Somatic Features. The tetrad of findings – short stature, obesity, hypogonadism, and severe intellectual disability – are present in most affected males. Hypogonadism is manifest by small penis and testes and absent or scant body hair. Facial hair is present and gynecomastia conspicuously absent. The fingers are tapered and strength is diminished. Obesity is constant. Hormone levels – FSH, LH, testosterone – are normal.

Growth and Development. Prenatal growth is not known. Adult height varies between 145 centimeters and 177 centimeters, weight between 80 kilograms and 120 kilograms.

Cognitive Function. IQ scores ranged between 40 and 50.

Heterozygote Expression. No intellectual impairment.

Comment. This X-linked hypogonadism syndrome most resembles Wilson-Turner syndrome, which maps to the same region. Gynecomastia is typically present in Wilson-Turner syndrome and absent in Ahmad syndrome. Borjeson-Forssman-Lehmann and MEHMO syndromes map outside the linkage region.

REFERENCE

Ahmad W. De Fusco M, ul Haque MF, et al.: Linkage mapping of a new syndromic form of X-linked mental retardation, MRXS7, associated with obesity. Eur J Hum Genet 7:828, 1999.

DIFFERENTIAL MATRIX

Syndrome	Short Stature	Hypogonadism	Obesity	Comments
Ahmad	+	+	+	Tapered fingers
Börjeson-Forssman-Lehmann	+	+	+	Microcephaly, coarse face, large ears, gynecomastia, narrow sloped shoulders, visual impairment, tapered digits, hypotonia
Urban	+	+	+	Small hands and feet, digital contractures, osteoporosis, hypotonia
Vasquez	+	+	+	Microcephaly, gynecomastia, hypotonia
XLID-Hypogonadism-Tremor	+	+	+	Prominent lower lip, muscle wasting of legs, abnormal gait, seizures, tremor
Young-Hughes	+	+	+	Small palpebral fissures, cupped ears, ichthyosiform scaling, hypogenitalism
ATRX-Associated XLID	+	+	0	Microcephaly, telecanthus/hypertelorism, small triangular nose, tented upper lip, open mouth, wide spacing of teeth, abnormal genitalia, minor musculoskeletal anomalies, hypotonia, erythrocyte HbH inclusions in some
Wilson-Turner	0	+	+	Normal growth, small hands and feet, tapered digits, gynecomastia, emotional lability, hypotonia

AICARDI SYNDROME

(AGENESIS OF CORPUS CALLOSUM-LACUNAR CHORIORETINOPATHY SYNDROME)

OMIM 304050

Xp22.3-p22.2 (TENTATIVE)

Definition. XLID with agenesis of the corpus callosum, lacunar chorioretinopathy, costovertebral anomalies, and seizures in females. The tentative location of the responsible gene is based on an X:3 translocation with the X breakpoint at p22.3-22.2.

Somatic Features. More than any other manifestation, lacunar chorioretinopathy serves to distinguish Aicardi syndrome from other conditions with agenesis of the corpus callosum and seizures. Bilateral punched-out areas of pigment epithelium occur near the optic disc, appear yellow-white, and have little surrounding pigment deposition. Deposition of pigment around and within the lacunae increases with age. Microphthalmia, iris synechiae, optic atrophy, and colobomas may occur as well. Cranial size varies depending on whether enlarged ventricles are present. Isolated cortical heterotopias occur in at least half of cases. Hemivertebrae, scoliosis, and absent or malformed ribs are found in one-third of those affected. Cleft lip and cleft palate, hiatal hernia, and hip dysplasia have been described in a few cases.

Growth and Development. Normal intrauterine and postnatal growth is the rule. Cephalic growth may slow resulting in microcephaly. Developmental milestones are globally delayed.

Cognitive Function. Severe impairment, with few achieving the rudiments of speech.

Neurological Findings. Severe impairment of neurological function is obvious from early infancy. Seizures of a wide variety (infantile spasms, generalized seizures, staring spells) occur, in some cases beginning as early as the first day of life. The EEG shows the characteristic burst-suppression pattern of hypsarrhythmia, other seizure discharges, and asynchrony between the cerebral hemispheres.

Imaging. Agenesis of the corpus callosum, cerebral asymmetry with cortical dysplasia, neuronal migration abnormalities, enlarged lateral ventricles, choroid plexus cysts, cerebellar hypoplasia, and posterior fossa cysts may be demonstrated.

Comment. Microcephaly, chorioretinopathy, seizures, and developmental delay calls to mind prenatal infection, especially prenatal toxoplasmosis. The distinctive lacunar retinopathy serves best to distinguish Aicardi syndrome from these infections. As a rule, Aicardi syndrome occurs sporadically and only in females. No affected female has reproduced. Consideration that the syndrome is X-linked

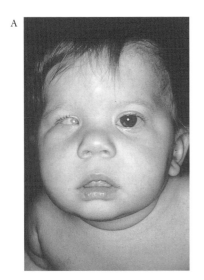 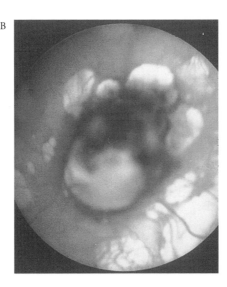 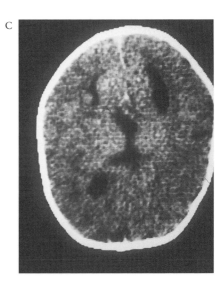

Aicardi syndrome. One-year-old female with microphthalmia (A); lacunar choreoretinopathy (B); cranial CT showing high third ventricle consistent with agenesis of the corpus callosum (C). Courtesy of Dr. Alan Donnenfeld, Pennsylvania Hospital, Philadelphia.

dominant with expression in females and gestational lethality in males is based on the increased abortions and decreased male:female ratio in at risk sibships. An increase in skewing of X-inactivation has been reported. The few males reported have had atypical chorioretinal findings, lissencephaly or other structural brain anomalies, may represent phenocopies, or may result from somatic mosaicism. In some cases, a 47, XXY karyotype has been demonstrated.

REFERENCES

Aicardi J: Aicardi syndrome. Brain Dev 27:164, 2005.

Aicardi J, Chevrie J-J, Rousselie F: le syndrome spasmes en flexion, agenesie calleuse, anomalies chorio-retiniennes. Arch Franc Ped 26:1103, 1969.

Aicardi J, Lefebvre J, Lerique A: Spasms in flexion, callosal agenesis, ocular abnormalities: a new syndrome. Electroenceph Clin Neurophysiol 19:609, 1965.

Chen T-H, Chao M-C, Lin L-C, et al.: Aicardi syndrome in a 47,XXY male neonate with lissencephaly and holoprosencephaly. J Neurol Sci 278:138, 2009.

Donnenfeld AE, Packer RJ, Zackai EH, et al.: Clinical, cytogenetic, and pedigree findings in 18 cases of Aicardi syndrome. Am J Med Genet 32:461, 1989.

Kroner BL, Preiss LR, Ardini M-A, et al.: New incidence, prevalence, and survival of Aicardi syndrome from 408 cases. J Child Neurol 23:531, 2008.

Sutton VR, Hopkins BJ, Eble TN, et al.: Facial and physical features of Aicardi syndrome: infants to teenagers. Am J Med Genet 138A:254, 2005.

Willis J, Rosman NP: The Aicardi syndrome versus congenital infection: diagnostic considerations. J Pediatr 96:235, 1980.

DIFFERENTIAL MATRIX

Syndrome	Ocular Abnormality	CNS Anomalies	Vertebral or Rib Defects	Comments
Aicardi	+	+	+	Lacunar retinopathy, costovertebral anomalies, agenesis of corpus callosum, seizures
Cerebro-Cerebello-Coloboma	+	+	0	Hydrocephaly, cerebellar vermis hypoplasia, retinal coloboma, hypotonia, seizures, abnormal respiratory pattern
Cerebro-Oculo-Genital	+	+	0	Microcephaly, hydrocephaly, short stature, agenesis of corpus callosum, microphthalmia, ptosis, hypospadias, cryptorchidism, clubfoot, spasticity
MIDAS	+	+	0	Microphthalmia, corneal opacification, dermal aplasia, dysgenesis of corpus callosum, cardiac defects, cardiomyopathy
Chassaing-Lacombe Chondrodysplasia	+	0	+	Spondylometaphyseal dysplasia, hydrocephaly, and microphthalmia in males. Spondylometaphyseal dysplasia with rhizomelic shortening of limbs and learning disability in females
Lenz Microphthalmia	+	0	+	Microcephaly, microphthalmia, malformed ears, cleft lip/palate, cardiac and genitourinary anomalies, thumb duplication or hypoplasia, narrow shoulders
Roifman	+	0	+	Microcephaly, short stature, spondyloepiphyseal dysplasia, retinal pigmentary deposits, antibody deficiency, eczema, hypotonia

ALLAN-HERNDON-DUDLEY SYNDROME

(ALLAN-HERNDON SYNDROME)

OMIM 300523

Xq13.2

SLC16A2 (MCT8)

Definition. XLID with generalized muscle hypoplasia, childhood hypotonia, ataxia, athetosis, dysarthria, and spastic paraplegia. The gene (*SLC16A2*) is responsible for transporting triiodothyronine into neurons.

Somatic Features. Marked hypotonia and paucity of skeletal muscle mass permits diagnosis in infancy. Although the facies do not appear distinctive in childhood, there is a tendency in adult life toward elongation of the face, cupping or abnormal folding of the ears, and large ears. In one family, bitemporal narrowness and midface hypoplasia was noted. No malformations have been noted. Spastic paraplegia and contractures of the small and large joints become evident in adult life. Shallow pectus excavatum, ulnar deviation of the hand, scoliosis, and valgus position of the great toe may be seen. Excessive drooling and dysarthria continue into adult life, deep tendon reflexes become hyperactive, and clonus and Babinski signs may be seen. Fungal infections appear common.

Growth and Development. Some affected males never develop speech or independent ambulation. Adult stature and head circumference appears normal. Puberty occurs at the usual age, and external genitalia are normal.

Cognitive Function. Severe cognitive impairment and attentive friendly countenance.

Heterozygote Expression. None

Imaging. Magnetic resonance imaging of the brain in a 1-year-old was normal; in a 58-year-old showed prominence of the cortical sulci and mild dilation of the ventricular system.

Laboratory. Peripheral nerve (peroneal) conduction in one affected male was mildly impaired and showed some spontaneous motor potential, but muscle microscopy showed no pathologic changes. Serum free and total T_3 are elevated, and T_4 may be in the low normal range. TSH is normal.

Treatment. Several patients have been treated with T_4 and propylthiouracil without psychomotor improvement.

Comment. Allan-Herndon-Dudley syndrome is one of several XLID syndromes that present initially with hypotonia and later transition to spasticity. Although the T_3 is elevated, there are no systemic signs of thyroid dysfunction.

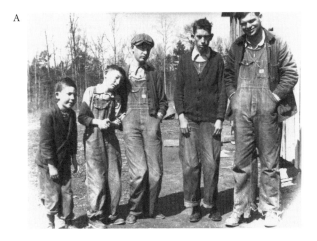
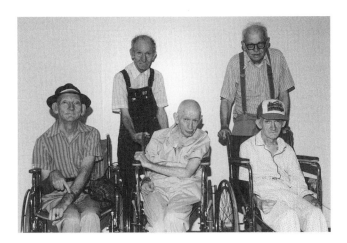

Allen-Herndon-Dudley Syndrome. Five affected males from original family in childhood and late adult life (A).

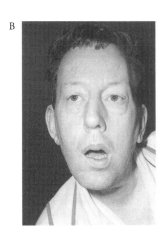

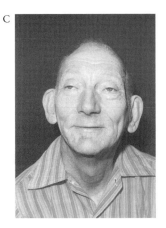

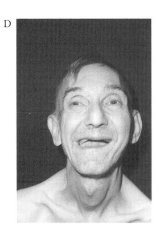

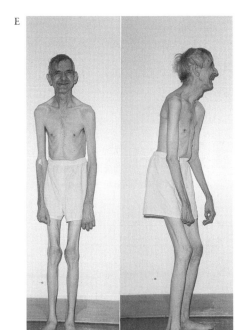

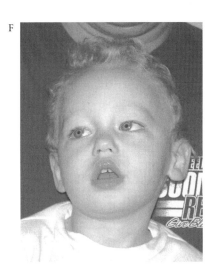

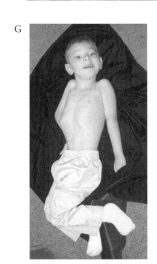

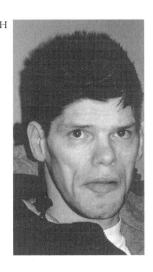

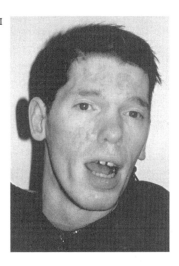

Forty-nine-year-old with long face, bitemporal narrowing, flat midface, and myopathic appearance (B); 61-year-old with bitemporal narrowing, midface hypoplasia, and simple cupped ears (C); and 65-year-old with bitemporal narrowing, cupped ears, and marked hypoplasia of musculature (D,E); Two cousins and their uncles from another family showing hypotonic face in 22-month-old child (F); muscle hypoplasia and spasticity in 4-year-old cousin (G); gaunt face in 38-year-old uncle (H), and gaunt face and open mouth in 39-year-old uncle (I).

REFERENCES

Allan W, Herndon CN, Dudley FC: Some examples of the inheritance of mental deficiency: Apparently sex-linked idiocy and microcephaly. Am J Ment Defic 48:325, 1944.

Bialer MG, Lawrence L, Stevenson RE, et al.: Allan-Herndon-Dudley syndrome: Clinical and linkage studies on a second family. Am J Med Genet 43:491, 1992.

Dumitrescu AM, Liao X-H, Best TB, et al.: A novel syndrome combining thyroid and neurological abnormalities is associated with mutations in a monocarboxylate transporter gene. Am J Hum Genet 74:168, 2004.

Friesema ECH, Grueters A, Biebermann H, et al.: Association between mutations in a thyroid hormone transporter and severe X-linked psychomotor retardation. Lancet 364:1435, 2004.

Schwartz CE, May MM, Carpenter NJ, et al.: Allan-Herndon-Dudley syndrome and the monocarboxylate transporter 8 (MCT8) gene. Am J Hum Genet 77:41, 2005.

Schwartz CE, Ulmer J, Brown A, et al.: Allan-Herndon syndrome. II. Linkage to DNA markers in Xq21. Am J Hum Genet 47:454, 1990.

Stevenson RE, Goodman HO, Schwartz CE, et al.: Allan-Herndon syndrome. I. Clinical studies. Am J Hum Genet 47:446, 1990.

Wémeau JL, Pigeyre M, Proust-Lemoine E, et al.: Beneficial effects of propylthiouracil plus L-thyroxine treatment in a patient with a mutation in MCT8. J Clin Endocrinol Metab 93:2084, 2008.

DIFFERENTIAL MATRIX

Syndrome	Ataxia	Spastic Paraplegia	Muscle Hypoplasia	Comments
Allan-Herndon-Dudley	+	+	+	Childhood hypotonia, dysarthria, athetosis, large ears with cupping or abnormal architecture, contractures
Apak Ataxia-Spastic Diplegia	+	+	+	Short stature, clubfoot, dysarthria, nystagmus
Goldblatt Spastic Paraplegia	+	+	+	Optic atrophy, exotropia, nystagmus, dysarthria, contractures
XLID-Spastic Paraplegia-Athetosis	+	+	+	Nystagmus, weakness, dysarthria, muscle wasting, contractures
Adrenoleukodystrophy	+	+	0	Adrenal insufficiency, diffuse skin pigmentation, progressive neurologic deterioration and dementia, elevated very-long-chain fatty acids in plasma
Hydrocephaly-MASA Spectrum	+	+	0	Ophthalmoplegia, lack of speech and ambulation, incontinence
Pelizaeus-Merzbacher	+	+	0	Optic atrophy, nystagmus, hypotonia, dystonia, CNS dysmyelination
Pettigrew	+	+	0	Microcephaly or hydrocephaly, long face with macrostomia and prognathism, Dandy-Walker malformation, small testes, contractures, choreoathetosis, iron deposits in basal ganglia, seizures
Ataxia-Deafness-Dementia, X-linked	+	+	0	Optic atrophy, deafness, hypotonia, hyperreflexia, recurrent episodes of choking and vomiting, seizures, childhood death
XLID-Ataxia-Dementia	+	+	0	Adult-onset dementia
XLID-Spastic Paraplegia, type 7	+	+	0	Nystagmus, reduced vision, absent speech and ambulation, bowel and bladder dysfunction
Arts	+	0	+	Growth deficiency, poor muscle development, hypotonia, areflexia, seizures, childhood death
Christianson	+	0	+	Microcephaly, short stature, long narrow face, contractures, seizures
XLID-Hypogonadism-Tremor	+	0	+	Short stature, prominent lower lip, muscle wasting of legs, abnormal gait, hypogonadism, obesity, seizures, tremor
Fitzsimmons	0	+	+	Pes cavus, hyperkeratosis of palms and soles, dystrophic nails

ALPHA-THALASSEMIA INTELLECTUAL DISABILITY (*SEE ALSO ATRX*-ASSOCIATED XLID)

(XLID-HYPOTONIC FACIES SYNDROME, CEREBROFACIOGENITAL SYNDROME, ATR-X, CHUDLEY-LOWRY SYNDROME, CARPENTER-WAZIRI SYNDROME, HOLMES-GANG SYNDROME, XLID-ARCH FINGERPRINTS-HYPOTONIA)

OMIM 301040, 309580

Xq21.1

ATRX (XNP)

Definition. XLID with short stature, microcephaly, hypotonic facies with hypertelorism, small nose, open mouth and prominent lips, brachydactyly, genital anomalies, hypotonia, and, in some cases, hemoglobin H inclusions in erythrocytes.

Somatic Features. Most somatic manifestations can be noted from birth and in part may appear more distinctive in early childhood than later in life. Microcephaly is the rule and is often present at birth. Facial characteristics include telecanthus or hypertelorism, epicanthus, flat nasal bridge, maxillary hypoplasia, small triangular nose, anteverted nares, open mouth with prominent lips, and wide spacing of the incisors. There is a tendency toward coarsening of the facial features with age. Many minor anomalies of the skeleton may be noted: brachydactyly, tapering fingers, clinodactyly, digital contractures, overlapping digits, pes planus, varus and valgus foot deformations, kyphosis, scoliosis, pectus carinatum, and dimples over the lower spine. Undifferentiated genitalia or sex reversal occur

uncommonly, but most cases have some genital anomaly including hypospadias, cryptorchidism, or genital hypoplasia. Major malformations are rare, but cleft palate and cardiac septal defects have been described.

Growth and Development. Most patients will ultimately have short stature. In some cases it is apparent from birth and in others appears to begin or become more pronounced at puberty. Puberty is often delayed. Development is globally and profoundly delayed. Walking is delayed until late childhood and other motor skills come late as well. Speech is absent or severely limited.

Behavior. Generally described as affectionate but some suggestion of outbursts of laughter or crying.

Neurological Findings. Hypotonia dominates the neuromuscular phenotype and undoubtedly contributes to the somatic appearance as well.

Heterozygote Expression. Although hypertelorism and maxillary hypoplasia have been noted, there is little evidence for expression in carrier females. Carriers may, in some cases, be identified by rare HbH inclusions in erythrocytes. The usual absence of manifestations in carriers

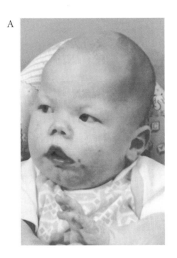
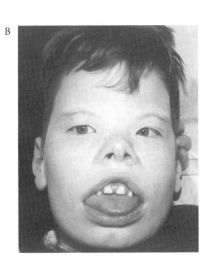

Alpha-Thalassemia Intellectual Disability. Microcephaly, hypertelorism, telecanthus, depressed nasal bridge, short triangular nose, anteverted nostrils, full lips, and tented upper lip at age 6 months (**A**) and 21 years (**B**).

serves as an important means of clinical differentiation from Coffin-Lowry syndrome. Carriers typically have marked skewing of X-chromosome inactivation with preferential inactivation of the chromosome carrying the *ATRX* mutation.

Natural History. Affected males are obviously and profoundly affected from birth. In addition to the slow developmental progress, infancy is compromised by poor feeding, vomiting and esophageal reflux, recurrent respiratory and urinary infections, apneic or cyanotic spells, and constipation. Most do not develop meaningful speech and motor skills are markedly impaired.

Laboratory. A mild microcytic anemia may be present. Inclusions in erythrocytes stained with brilliant cresyl blue for hemoglobin H (β_4 tetramers) or hemoglobin electrophoresis offer convenient methods for screening for Alpha-Thalassemia Intellectual Disability syndrome. However, many cases do not have significant enough levels of HbH to be detected by electrophoresis and erythrocyte inclusions may be rare, necessitating repeated screening. Other cases may lack hemoglobin abnormalities altogether. Diagnostic confirmation depends on mutational analysis of the responsible gene.

Comment. Although the first cases of Alpha-Thalassemia Intellectual Disability syndrome were ascertained because of mild hematologic abnormalities, subsequent cases were identified because of somatic manifestations. Four other named XLID syndromes (Chudley-Lowry, Carpenter-Waziri, Holmes-Gang, and XLID-Arch Fingerprints-Hypotonia syndromes) have been shown to have mutations of *ATRX*, as have individuals with intellectual disability and spastic paraplegia and individuals with nonsyndromal XLID. Previously, Juberg-Marsidi was considered to be an allelic condition but now is known to be caused by mutations in *HUWE1*. Smith-Fineman-Myers syndrome has also been considered to be allelic, but an *ATRX* mutation has not been confirmed in the original family.

Coffin-Lowry syndrome may be easily confused with the Alpha-Thalassemia Intellectual Disability syndrome, especially in early childhood. The frequent presence of carrier manifestations, large fleshy hands and fingers, and skeletal abnormalities as well as absence of genital anomalies in Coffin-Lowry syndrome serve as distinguishing features.

Mutational analysis – *ATRX* in Alpha-Thalassemia Intellectual Disability syndrome and *RSK2* in Coffin-Lowry – can confirm the correct diagnosis in most cases.

REFERENCES

Abidi FE, Cardoso C, Lossi AM, et al.: Mutation in the 5' alternatively spliced region of the XNP/ATR-X gene causes Chudley-Lowry syndrome. Eur J Hum Genet 13:176, 2005.

Chudley AE, Lowry RB, Hoar DI: Mental retardation, distinct facial changes, short stature, obesity, and hypogonadism: a new X-linked mental retardation syndrome. Am J Med Genet 31:741, 1988.

Donnai D, Clayton-Smith J, Gibbons RJ, et al.: The non-deletion α-thalassaemia/mental retardation syndrome. Further support for X linkage. J Med Genet 28: 742, 1991.

Gibbons RJ, Brueton L, Buckle VJ, et al.: Clinical and hematologic aspects of the X-linked α-thalassemia/mental retardation syndrome (ATR-X). Am J Med Genet 55:288, 1995.

Gibbons RJ, Picketts DJ, Villard L, et al.: Mutations in a putative global transcriptional regulator cause X-linked mental retardation with α-thalassemia (ATR-X syndrome). Cell 80:837, 1995.

Gibbons RJ, Suthers GK, Wilkie AOM, et al.: X-linked α-thalassemia/mental retardation (ATR-X) syndrome: Localization to Xq12-q21.31 by X inactivation and linkage analysis. Am J Hum Genet 51:1136, 1992.

Gibbons RJ, Wada T, Fisher CA, et al.: Mutations in the chromatin-associated protein ATRX. Hum Mutat 29:796, 2008.

Guerrini R, Shanahan JL, Carrozzo R, et al.: A nonsense mutation of the ATRX gene causing mild mental retardation and epilepsy. Ann Neurol 47:117, 2000.

Martínez F, Tomás M, Millán JM, et al.: Genetic localisation of mental retardation with spastic diplegia to the pericentromeric region of the X chromosome: X inactivation in female carriers. J Med Genet 35:284, 1998.

Stevenson RE, Häne B, Arena JF, et al.: Arch fingerprints, hypotonia, and areflexia associated with X linked mental retardation. J Med Genet 34:465, 1997.

Villard L, Gecz J, Mattei JF, et al.: XNP mutation in a large family with Juberg-Marsidi syndrome. Nat Genet 12:359, 1996.

Wilkie AOM, Gibbons RJ, Higgs DR, et al.: X-linked α-thalassemia/mental retardation: spectrum of clinical features in three related males. J Med Genet 28:738, 1991.

Yntema HG, Poppelaars FA, Derksen E, et al.: Expanding phenotype of XNP mutations: mild to moderate mental retardation. Am J Med Genet 110:243, 2002.

DIFFERENTIAL MATRIX

Syndrome	Microcephaly	Hypotonic Facies	Urogenital Anomalies	Comments
Alpha-Thalassemia Intellectual Disability (*ATRX*-Associated XLID)	+	+	+	Short stature, telecanthus, small triangular nose, tented upper lip, open mouth, wide spacing of teeth, genital anomalies, musculoskeletal anomalies, hemoglobin H inclusions in erythrocytes
Proud (*ARX*-Associated XLID)	+	+	+	Hearing loss, vision loss, agenesis of corpus callosum, cryptorchidism, inguinal hernias, ataxia, spasticity, seizures
Coffin-Lowry	+	+	0	Short stature, hypertelorism, anteverted nares, tented upper lip, prominent lips and large mouth, large ears, soft hands with tapered digits, pectus carinatum
Miles-Carpenter	+	+	0	Short stature, ptosis, small palpebral fissures, open mouth, pectus excavatum, scoliosis, long hands, camptodactyly, rockerbottom feet, arch fingerprints, spasticity, unsteady gait
Smith-Fineman-Myers	+	+	0	Ptosis, flat philtrum, scoliosis, midfoot varus, narrow feet, seizures, hypotonia
Vasquez	+	0	+	Short stature, gynecomastia, obesity, hypotonia, hypogonadism
XLID-Hypogonadism-Tremor	+	0	+	Short stature, prominent lower lip, muscle wasting of legs, abnormal gait, hypogonadism, obesity, seizures, tremor
XLID-Hypospadias	+	0	+	Trigonocephaly, synophrys, beaked nose, dysplastic ears, joint hyperextensibility, hypotonia
XLID-Microcephaly-Testicular Failure	+	0	+	Short stature, prominent supraorbital ridges, high nasal bridge, prominent nose, macrostomia, hypogonadism
XLID-Psoriasis	0	+	+	Hypertelorism, strabismus, large ears, macrostomia, psoriasis, seizures

AP1S2-ASSOCIATED XLID

(MRX59, *AP1S2* SPECTRUM, TURNER XLID SYNDROME, FRIED SYNDROME,
XLID-HYDROCEPHALY-BASAL GANGLIA CALCIFICATION)

OMIM 300630

Xp22.2

AP1S2

Definition. Three XLID entities have been found to have *AP1S2* mutations: Turner XLID, Fried syndrome, and MRX59. Because of phenotypic differences, Turner XLID and X-linked Hydrocephaly-Basal Ganglia Calcifications (Fried syndrome) are briefly summarized here and have separate entries in this Atlas.

Turner et al. (2003) reported a kindred in which seven males had mild to moderate intellectual disability, microcephaly, hypotonia, absent or minimal speech, and bouts of aggressiveness. One male had hydrocephalus. A kindred with four affected males with similar degree of disability and hypotonia, but without microcephaly and less frequent speech limitations and aggressive outbursts, was included in the report of Tarpey et al. (2006).

Fried (1973) reported a kindred in which six affected males had hydrocephaly, calcification of the basal ganglia, awkward gait, and spastic paraplegia. Only one had microcephaly and two had head enlargement caused by hydrocephaly. A second family was reported by Saillour et al. in 2007. In neither family was a tendency to aggressive behavior reported.

The five affected males in the MRX59 family had variable (mild to severe) intellectual disability, head circumference (<3rd centile to >50th centile), speech acquisition (absent to delayed, but present), and aggressive behavior. Hypotonia was consistently present.

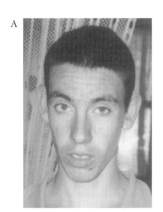 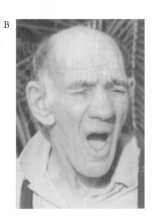 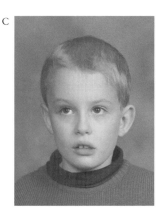 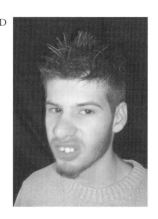

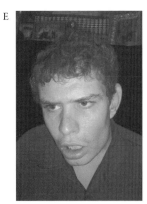 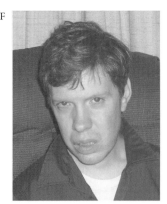 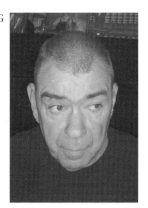

AP1S2-Associated XLID. Fifteen-year-old male and 70-year-old uncle with prominent forehead, long nose and face, narrow jaw, and prominent ears (**A, B**). Eleven-year-old male (**C**), his 17-year-old cousin (**D**), 30-year-old uncle (**E**), 41-year-old uncle (**F**), and 62-year-old great uncle (**G**) with variable facial features including long face, prominent lips, and small jaw from family reported by Carpenter et al. as MRX59 (Am J Med Genet 85:266, 1999).
Illustrations A and B courtesy of Dr. Gillian Turner, New South Wales, Australia.

REFERENCES

Carpenter NJ, Brown WT, Qu Y, et al.: Regional localization of a nonspecific X-linked mental retardation gene (MRX59) to Xp21.2-p22.2. Am J Med Genet 85:266, 1999.

Fried K: X-linked mental retardation and-or hydrocephalus. Clin Genet 3:258, 1972.

Saillour Y, Zanni G, Des Portes V, et al.: Mutations in the AP1S2 gene encoding the sigma 2 subunit of the adaptor protein 1 complex are associated with syndromic X-linked mental retardation with hydrocephalus and calcifications in basal ganglia. J Med Genet 44:739, 2007.

Strain L, Wright AF, Bonthron DT: Fried syndrome is a distinct X linked mental retardation syndrome mapping to Xp22. J Med Genet 34:535, 1977.

Turner G, Gedeon A, Kerr B, et al.: Syndromic form of X-linked mental retardation with marked hypotonia in early life, severe mental handicap, and difficult adult behavior maps to Xp22. Am J Med Genet A 117A:245, 2003.

DIFFERENTIAL MATRIX

Syndrome	Iron Deposits or Calcification of Basal Ganglia	Spastic Paraplegia	Muscle Hypoplasia	Comments
AP1S2-Associated XLID	+	+	+	Hydrocephaly, sensory impairment
Gustavson	+	+	+	Microcephaly, short stature, optic atrophy with blindness, large ears, deafness, joint contractures, rockerbottom feet, brain undergrowth, hydrocephaly, cerebellar hypoplasia, seizures
Pelizaeus-Merzbacher	+	+	+	Optic atrophy, nystagmus, hypotonia, ataxia, spasticity, dystonia, CNS dysmyelination
Schimke	+	+	0	Microcephaly, sunken eyes, downslanting palpebral fissures, narrow nose, wide spacing of teeth, cupped ears, hypotonia, abducens palsy, hearing loss, vision loss, choreoathetosis, contractures

APAK ATAXIA-SPASTIC DIPLEGIA SYNDROME

Definition. XLID with short stature, muscle hypoplasia, nystagmus, ataxia, and spasticity. The gene has not been mapped.

Somatic Features. The head circumference is normal, and facial abnormalities are not described. The musculature – especially the peroneal muscles – are hypoplastic; clubfoot and other foot contractures occur.

Growth and Development. Short stature is obvious in childhood.

Cognitive Function. Specific testing is not available, but comprehension appears better than limited speech and motor skills suggest.

Neurological Findings. Males never learn to walk and speech is dysarthric. Ataxia is manifested as head and truncal instability, nystagmus, dysmetria, and adiadochokinesis. The ability to sit may be gained by age 2 years but is lost within a few years. Spasticity is manifested by impaired fine motor skills, increased deep tendon reflexes, Babinski signs, and contracture of the joints. Sensation appears normal. Neurological signs appear early with nystagmus in early months, spasticity by the end of the first year, truncal ataxia at age 2 to 3 years, and dysarthric speech at age 3 to 4 years. Death from infections occurs in the third or fourth decade.

Heterozygote Expression. One carrier female had hyperactive deep tendon reflexes.

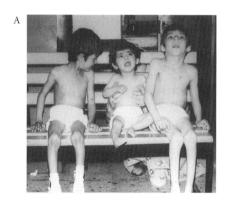

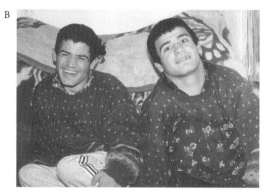

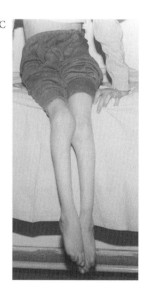

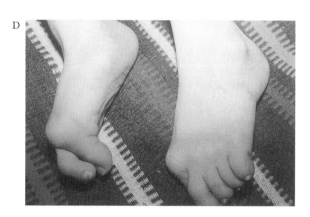

Apak Ataxia-Spastic Diplegia Syndrome. Affected brothers at ages 6, 2, and 8 years (**A**); maternal uncles as young adults (**B**); muscle hypoplasia of lower limbs in an 8-year-old (**C**); foot contractures in a young adult (**D**).   Courtesy of Dr. Selcuk Apak, Institute of Child Health, University of Istanbul, Turkey.

Imaging. CT was normal in one case at age 9 years.

Laboratory. EEG, EMG, and nerve conduction velocity were normal in one case.

Comment. Apak syndrome, represented by a single family, is set aside as a distinct syndrome because it differs in some respects from other X-linked cerebellar ataxias and spastic diplegias. Cerebellar and pyramidal signs become obvious in the initial years of life, cognitive function is impaired, neurological dysfunction progresses to total disability in the teen years, and lifespan is shortened. Linkage studies were not successful in mapping the gene location. The relationship to X-linked olivopontocerebellar atrophy (MIM 302500) is not known.

REFERENCE

Apak S, Yüksel M, Özmen M, et al.: Heterogeneity of X-linked recessive (spino)cerebellar ataxia with or without spastic diplegia. Am J Med Genet 34:155, 1989.

DIFFERENTIAL MATRIX

Syndrome	Ataxia	Spastic Paraplegia	Muscle Hypoplasia	Comments
Apak Ataxia-Spastic Diplegia	+	+	+	Short stature, nystagmus, dysarthria, contractures
Allan-Herndon-Dudley	+	+	+	Childhood hypotonia, dysarthria, athetosis, large ears with cupping or abnormal architecture, contractures
Goldblatt Spastic Paraplegia	+	+	+	Optic atrophy, exotropia, nystagmus, dysarthria, contractures
XLID-Spastic Paraplegia-Athetosis	+	+	+	Nystagmus, weakness, dysarthria, muscle wasting, contractures
Adrenoleukodystrophy	+	+	0	Adrenal insufficiency, diffuse skin pigmentation, progressive neurologic deterioration and dementia, elevated very-long-chain fatty acids in plasma
Hydrocephaly-MASA Spectrum	+	+	0	Hydrocephaly, adducted thumbs, dysgenesis of corpus callosum
Pelizaeus-Merzbacher	+	+	0	Optic atrophy, nystagmus, hypotonia, dystonia, CNS dysmyelination
Pettigrew	+	+	0	Microcephaly or hydrocephaly, long face with macrostomia and prognathism, Dandy-Walker malformation, small testes, contractures, choreoathetosis, iron deposits in basal ganglia, seizures
Ataxia-Deafness-Dementia, X-linked	+	+	0	Optic atrophy, vision loss, hearing loss, hypotonia, seizures, childhood death
XLID-Ataxia-Dementia	+	+	0	Adult-onset dementia
XLID-Spastic Paraplegia, type 7	+	+	0	Nystagmus, reduced vision, absent speech and ambulation, bowel and bladder dysfunction
Arts	+	0	+	Growth deficiency, poor muscle development, hypotonia, areflexia, seizures, childhood death
Christianson	+	0	+	Microcephaly, short stature, long narrow face, contractures, seizures
XLID-Hypogonadism-Tremor	+	0	+	Short stature, prominent lower lip, muscle wasting of legs, abnormal gait, hypogonadism, obesity, seizures, tremor
Fitzsimmons	0	+	+	Pes cavus, hyperkeratosis of palms and soles, dystrophic nails

ARMFIELD SYNDROME

(XLID-GLAUCOMA-CLEFTING)

OMIM 300261

Xq28

Definition. XLID with short stature, small hands and feet, glaucoma, cleft palate, and seizures.

Somatic Features. Facial characteristics include prominent forehead, epicanthus, downslanting palpebral fissures, midface hypoplasia, large ears, cleft palate, and micrognathia. Cataracts and glaucoma may develop in adult life. The head circumference is quite variable, from below the 3rd centile to above the 97th centile, the latter probably secondary to hydrocephaly. Short stature is typical. The hands and feet are small, and there is stiffness of large and small joints. Other variable features include facial asymmetry, cupped ears, inguinal hernias, and undescended testes.

Growth and Development. Short stature with onset prenatally.

Cognitive Function. Severe impairment with IQs of 20 to 50.

Neurological Findings. Seizures, with onset in infancy or early childhood, are a consistent sign.

Heterozygote Expression. None

Imaging. Hydrocephaly was documented in two males, one of which also had a cystic fourth ventricle.

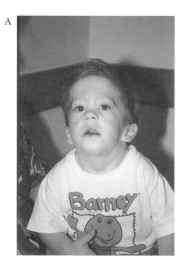

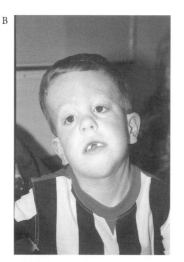

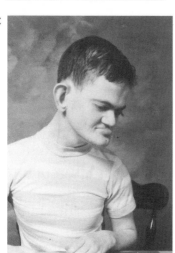

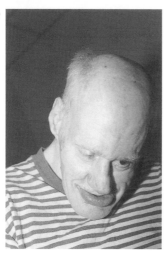

Armfield Syndrome. Brothers at ages 4 years (A) and 8 years (B) showing macrocephaly, ptosis, hypertelorism, downslanting palpebral fissures, and upfolded earlobes; uncles age 23 years (C) and 62 years (D) showing tall forehead, cupped ears, depressed midface, short philtrum, and patulous lower lip.

Laboratory. Low somatomedin C was found in two patients.

Comment. Xq28 is the most densely mapped region of the human genome. Fifteen XLID syndromes, exhibiting a broad spectrum of clinical phenotypes, have been mapped there, as have nonsyndromal XLID caused by *AFF2 (FRAXE)*, *GDI1*, and *RAB39B* mutations. Cleft palate and adult-onset glaucoma or cataracts serve to distinguish Armfield syndrome from the others.

REFERENCE

Armfield K, Schwartz CE, Lubs HA, et al.: An XLMR syndrome with short stature, small hands and feet, seizures, cleft palate, and glaucoma is linked to Xq28. Am J Med Genet 85:236, 1999.

DIFFERENTIAL MATRIX

Syndrome	Ocular Abnormality	Orofacial Clefting	Seizures	Comments
Armfield	+	+	+	Short stature, cataracts or glaucoma, dental anomalies, small hands and feet, hydrocephaly, joint stiffness
Cerebro-Cerebello-Coloboma	+	O	+	Hydrocephaly, cerebellar vermis hypoplasia, retinal coloboma, hypotonia, abnormal respiratory pattern
Cerebro-Oculo-Genital	+	O	+	Microcephaly, hydrocephaly, short stature, agenesis of corpus callosum, microphthalmia, ptosis, hypospadias, cryptorchidism, clubfoot, spasticity
Incontinentia Pigmenti	+	O	+	Cutaneous vesicles, verrucous lesions, irregular hyperpigmentation, microcephaly, oligodontia, abnormally shaped teeth, spasticity
Lowe	+	O	+	Short stature, cataracts, hypotonia, aminoaciduria, progressive renal disease
Wittwer	+	O	+	Microcephaly, short stature, microphthalmia, hearing loss, vision loss, hypertelorism, genitourinary anomalies, hypotonia
Oral-Facial-Digital I	O	+	+	Sparse scalp hair, dystopia canthorum, flat midface, hypoplastic alae nasi, lingual hamartomas, syndactyly, clinodactyly, structural brain anomalies, polycystic kidneys
Pallister W	O	+	+	Short stature, prominent forehead, wide nasal tip, incomplete cleft lip/palate, spasticity, contractures

ARTS SYNDROME

(LETHAL XLID-ATAXIA-DEAFNESS)

OMIM 301835

Xp22.3

PRPS1

Definition. XLID with impaired growth, paucity of muscles, and progressive neurological deterioration with ataxia, deafness, vision loss, seizures, and areflexia. Mutations in the phosphoribosyl pyrophosphate synthetase 1 gene have been demonstrated.

Somatic Features. No craniofacial features have been described. Neuromuscular findings predominate. There is a generalized paucity of muscles. From birth, males are hypotonic, weak, and areflexic. Motor development appears to worsen following respiratory infection in early childhood. In particular, truncal and limb ataxia develop and progressively worsen. Hearing appears severely impaired, in some cases from birth. None has developed speech. Vision may be normal initially but, if so, deteriorates with pallor of the discs and nystagmus within the first few years. Seizures – tonic-clonic or complex types – further complicate the childhood course.

Neurological Findings. A relentless neuromuscular deterioration leads to death in early childhood (ages newborn to 5 years). Neurological findings appear to accentuate following childhood infection. Generalized muscle underdevelopment is reflected in hypotonia and weakness. Reflexes are absent. Truncal and limb ataxia are present from infancy. Deafness, loss of vision, and seizures are further manifestations of the deterioration.

Heterozygote Expression. Carrier females frequently have hearing impairment in early adulthood. One obligate carrier had clubfoot, ataxia, hypotonia, hyperreflexia, and Babinski signs. Two other possible carriers had similar findings.

Neuropathology. Diffuse slowing or seizure discharges were present on EEG. EMG and muscle histology showed signs of denervation (usually with grouping of type 1 fibers). Visual stimulation showed increased transmission latency in one case and absence of occipital response in another. On postmortem examination of one case, the brainstem, cerebrum, and cerebellum were normal. The dorsal columns and dorsal nerve roots lacked axonal myelination, a finding similar to that seen in Friedreich ataxia.

Laboratory. A wide range of studies were normal, including renal function, thyroid hormones, serum and CSF pyruvate and lactate, carnitine, very-long-chain fatty acids, phytanic acid, cranial MRI, and lysosomal enzymes. Serum immunoglobulins were normal but with low-normal IgA.

Comment. Childhood lethality may serve as a measure of the overall severity of the biological insult resulting from mutation of X-linked genes. Lethality in the XLID syndromes appears more commonly associated with impaired nervous system function than with specific malformations or manifestations in essential organs such as the heart or kidneys. XLID syndromes with severely impaired nervous system function and childhood lethality include Arts, Bertini, Gustavson, Holmes-Gang, Hydrocephaly-Cerebellar Agenesis, Hereditary Bullous Dystrophy, Pai (MRX64), Paine, VACTERL-Hydrocephalus, X-Linked Ataxia-Deafness-Dementia, and X-linked Lissencephaly. Childhood lethality may also be associated with metabolic insults (e.g., Ornithine Transcarbamoylase Deficiency, Pyruvate Dehydrogenase Deficiency, Adrenoleukodystrophy).

Some individuals with superactivity of phosphoribosyl pyrophosphate synthetase 1 have shown deafness, developmental delay, and neurologic signs in males.

REFERENCES

Arts WFM, Loonen MCB, Sengers RCA, et al. X-linked ataxia, weakness, deafness, and loss of vision in early childhood with a fatal course. Ann Neurol 33:535, 1993.

Christen HJ, Hansfeld P, Duley JA, et al.: Distinct neurological syndromes in two brothers with hyperuricaemia. Lancet 340:1167, 1992.

De Brouwer APM, Williams KL, Duley JA, et al.: Arts syndrome is caused by loss-of-function mutations in *PRPS1*. Am J Hum Genet 81:507, 2007.

Kremer H, Hamel BCJ, van den Helm B, et al.: Localization of the gene (or genes) for a syndrome with X-linked mental retardation, ataxia, weakness, hearing impairment, loss of vision and a fatal course in early childhood. Hum Genet 98:513, 1996.

Syndrome	Ataxia	Vision Loss	Hearing Loss	Comments
Arts	+	+	+	Growth deficiency, poor muscle development, hypotonia, areflexia, seizures, childhood death
Mohr-Tranebjaerg	+	+	+	Neurological deterioration with childhood onset, dystonia, spasticity
Ataxia-Deafness-Dementia, X-linked	+	+	+	Optic atrophy, spastic paraplegia, hypotonia, seizures, childhood death
Bertini	+	+	0	Macular degeneration, hypotonia, seizures, childhood death, hypoplasia of cerebellar vermis and corpus callosum, developmental delays and regression, postnatal growth impairment
Goldblatt Spastic Paraplegia	+	+	0	Optic atrophy, exotropia, nystagmus, spastic paraplegia, dysarthria, muscle hypoplasia, contractures
Optic Atrophy, X-linked	+	+	0	Optic atrophy, tremors, areflexia, emotional lability
Gustavson	0	+	+	Microcephaly, short stature, optic atrophy with blindness, large ears, joint contractures, rockerbottom feet, brain undergrowth, hydrocephaly, cerebellar hypoplasia, spasticity, seizures
Norrie	0	+	+	Ocular dysplasia and degeneration, adult-onset hearing loss
Paine	0	+	+	Microcephaly, short stature, optic atrophy, spasticity, seizures
Proud (*ARX*-Associated XLID)	0	+	+	Spasticity, seizures, short stature, microcephaly, agenesis of corpus callosum, cryptorchidism, inguinal hernias
Schimke	0	+	+	Microcephaly, sunken eyes, downslanting palpebral fissures, narrow nose, wide spacing of teeth, cupped ears, hypotonia, abducens palsy, spasticity, choreoathetosis, contractures
Wittwer	0	+	+	Microcephaly, short stature, microphthalmia, hypertelorism, genitourinary anomalies, hypotonia, seizures

ARX-ASSOCIATED XLID

(ARX-SPECTRUM, ARX-RELATED XLID, PARTINGTON SYNDROME, INTELLECTUAL
DISABILITY-TONIC SEIZURES-DYSTONIA, XLID-MYOCLONIC EPILEPSY, WEST
SYNDROME, INFANTILE EPILEPTIC-DYSKINETIC ENCEPHALOPATHY, OHTAHARA
SYNDROME OR EARLY INFANTILE EPILEPTIC ENCEPHALOPATHY, PROUD SYNDROME,
HYDRANENCEPHALY WITH ABNORMAL GENITALIA, X-LINKED LISSENCEPHALY
WITH ABNORMAL GENITALIA)

OMIM 300004, 300215, 300419, 308350,
309510

Xp21.3

ARX

Definition. Ten phenotypes, linked by having intellectual disability in common, are subsumed under this rubric. These phenotypes include a seizure subgroup (West syndrome or XLID-Infantile Spasms, X-linked Myoclonic Epilepsy, Infantile Epilepsy-Dyskinesia, Ohtahara syndrome or Early Infantile Epileptic Encephalopathy), a brain malformation subgroup (Proud syndrome or Agenesis of the Corpus Callosum with Abnormal Genitalia, X-linked Lissencephaly with Abnormal Genitalia and Hydranencephaly with Abnormal Genitalia), a dystonia subgroup (Partington syndrome and Tonic Seizures with Dystonia), and nonsyndromal XLID. Among these disorders, the nonsyndromal XLID presentation is most common, accounting for more than one-third of cases. Next in order of frequency are X-linked Lissencephaly with Abnormal Genitalia, West syndrome, and Partington syndrome. Separate entries are maintained in this Atlas for the more common syndromal subtypes and a phenotype summary is provided here. The *ARX* gene has four polyalanine tracts, and expansions of the first two tracts account for more than half of the disease-associated mutations.

Lissencephaly with Abnormal Genitalia, X-Linked (OMIM 300215). Microcephaly, intractable seizures with onset soon after birth, poor temperature regulation, chronic diarrhea, and abnormal genitalia comprise the clinical phenotype. Agenesis of the corpus callosum and lissencephaly with excessive thinness of the cerebral cortex is demonstrated by brain imaging. The *ARX* mutations predominantly truncate the protein, although missense mutations affecting different domains have been found in one-fourth of cases.

West Syndrome (XLID-Infantile Spasms, OMIM 308350). Seizures, usually in the form of infantile spasms,

herald the symptomatic phase of West syndrome by age 6 months. There follows a period with slowing of development and then loss of skills. Early childhood death is not uncommon. Most cases are caused by expansion of one of the two polyalanine tracts.

Partington Syndrome (MRXS1, XLID-Dystonia Syndrome, OMIM 309510). Involuntary movements – particularly dystonia – dominate the clinical phenotype. Dysarthria and dystonic spasms of the hands develop prior to school age and progress slowly, if at all. The gait may be awkward, and scoliosis, flexed posturing, and hyper-reflexia may occur. Malformations and consistent craniofacial dysmorphism do not occur. All cases have resulted from expansion of the second polyalanine tract.

REFERENCES

Bienvenu T, Poirier K, Friocourt G, et al.: ARX, a novel Prd-class-homeobox gene highly expressed in the telencephalon, is mutated in X-linked mental retardation. Hum Molec Genet 11:981, 2002.

Kato M, Das S, Petras K, et al.: Mutations of ARX are associated with striking pleiotropy and consistent genotype-phenotype correlation. Hum Mutat 23:147, 2004.

Kato M, Saitoh S, Kamei A, et al.: A longer polyalanine expansion mutation in the ARX gene causes early infantile epileptic encephalopathy with suppression-burst pattern (Ohtahara syndrome). Am J Hum Genet 81:361, 2007.

Kitamura K, Yanazawa M, Sugiyama N, et al.: Mutation of ARX causes abnormal development of forebrain and testes in mice and X-linked lissencephaly with abnormal genitalia in humans. Nat Genet 32:359, 2002.

Nawara M, Szczaluba K, Poirier K, et al.: The ARX mutations: a frequent cause of X-linked mental retardation. Am J Med Genet A 140:727, 2006.

Partington MW, Mulley JC, Sutherland GR, et al.: X-linked mental retardation with dystonic movements of the hands. Am J Med Genet 30:251, 1988.

Partington MW, Turner G, Boyle J, et al.: Three new families with X-linked mental retardation caused by the 428–451dup(24bp) mutation in ARX. Clin Genet 66:39, 2004.

Proud VK, Levine C, Carpenter NJ: New X-linked syndrome with seizures, acquired micrencephaly, and agenesis of the corpus callosum. Am J Med Genet 43:458, 1992.

Shoubridge C, Fullston T, Gecz J: ARX spectrum disorders: making inroads into the molecular pathology. Hum Mutat 31:889, 2010.

Strømme P, Mangelsdorf ME, Shaw MA, et al.: Mutations in the human ortholog of Aristaless cause X-linked mental retardation and epilepsy. Nat Genet 30:441, 2002.

Turner G, Partington M, Kerr B, et al.: Variable expression of mental retardation, autism, seizures, and dystonic hand movements in two families with an identical ARX gene mutation. Am J Med Genet 112:405, 2002.

DIFFERENTIAL MATRIX

Syndrome	Neuronal Migration Disturbances	Dysgenesis of Corpus Callosum	Seizures	Comments
ARX-Associated XLID	+	+	+	Dystonia, dysarthria, infantile spasms, seizures of various types, abnormal genitalia
Aicardi	+	+	+	Lacunar retinopathy, costovertebral anomalies, agenesis of corpus callosum, ocular abnormality, CNS anomalies, vertebral or rib defects
CK	+	0	+	Microcephaly, asthenic build, hypotonia, long thin face, scoliosis, behavior problems
Bertini	0	+	+	Developmental delays and regression, postnatal growth impairment, macular degeneration, ataxia, cerebellar hypoplasia, hypotonia
Juberg-Marsidi-Brooks	0	+	+	Microcephaly and hydrocephaly, short stature, deep-set eyes, blepharophimosis, cupped ears, bulbous nose, small mouth, thin upper lip, pectus excavatum, flexion contractures, spasticity
Kang	0	+	+	Frontal prominence, telecanthus, small nose, short hands, downslanted mouth, brachydactyly, microcephaly, spastic paraplegia
Pyruvate Dehydrogenase Deficiency	0	+	+	Microcephaly, ataxia, dysarthria, structural brain anomalies, hypotonia, lactic acidosis

ATAXIA-DEAFNESS-DEMENTIA, X-LINKED

(XLID-ATAXIA-DEAFNESS, SCHMIDLEY SYNDROME,
SPINOCEREBELLAR ATAXIA, X-LINKED 3)

OMIM 301790

Definition. XLID with optic atrophy, deafness, hypotonia, progressive ataxia, and seizures. Fatal during the first decade. The condition has not been mapped.

Somatic Features. No distinctive somatic features have been described. Optic atrophy is demonstrable during the first year. Neurological signs appear in early infancy and progress steadily to demise in mid-childhood.

Growth and Development. Developmental milestones lag from the outset. Affected boys fail to walk independently and have little or no speech. Growth parameters have not been described.

Neurological Findings. Recurrent episodes of choking, dysphagia, or vomiting with lethargy, weakness, and incoordination lasting several days punctuate a course of poor developmental progress and neurological deterioration. Deafness, optic atrophy, and esotropia are noted by age 1 year. Paralysis of ocular movements may occur late in the course. Neuromuscular findings include ataxia of head, trunk, and limbs; dysmetria; tremors; head titubation; depressed deep tendon reflexes; and hypotonia. Seizures develop after a few years, and death from pneumonia occurs by age 2 years. Spasticity may be a late manifestation.

Heterozygote Expression. One mother had two episodes in adult life with ataxia and confusion. Brain imaging showed cerebellar atrophy and enlargement of the fourth ventricle.

Neuropathology. Post mortem examination has shown neuronal loss and gliosis in the brainstem and cerebellum. The dentate nucleus and inferior olive are invariably involved. Diffuse gliosis was present in the cerebellum with loss of myelinated fibers in the white matter and loss of Purkinje and granule cells in the cortex.

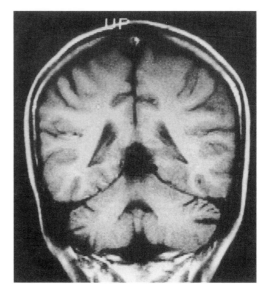

Ataxia-Deafness-Dementia, X-linked. Magnetic resonance image showing prominent cerebellar folia and enlarged fourth ventricle.   Courtesy of Dr. Morris Levinsohn, Beachwood, Ohio.

Comment. Although the recurrence of vomiting, lethargy, and incoordination suggests a metabolic disturbance, none has been found. A similar course – but without deafness and recurrent episodes of vomiting, lethargy, and incoordination – has been reported by Malamud and Cohen (1958).

REFERENCES

Malamud N, Cohen P: Unusual form of cerebellar ataxia with X-linked inheritance. Neurology 8:261, 1958.
Schmidley JW, Levinsohn MW, Manetto V: Infantile X-linked ataxia and deafness: A new clinicopathologic entity? Neurology 37:1344, 1987.

Syndrome	Ataxia	Hearing Loss	Vision Loss	Comments
Ataxia-Deafness-Dementia, X-linked	+	+	+	Optic atrophy, spastic paraplegia, hypotonia, childhood death
Arts	+	+	+	Growth deficiency, poor muscle development, hypotonia, areflexia, seizures, childhood death
Gustavson	+	+	+	Microcephaly, short stature, optic atrophy with blindness, large ears, joint contractures, rockerbottom feet, brain undergrowth, hydrocephaly, cerebellar hypoplasia, spasticity, seizures
Mohr-Tranebjaerg	+	+	+	Neurologic deterioration with childhood onset, dystonia, spasticity
Proud (*ARX*-Associated XLID)	+	+	+	Microcephaly, agenesis of corpus callosum, cryptorchidism, inguinal hernias, spasticity, seizures
Goldblatt Spastic Paraplegia	+	0	+	Optic atrophy, exotropia, nystagmus, spastic paraplegia, dysarthria, muscle hypoplasia, contractures
Pelizaeus-Merzbacher	+	0	+	Optic atrophy, nystagmus, hypotonia, spasticity, dystonia, CNS dysmyelination
Adrenoleukodystrophy	0	+	+	Adrenal insufficiency, diffuse skin pigmentation, spastic paraplegia, progressive neurologic deterioration and dementia, elevated long chain fatty acids in plasma
Paine	0	+	+	Microcephaly, short stature, optic atrophy, spasticity, seizures
Schimke	0	+	+	Microcephaly, sunken eyes, downslanting palpebral fissures, narrow nose, wide spacing of teeth, cupped ears, hypotonia, abducens palsy, spasticity, choreoathetosis, contractures
Wittwer	0	+	+	Microcephaly, short stature, microphthalmia, hypertelorism, genitourinary anomalies, hypotonia, seizures

ATKIN-FLAITZ SYNDROME
(ATKIN SYNDROME)

OMIM 300431

Definition. XLID with short stature, macrocephaly, coarse facial features, broad short hands with tapered fingers, macro-orchidism and seizures. The gene has not been mapped.

Somatic Features. Macrocephaly, large forehead, prominent supraorbital ridges, hypertelorism, broad nasal tip with anteverted nostrils, and thick lower lip give the distinctive facial appearance. Large ears, downslanted palpebral fissures and micrognathia may also be present. Intraoral findings include an upper midline diastema, small upper lateral incisors, palatal torus or prominent raphe, and prominent median furrow of the tongue. The former two findings, as well as macrocephaly and micrognathia, may represent familial characteristics within the first reported family. Other than short stature, short hands, and a tendency to postpubertal obesity, there are no musculoskeletal findings. The hands, although short and broad with tapered fingers, do not have the doughy consistency found in the Coffin-Lowry syndrome. The testes are large, a finding noted also in nonaffected males. Seizures occur in a minority.

Cognitive Function. Moderate impairment

Neurological Findings. Seizures occur in a minority. Although facial structures suggest muscular hypotonia, it has not been described.

Heterozygote Expression. Carrier females are less severely affected, having mild cognitive impairment, large forehead with prominent supraorbital ridges, hypertelorism, broad nasal tip, and thick lower lip. They are short and tend to be obese.

Comment. Although the facial coarseness suggests the Coffin-Lowry syndrome, the presence of macrocephaly and macro-orchidism and the absence of soft doughy hands and skeletal abnormalities should provide easy distinction. Clark and Baraitser have described a mother and two sons with similar features with the exception that they lacked hypertelorism and short stature.

A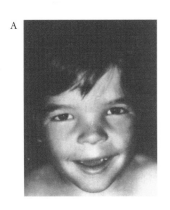
B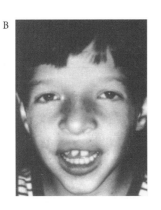
C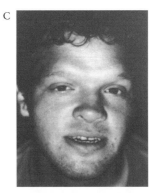

D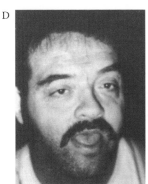
E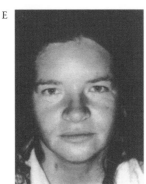
F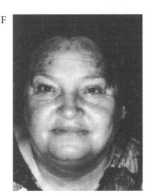

Atkin-Flaitz Syndrome. Coarse facial features with macrocephaly, hypertelorism, broad nasal tip, and prominent lips in affected males ages 6, 8, 21, and 39 years **(A, B, C, D)**; and in carrier females at ages 28 and 53 years **(E, F)**.   Courtesy of the *American Journal of Medical Genetics*, Copyright 1985, Alan R. Liss, Inc.

32

REFERENCES

Atkin JF, Flaitz K, Patil S, et al.: A new X-linked mental retardation syndrome. Am J Med Genet 21:697, 1985.

Baraitser M, Reardon W, Vijeratnam S: Nonspecific X-linked mental retardation with macrocephaly and obesity. Am J Med Genet 57:380, 1995.

Clark RD, Baraitser M: Letter to the Editor: A new X-linked mental retardation syndrome. Am J Med Genet 26:13, 1987.

DIFFERENTIAL MATRIX

Syndrome	Short Stature	Coarse Facial Features	Obesity	Comments
Atkin-Flaitz	+	+	+	Macrocephaly, hypertelorism, downslanting palpebral fissures, broad nasal tip, thick lower lip, brachydactyly, seizures
Börjeson-Forssman-Lehmann	+	+	+	Hypotonia, hypogonadism, microcephaly, large ears, gynecomastia, narrow sloped shoulders, visual impairment, tapered digits
XLID-Hypogonadism-Tremor	+	+	+	Prominent lower lip, muscle wasting of legs, abnormal gait, hypogonadism, obesity, seizures, tremor
Coffin-Lowry	+	+	0	Microcephaly, hypertelorism, anteverted nares, tented upper lip, prominent lips, and large mouth, large ears, soft hands with tapered digits, pectus carinatum, hypotonia
Mucopolysaccharidosis II	+	+	0	Macrocephaly, hepatosplenomegaly, hernias, joint stiffness, thick skin, hirsutism, behavioral disturbance
Ahmad	+	0	+	Hypogonadism, tapered fingers
Clark-Baraitser	0	+	+	Macrocephaly, large stature, dental abnormalities, broad nasal tip, thick lower lip, macro-orchidism

ATRX-ASSOCIATED XLID

(*ATRX* SPECTRUM, α-THALASSEMIA INTELLECTUAL DISABILITY, XLID-HYPOTONIC FACIES, CEREBROFACIOGENITAL SYNDROME, CHUDLEY-LOWRY SYNDROME, CARPENTER-WAZIRI SYNDROME, HOLMES-GANG SYNDROME, XLID-ARCH FINGERPRINTS-HYPOTONIA)

OMIM 301040, 309580

Xq21.1

ATRX (XNP, XH2)

Definition. A number of more-or-less distinct phenotypes, all with intellectual disability and most with growth impairment and craniofacial manifestations, comprise the *ATRX*-Associated XLID syndromes. Alpha-Thalassemia Intellectual Disability, the prototype, occupies the most severe end of the spectrum, nonsyndromal XLID the least severe extreme, and several intermediate phenotypes the remaining interval. The named XLID syndromes with *ATRX* mutations are retained as individual entries in this Atlas and a capsule of the phenotype for each of the syndromal subtypes is provided here.

Alpha-Thalassemia Intellectual Disability (OMIM 301040). Short stature, microcephaly, hypotonic facies with hypertelorism, small triangular nose, open mouth, spacing of the teeth, prominent lips, brachydactyly, genital anomalies, and hemoglobin H inclusions in erythrocytes are the typical findings. The craniofacial findings are generally obvious from infancy and may persist or become less obvious in adult life. Minimal skeletal anomalies (tapering digits, clinodactyly, overlapping digits, foot deformations, kyphosis, and scoliosis) are common. Underdevelopment of the genitalia, undescended testes, or hypospadias occurs in

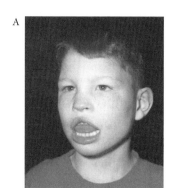
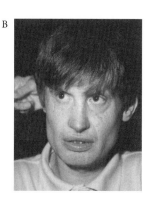
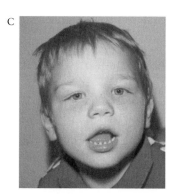
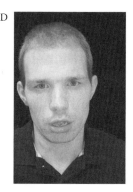
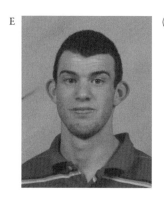
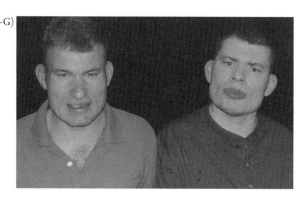

ATRX-Associated XLID. Six-year-old with typical craniofacial findings – microcephaly, small nose, large open mouth with tented upper lip (**A**); 33-year-old affected uncle with normal head circumference, long nose, short philtrum, and absence of typical facial findings (**B**). Four members of another family: 8-year-old male with microcephaly, hypertelorism, downslanting palpebral fissures, open mouth with tented upper lip, and wide spacing of the teeth (**C**); same male at age 26 years (**D**); a cousin at age 23 years with normal head circumference, cupped ears, and upslanting palpebral fissures (**E**); twin uncles with normal head circumference, square face, sunken eyes, flat midface, cupped ears, and cleft chin at age 37 years (**F, G**).

most cases. Cleft palate, cardiac defects, and undifferentiated genitalia are uncommon structural defects.

Holmes-Gang Syndrome (OMIM 309580). A single family with this severe phenotype has been reported. The infants had microcephaly, large fontanelles, and hypotonic face with hypertelorism, small nose, tented upper lip, and short philtrum. The feet were clubbed. Renal dysplasia was present in one case. Development was profoundly delayed, and death occurred in infancy or early childhood.

Chudley-Lowry Syndrome (XLID-Hypotonia-Hypogonadism) (OMIM 309580). In a single family reported, almond-shaped eyes, small nose with depressed nasal bridge, open mouth, short philtrum, and tented upper lip combined to give a distinctively hypotonic appearing face. Other manifestations included narrow bitemporal diameter, short neck, brachydactyly with tapered fingers and an excessive number of arch fingerprints, fifth finger camptodactyly, small or undescended testes, and genu valgum. Statural growth and head circumference fell in the lower centiles; weight fell in the upper centiles.

Carpenter-Waziri Syndrome (OMIM 309580). Six affected males in the single family reported shared short stature, hypotonic facies, spacing of the teeth, and brachydactyly. Minor skeletal anomalies were present. Microcephaly was present in some, but in others the head circumference measured in the lower centiles.

XLID-Arch Fingerprints-Hypotonia (OMIM 309580). Four affected males in a single family had a square facial appearance, tented upper lip, and thickening of the helices, upper eyelids, and alae nasi. Prenatal and postnatal growth parameters, including head circumference, were normal. Other findings included hypotonia, tapered fingers, excessive arches or low ridge-count fingerprints, genu valgum, and absent reflexes.

REFERENCES

Abidi F, Schwartz CE, Carpenter NJ, et al.: Carpenter-Waziri syndrome results from a mutation in XNP. Am J Med Genet 85:249, 1999.

Abidi FE, Cardoso C, Lossi AM, et al.: Mutation in the 5' alternatively spliced region of the XNP/ATR-X gene causes Chudley-Lowry syndrome. Eur J Hum Genet 13:176, 2005.

Carpenter NJ, Qu Y, Curtis M, et al.: X-linked mental retardation syndrome with characteristic "coarse" facial appearance, brachydactyly, and short stature maps to proximal Xq. Am J Med Genet 85:230, 1999.

Carpenter NJ, Waziri M, Liston J, et al.: Studies on X-linked mental retardation: Evidence for a gene in the region Xq11-q22. Am J Hum Genet 43:A139, 1988.

Chudley AE, Lowry RB, Hoar DI: Mental retardation, distinct facial changes, short stature, obesity, and hypogonadism. A new X-linked mental retardation syndrome. Am J Med Genet 31:741, 1988.

Donnai D, Clayton-Smith J, Gibbons RJ, et al.: The non-deletion α-thalassaemia/mental retardation syndrome. Further support for X linkage. J Med Genet 28: 742, 1991.

Gibbons RJ, Brueton L, Buckle VJ, et al.: Clinical and hematologic aspects of the X-linked α-thalassemia/mental retardation syndrome (ATR-X). Am J Med Genet 55:288, 1995.

Gibbons RJ, Picketts DJ, Villard L, et al.: Mutations in a putative global transcriptional regulator cause X-linked mental retardation with α-thalassemia (ATR-X syndrome). Cell 80:837, 1995.

Gibbons RJ, Suthers GK, Wilkie AOM, et al.: X-linked α-thalassemia/mental retardation (ATR-X) syndrome: Localization to Xq12-q21.31 by X inactivation and linkage analysis. Am J Hum Genet 51:1136, 1992.

Gibbons RJ, Wada T, Fisher CA, et al.: Mutations in the chromatin-associated protein ATRX. Hum Mutat 29:796, 2008.

Holmes LB, Gang DL: Brief clinical report: An X-linked mental retardation syndrome with craniofacial abnormalities, microcephaly and club foot. Am J Med Genet 17:375, 1984.

Stevenson RE, Abidi F, Schwartz CE, et al.: Holmes-Gang syndrome is allelic with XLMR-hypotonic face syndrome. Am J Med Genet 94:383, 2000.

Stevenson RE, Häne B, Arena JF, et al.: Arch fingerprints, hypotonia, and areflexia associated with X linked mental retardation. J Med Genet 34:465, 1997.

Wilkie AOM, Gibbons RJ, Higgs DR, et al.: X-linked α-thalassemia/mental retardation: spectrum of clinical features in three related males. J Med Genet 28:738, 1991.

DIFFERENTIAL MATRIX

Syndrome	Microcephaly	Hypotonic Facies	Urogenital Anomalies	Comments
ATRX-Associated XLID	+	+	+	Short stature, telecanthus, small triangular nose, tented upper lip, open mouth, wide spacing of teeth, genital anomalies, musculoskeletal anomalies, hemoglobin H inclusions in erythrocytes
Proud (*ARX*-Associated XLID)	+	+	+	Hearing loss, vision loss, agenesis of corpus callosum, cryptorchidism, inguinal hernias, ataxia, spasticity, seizures
Smith-Fineman-Myers	+	+	0	Ptosis, flat philtrum, scoliosis, midfoot varus, narrow feet, seizures, hypotonia
Coffin-Lowry	+	+	0	Short stature, hypertelorism, anteverted nares, tented upper lip, prominent lips and large mouth, large ears, soft hands with tapered digits, pectus carinatum
Miles-Carpenter	+	+	0	Short stature, ptosis, small palpebral fissures, open mouth, pectus excavatum, scoliosis, long hands, camptodactyly, rockerbottom feet, arch fingerprints, spasticity, unsteady gait
Vasquez	+	0	+	Short stature, gynecomastia, obesity, hypotonia, hypogonadism
XLID-Hypospadias	+	0	+	Trigonocephaly, synophrys, beaked nose, dysplastic ears, joint hyperextensibility, hypotonia
XLID-Microcephaly-Testicular Failure	+	0	+	Short stature, prominent supraorbital ridges, high nasal bridge, prominent nose, macrostomia, hypogonadism
XLID-Psoriasis	0	+	+	Hypertelorism, strabismus, large ears, macrostomia, psoriasis, seizures

BERGIA CARDIOMYOPATHY

(X-LINKED FAMILIAL LETHAL CARDIOMYOPATHY)

Definition. XLID with myopia, slowly progressive scapuloperoneal muscular dystrophy, and hypertrophic cardiomyopathy. The gene has not been mapped.

Somatic Features. Major malformations or distinctive craniofacial characteristics do not occur. There is a slowly progressive muscular dystrophy with predominant humeroperoneal weakness. The clinical course is dominated by the cardiomyopathy, manifested by subendocardial and patchy subepicardial fibrosis, vacuolization, and fatty deposition in myocytes, all of which lead to limited exercise tolerance, syncope, heart failure, arrhythmias, and death by early adult life. Marked myopia may be a feature.

Growth and Development. Childhood growth proceeds normally. Muscle hypertrophy does not occur; rather, muscles show progressive wasting. Early childhood development milestones may be achieved at the usual times.

Cognitive Function. Impairment of cognitive function is first noted at age 5 to 6 years and may be progressive.

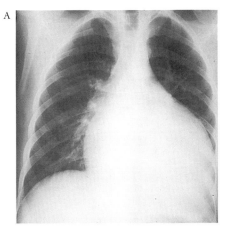

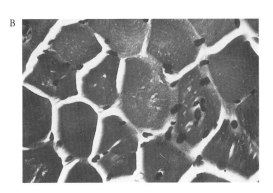

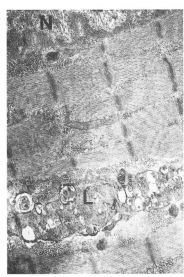

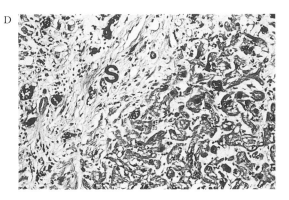

Bergia Cardiomyopathy. Chest radiograph of 17-year-old male showing cardiomegaly **(A)**. Light microscopy of quadriceps biopsy revealing variable fiber size and shape and internalization of nuclei **(B)**; electron microscopy of quadriceps showing increased lysosomes [L] containing necrotic fibers **(C)**; light microscopy of left ventricle with increased interstitial connective tissue and fibrosis [S] **(D)**.   Courtesy of Dr. Ian Butler, University of Texas Health Science Center, Houston.

Neurological Findings. Incoordination becomes notable as ambulation is acquired. Deep tendon reflexes are normal. Weakness is best demonstrated in humeral and peroneal muscles. Incoordination may be secondary to the weakness. Distal muscle wasting and winging of the scapula may be present. Nerve conduction appears normal. Electromyography is consistent with a myopathy. Electroencephalography, brainstem auditory-evoked responses, and visual-evoked responses may be abnormal.

Heterozygote Expression. Dilation and poor function of the left ventricle has been described in one carrier female. There was no evidence for dystrophy of skeletal muscles or impairment of cognitive function.

Laboratory. Muscle biopsy shows a dystrophic process with variation in fiber size, internalization of nuclei, and slight increase in fibrosis and fatty infiltration. Although increased glycogen may be present in muscle cells, enzymes involved in glycogen metabolism have been normal. Creatine kinase and other muscle enzymes are elevated.

Comment. Cardiac disease occurs uncommonly among the XLID syndromes and even more rarely is responsible for childhood demise. Structural heart defects have been described in Alpha-Thalassemia Intellectual Disability, Hereditary Bullous Dystrophy, Opitz FG, Telecanthus-Hypospadias, Renpenning (Cerebro-Palato-Cardiac, Golabi-Ito-Hall), Lenz, MIDAS and Simpson-Golabi-Behmel syndromes. X-linked cardiomyopathies are also few in number: Duchenne Muscular Dystrophy, Myotubular Myopathy, and Bergia Cardiomyopathy. The relationship of Bergia Cardiomyopathy to Danon Disease (OMIM 300257), a vacuolar cardiomyopathy and variable intellectual disability caused by mutations in the lysosome-associated membrane protein 2 (*LAMP2*), is not known.

REFERENCES

Bergia B, Sybers HD, Butler IJ: Familial lethal cardiomyopathy with mental retardation and scapuloperoneal muscular dystrophy. J Neurol Neurosurg Psychiatry 49:1423, 1986.

van der Kooi AJ, van Langen IM, Aronica E, et al.: Extension of the clinical spectrum of Danon disease. Neurology 70:1358, 2008.

DIFFERENTIAL MATRIX

Syndrome	Cardiomyopathy	Muscle Wasting	Childhood Death	Comments
Bergia Cardiomyopathy	+	+	+	Scapuloperoneal muscle atrophy, limited exercise tolerance, arrhythmias
Duchenne Muscular Dystrophy	+	+	+	Hypertrophy of calf muscles, elevated muscle enzymes, progressive weakness, loss of reflexes, contractures
Myotubular Myopathy	+	+	+	Hypotonic facies, open mouth, tented upper lip, hydrocephaly, long digits, cryptorchidism, hypotonia, weakness, areflexia

BERTINI SYNDROME

(BERTINI-DES PORTES SYNDROME, XLID-MYOCLONUS-MACULAR DEGENERATION)

Xpter-p22.33

Definition. XLID with hypotonia, ataxia, myoclonus, and macular degeneration.

Somatic Features. Facial or musculoskeletal features are not described; imaging studies document hypoplasia of the cerebellar vermis and of the corpus callosum.

Growth and Development. Intrauterine growth is normal or nearly so, but slow statural and cephalic growth becomes obvious postnatally. Development skills are acquired slowly and are lost during late childhood.

Cognitive Function. Development is globally delayed and cognitive function markedly impaired.

Neurological Findings. Males appear severely affected from birth with hypotonia and ataxia. They suck poorly and development progresses slowly. Death often occurs from infections in infancy, and survivors follow a relentless course of deterioration with seizures, macular degeneration, and death by late childhood.

Neuropathology. Partial brain examination in one case showed no neuronal loss or storage products.

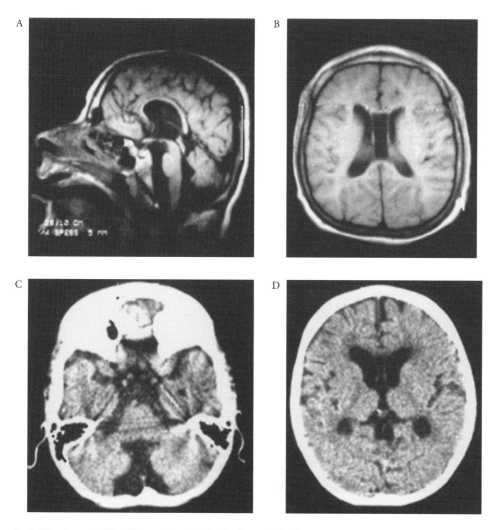

Bertini Syndrome. MRI of 10-year-old male showing hypoplasia of cerebellar vermis, hypoplasia of corpus callosum, and septum pellucidum cyst **(A, B)**; cranial tomography of 10-year-old cousin showing hypoplasia of cerebellar vermis, cyst of the septum pellucidum, and persistent cavum vergae **(C, D)**. Courtesy of the *American Journal of Medical Genetics*, Copyright 1992, Wiley-Liss, Inc.

Comment. Although the course mimics storage disease, extensive search for such an underlying disorder has not been found. Several other XLID syndromes with hypoplasia of the cerebellum and agenesis of the corpus callosum have been recognized, but none maps to the same region of Xp.

REFERENCES

Bertini E, Cusmai R, de Saint Basile G, et al.: Congenital X-linked ataxia, progressive myoclonic encephalopathy, macular degeneration and recurrent infections. Am J Med Genet 43:443, 1992.

des Portes V, Bachner L, Brüls T, et al.: X-linked neurodegenerative syndrome with congenital ataxia, late-onset progressive myoclonic encephalopathy and selective macular degeneration, linked to Xp22.33-pter. Am J Med Genet 64:69, 1996.

DIFFERENTIAL MATRIX

Syndrome	Ataxia	Cerebellar Hypoplasia	Hypotonia	Comments
Bertini	+	+	+	Developmental delays and regression, postnatal growth impairment, macular degeneration, seizures
Cerebro-Cerebello-Coloboma	+	+	+	Hydrocephaly, retinal coloboma, hypotonia, seizures, abnormal respiratory pattern
Pettigrew	+	+	+	Dandy-Walker malformation, spasticity, microcephaly or hydrocephaly, long face with macrostomia and prognathism, small testes, contractures, choreoathetosis, iron deposits in basal ganglia, seizures
Christianson	+	+	0	Short stature, microcephaly, general asthenia, contractures, seizures, ophthalmoplegia
Pelizaeus-Merzbacher	+	+	+	Optic atrophy, hypotonia, dystonia, CNS dysmyelination, spastic paraplegia, nystagmus
Schimke	0	+	+	Microcephaly, sunken eyes, downslanting palpebral fissures, narrow nose, wide spacing of teeth, cupped ears, abducens palsy, hearing loss, vision loss, spasticity, choreoathetosis, contractures

BÖRJESON-FORSSMAN-LEHMANN SYNDROME

(BFL SYNDROME)

OMIM 301900

Xq26

PHF6

Definition. XLID with variable stature and head size, angular face with prominent cheekbones, deep-set eyes, large and thick ears, gynecomastia, small or undescended testes, obesity and hypotonia. Missense and truncating mutations in the zinc finger gene, *PHF6*, have been reported.

Somatic Features. The midface is most characteristic, the face appearing heavy and angular with prominent supraorbital ridges and cheekbones, dense eyebrows, deeply set eyes, ptosis, epicanthus and large fleshy ears. There is a tendency to visual impairment with pale optic discs, hyperopia, nystagmus and cataract formation. The nose is small and triangular with anteverted nares. The mouth may have a tented upper lip. The angular nature of the face may be softened to variable degree by fat deposition and hypotonia. Shoulders are narrow and may be excessively sloped. The fingers taper and have hyperextensible joints. There is shortness of the toes, some of which may be flexed. Otherwise, patients have short stature, microcephaly, generalized obesity with notable fat deposition in the breasts, hypotonia, small genitalia with hypogonadism, and seizures. The skin feels soft and doughy and acne is common. A milder phenotype with normal head circumference, normal stature, and less severe intellectual disability is present in some patients with documented *PHF6* mutations.

Growth and Development. Birth weight is normal, but generalized obesity appears early in childhood. Other growth parameters show considerable variability, but microcephaly and short stature are typical. All developmental milestones lag.

Cognitive Function. Cognitive function parallels the somatic phenotype with those having the most pronounced somatic manifestations having the most severe cognitive impairment. A friendly disposition is noted, but with challenging behavior prominent in some individuals.

Neurological Findings. Hypotonia is notable and evidenced during pregnancy by poor fetal movement. Some cases have vision loss with nystagmus and pale optic discs. Hyperreflexia occurs in many cases.

Heterozygote Expression. Carrier females tend to be short and heavy with broad midface, large ears and mild cognitive impairment. Some have impaired vision, hypotonia and soft skin, tapered digits, and short, flexed and widely-spaced toes.

Imaging. Mild ventricular dilation.

Laboratory. Both hypogonadotropic and hypergonadotropic hypogonadism have been documented. The EEG shows generalized low voltage with diminished alpha activity. Ardinger et al. (1984) have stressed radiographic features, thick calvarium, narrow cervical spinal cord, Scheuermann-like vertebral changes, and epiphyseal dysplasia with delayed bone maturation, short distal phalanges and small proximal heads of the femora and humeri.

Comment. Börjeson-Forssman-Lehmann is the prototype XLID syndrome with hypotonia, hypogonadism and obesity. The considerable interfamilial variability, particularly in regard to growth and cognitive function, has not been fully explained by correlation with the genotype.

REFERENCES

Ardinger HH, Hanson JW, Zellweger HU: Börjeson-Forssman-Lehmann syndrome. Am J Med Genet 19:653, 1984.

Börjeson M, Forssman H, Lehmann O: An X-linked recessively inherited syndrome characterized by grave mental deficiency, epilepsy and endocrine disorder. Acta Med Scand 171:13, 1962.

Carter MT, Picketss DJ, Hunter AG, et al.: Further clinical delineation of the Börjeson-Forssman-Lehmann syndrome in patients with PHF6 mutations. Am J Med Genet A 149A:246, 2009.

de Winter CF, van Dijk F, Stolker JJ, et al.: Behavioural phenotype in Börjeson-Forssman-Lehmann syndrome. J Intellect Disabil Res 53:319, 2009.

Dereymaeker AM, Fryns JP, Hoefnagels M, et al.: The Börjeson-Forssman-Lehmann syndrome. Clin Genet 29:317, 1986.

Gedeon AK, Kozman HM, Robinson H, et al.: Refinement of the background genetic map of Xq26-q27 and gene localisation for Börjeson-Forssman-Lehmann syndrome. Am J Med Genet 64:63, 1996.

Lower KM, Solders G, Bondeson ML, et al.: 1024C>T (R342X) is a recurrent PHF6 mutation also found in the original Börjeson-Forssman-Lehmann syndrome family. Eur J Hum Genet 12:787, 2004.

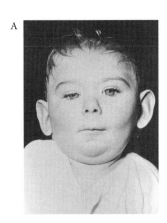 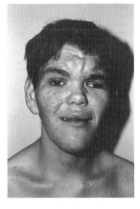 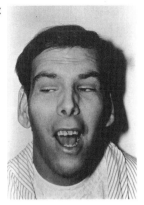

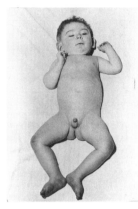 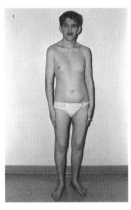 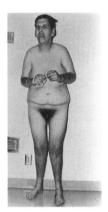

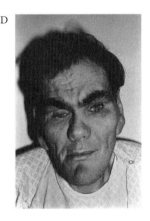 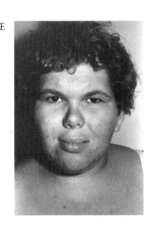

Börjeson-Forssman-Lehmann Syndrome. Ten-month-old male with microcephaly, large ears, depressed nasal bridge, ptosis, and hypotonia **(A)**; 24-year-old male with coarse facies and short stature **(B)**; 27-year-old male with ptosis, large ears, short stature, obesity, and hypogenitalism **(C)**; 40-year-old male with heavy cheekbones and sculpted facies **(D)**; 23-year-old female carrier with coarse facies, prominent supraorbital ridges, and large ears **(E)**.   Courtesy of Dr. Holly Hutchison Ardinger, University of Iowa Hospitals of Clinics, Iowa City.

Lower KM, Turner G, Kerr BA, et al.: Mutations in PHF6 are associated with Börjeson-Forssman-Lehmann syndrome. Nat Genet 32:661, 2002.

Mathews KD, Ardinger HH, Nishimura DY, et al.: Linkage localization of Börjeson-Forssman-Lehmann syndrome. Am J Med Genet 34:470, 1989.

Robinson LK, Jones KL, Culler F, et al.: The Börjeson-Forssman-Lehmann syndrome. Am J Med Genet 15:457, 1983.

Turner G, Gedeon A, Mulley J, et al.: Börjeson-Forssman-Lehmann syndrome: Clinical manifestations and gene localization to Xq26–27. Am J Med Genet 34:463, 1989.

Turner G, Lower KM, White SM, et al.: The clinical picture of the Börjeson-Forssman-Lehmann syndrome in males and heterozygous females with PHF6 mutations. Clin Genet 65: 226, 2004.

Visootsak J, Rosner B, Dykens E, et al.: Clinical and behavioral features of patients with Börjeson-Forssman-Lehmann syndrome with mutations in PHF6. J Pediatr 145:819, 2004.

Weber FT, Frias JL, Julius RL, et al.: Primary hypogonadism in the Börjeson-Forssman-Lehmann syndrome. J Med Genet 15:63, 1978.

DIFFERENTIAL MATRIX

Syndrome	Hypotonia	Hypogonadism	Obesity	Comments
Börjeson-Forssman-Lehmann	+	+	+	Short stature, microcephaly, coarse face, large ears, gynecomastia, narrow sloped shoulders, visual impairment, tapered digits
Vasquez	+	+	+	Microcephaly, short stature, gynecomastia
Wilson-Turner	+	+	+	Normal growth, small hands and feet, tapered digits, gynecomastia, emotional lability
ATRX-Associated XLID	+	+	0	Microcephaly, short stature, telecanthus/hypertelorism, small triangular nose, tented upper lip, open mouth, wide spacing of teeth, abnormal genitalia, minor musculoskeletal anomalies, erythrocyte HbH inclusions in some
Ahmad	0	+	+	Short stature, tapered fingers
Urban	0	+	+	Short stature, small hands and feet, digital contractures, osteoporosis
XLID-Hypogonadism-Tremor	0	+	+	Short stature, prominent lower lip, muscle wasting of legs, abnormal gait, seizures, tremor
Young-Hughes	0	+	+	Short stature, small palpebral fissures, cupped ears, ichthyosiform scaling

BRANCHIAL ARCH SYNDROME, X-LINKED
(TORIELLO BRANCHIAL ARCH SYNDROME)

OMIM 301950

Definition. XLID with microcephaly, branchial arch defects, hearing loss, and cryptorchidism. The condition has not been mapped.

Somatic Features. Microcephaly, hypertelorism, sparseness of lateral eyebrows, epicanthus, ptosis, downslanting palpebral fissures, flat malar area, high broad nasal bridge, anteverted nares, cupped and/or low-set ears, preauricular pits, high palate, long upper lip, flat philtrum, and micrognathia give a distinctive appearance. Facial and limb asymmetry, broad neck, and cryptorchidism may occur. The ear canals may be stenotic, and mixed hearing loss is typical.

Growth and Development. Head circumference is small, and stature tends to be in the lower percentiles.

Cognitive Function. No formal testing available, but cognitive function is considered mildly delayed.

Neurological Findings. Normal

Heterozygote Expression. None

Comment. The phenotype is based on a single family with three affected males. On the basis of pedigree structure, microcephaly, and cryptorchidism, they appear to differ from other branchial arch syndromes (Treacher Collins, Otofaciocervical, Branchioskeletogenital, Branchio-Oto-Renal, and Oculoauriculovertebral syndromes).

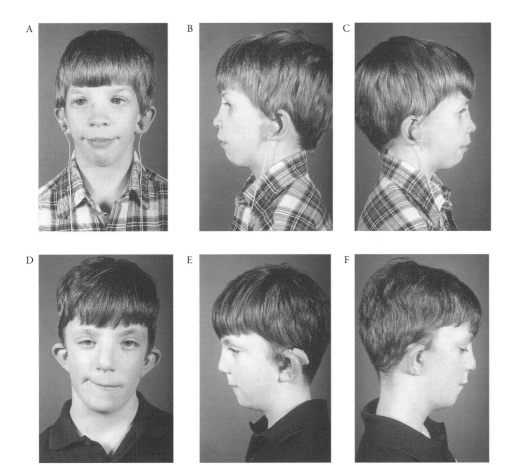

Branchial Arch Syndrome, X-linked. Microcephaly, triangular face, sparse lateral eyebrows, downslanting palpebral fissures, broad nasal bridge, malar hypoplasia, micrognathia, and cupped ears in a 10-year-old boy **(A-C)**; microcephaly, facial asymmetry, ptosis, high and broad nasal bridge, cupped ears, smooth philtrum with thin upper lip, epicanthus, sparse lateral eyebrows, and micrognathia in a 10-year-old cousin **(D-F)**. Courtesy of Dr. James Higgins, Spectrum Health, Grand Rapids, Michigan.

REFERENCES

Puri RD, Phadke SR: Further delineation of mandibulofacial dysostosis: Toriello type. Clin Dysmorphol 11:91, 2002.

Toriello HV, Higgins JV, Abrahamson J, et al.: X-linked syndrome of branchial arch and other defects. Am J Med Genet 21:137, 1985.

DIFFERENTIAL MATRIX

Syndrome	Microcephaly	Malformed Ears	Hearing Loss	Comments
Branchial Arch, X-linked	+	+	+	Branchial arch defects, micrognathia, facial and limb asymmetry
ATRX-Associated XLID	+	+	+	Short stature, telecanthus/hypertelorism, small triangular nose, tented upper lip, open mouth, wide spacing of teeth, abnormal genitalia, minor musculoskeletal anomalies, hypotonia, erythrocyte HbH inclusions in some
Coffin-Lowry	+	+	+	Short stature, bitemporal narrowing, almond-shaped eyes, depressed nasal bridge, tented upper lip, open mouth, hypogonadism, hypotonia, obesity
Gustavson	+	+	+	Short stature, optic atrophy with blindness, large ears, joint contractures, rockerbottom feet, brain undergrowth, hydrocephaly, cerebellar hypoplasia, spasticity, seizures
Lenz Microphthalmia	+	+	+	Microphthalmia, ocular dysgenesis, cleft lip/palate, cardiac and genitourinary anomalies, thumb duplication or hypoplasia, narrow shoulders
Proud (*ARX*-Associated XLID)	+	+	+	Vision loss, agenesis of corpus callosum, cryptorchidism, inguinal hernias, ataxia, spasticity, seizures
Schimke	+	+	+	Sunken eyes, downslanting palpebral fissures, narrow nose, wide spacing of teeth, hypotonia, abducens palsy, vision loss, spasticity, choreoathetosis, contractures
Paine	+	0	+	Short stature, optic atrophy, vision loss, spasticity, seizures
Pettigrew	+	0	+	Dandy-Walker malformation, spasticity, microcephaly or hydrocephaly, long face with macrostomia, small testes, contractures, choreoathetosis, iron deposits in basal ganglia, seizures
Wittwer	+	0	+	Short stature, microphthalmia, vision loss, hypertelorism, genitourinary anomalies, hypotonia, seizures

CANTU SYNDROME

(XLID-ALOPECIA-SHORT STATURE, XLID-KERATOSIS FOLLICULARIS)

OMIM 308830

Definition. XLID with short stature, microcephaly, alopecia, and seizures. The gene has not been localized.

Somatic Features. From birth, males are distinguished by near total absence of scalp hair, eyebrows, and eyelashes. The teeth erupt late. A generalized follicular keratosis occurs with greater prominence on the scalp, back, and limbs. Head growth is slow because of cortical atrophy. The face appears round, and the mandible is small.

Growth and Development. Intrauterine and postnatal growth is moderately impaired.

Neurological Findings. Seizures, beginning in early childhood, occurred in three of the four cases described.

Heterozygote Expression. None

Imaging. Pneumoencephalography demonstrated severe cortical atrophy.

Laboratory. Microscopy of scalp and skin biopsies shows normal dermis and keratosis follicularis. Hair appears normal.

Comment. Among XLID syndromes, near total alopecia is unique to Cantu syndrome and Hereditary Bullous Dystrophy, X-linked. Linkage studies have not been conducted in the single family with Cantu syndrome reported to date.

REFERENCE

Cantu J-M, Hernandez A, Larracilla J, et al.: A new X-linked recessive disorder with dwarfism, cerebral atrophy, and generalized keratosis follicularis. J Pediatr 84: 564, 1974.

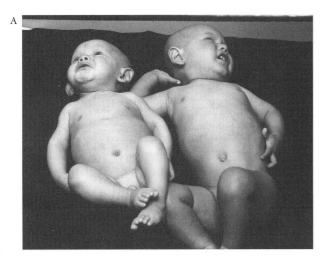

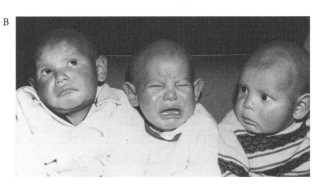

Cantu Syndrome. Brothers with scalp alopecia, sparse eyebrows and eyelashes, and keratosis follicularis of the scalp and forehead. Brothers shown in **A** are to the left in **B** but in reversed position.   Courtesy of Dr. Jose Marie Cantu, Latin American Human Genome Program, Guadalajara, Mexico.

DIFFERENTIAL MATRIX

Syndrome	Alopecia	Microcephaly	Seizures	Comments
Cantu	+	+	+	Short stature, follicular keratosis, cortical atrophy
Hereditary Bullous Dystrophy, X-linked	+	+	0	Short stature, bullous dystrophy, upslanting palpebral fissures, protruding ears, short and tapered digits, cardiac defects, small testes, early death from pulmonary infection
CK	0	+	+	Asthenic build, neuronal migration disturbance, hypotonia, long thin face, scoliosis, behavior problems

CARPENTER-WAZIRI SYNDROME (*SEE ALSO ATRX*-ASSOCIATED XLID)

(*ATRX* SPECTRUM)

OMIM 309580

Xq21.1

ATRX

Definition. XLID with short stature, small head, hypotonic facies, and brachydactyly. Carpenter-Waziri Syndrome is allelic to Alpha-Thalassemia Intellectual Disability (XLID-Hypotonic Facies), Chudley-Lowry, XLID-Arch Fingerprints-Hypotonia, and Holmes-Gang syndromes.

Somatic Features. Small cranium, thick eyebrows, depressed nasal bridge, wide nasal tip, small ears, open mouth with prominent lips and widely spaced teeth form a distinctive facial appearance. Upsweep of the frontal hair and epicanthus have also been described. Short stature is apparent in childhood, the hands are short with widened distal phalanges, and the thumbs are proximally placed. Hyperextension at the elbow, fifth finger clinodactyly, and syndactyly of toes 2 through 4 may occur. Genital abnormalities have not been described. Gallstones have occurred during childhood in one case.

Growth and Development. Although birth weight may be normal, short stature and microcephaly are usual during childhood. In some cases, the head circumference measures in the lower centiles.

Neurological Findings. None

Heterozygote Expression. None

Imaging. None

Comment. Phenotypic similarities to Alpha-Thalassemia Intellectual Disability and the pericentromeric localization have led to documentation of a missense mutation (I2056T) in helicase IV domain of the *ATRX* gene.

REFERENCES

Abidi F, Schwartz CE, Carpenter NJ, et al.: Carpenter-Waziri syndrome results from a mutation in XNP. Am J Med Genet 85:249, 1999.

Carpenter NJ, Qu Y, Curtis M, et al.: X-linked mental retardation syndrome with characteristic "coarse" facial appearance, brachydactyly, and short stature maps to proximal Xq. Am J Med Genet 85:230, 1999.

Carpenter NJ, Waziri M, Liston J, et al.: Studies on X-linked mental retardation: Evidence for a gene in the region Xq11-q22. Am J Hum Genet 43:A139, 1988.

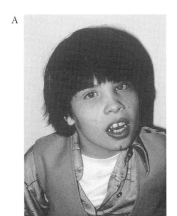 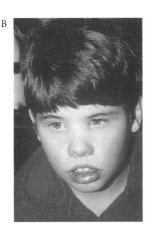 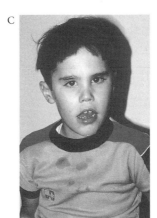 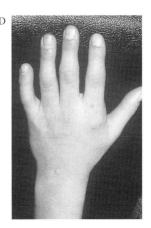

Carpenter-Waziri Syndrome. Microcephaly, depressed nasal bridge, tented upper lip, open mouth, prominent lower lip, and spacing of the teeth in brothers at ages 10 and 11 years (**A, B**); thick eyebrows, tented upper lip, open mouth, and prominent lower lip in 7-year-old maternal cousin of children shown in **A** and **B (C)**; brachydactyly affecting all digits (**D**).

Syndrome	Microcephaly	Hypotonic Facies	Brachydactyly	Comments
Carpenter-Waziri (*ATRX*-Associated XLID)	+	+	+	Short stature, telecanthus, small triangular nose, tented upper lip, open mouth, wide spacing of teeth, genital anomalies, musculoskeletal anomalies, hemoglobin H inclusions in erythrocytes
Coffin-Lowry	+	+	0	Short stature, hypertelorism, anteverted nares, tented upper lip, prominent lips and large mouth, large ears, soft hands with tapered digits, pectus carinatum
Miles-Carpenter	+	+	0	Short stature, ptosis, small palpebral fissures, open mouth, pectus excavatum, scoliosis, long hands, camptodactyly, rockerbottom feet, arch fingerprints, spasticity, unsteady gait
Proud (*ARX*-Associated XLID)	+	+	0	Hearing loss, vision loss, agenesis of corpus callosum, cryptorchidism, inguinal hernias, ataxia, spasticity, seizures
Smith-Fineman-Myers	+	+	0	Ptosis, flat philtrum, scoliosis, midfoot varus, narrow feet, seizures, hypotonia

CEREBRO-CEREBELLO-COLOBOMA SYNDROME

Definition. XLID with hydrocephaly, cerebellar vermis hypoplasia, retinal coloboma, hypotonia, seizures, and abnormal respiratory pattern.

Somatic Features. No consistent craniofacial abnormality is described, save the large head secondary to hydrocephaly. Marked hypotonia, absent reflexes, seizures, severe developmental failure, and irregular respiratory pattern of alternating apnea and tachypnea were the major clinical signs. Death occurred in early childhood.

Growth and Development. Intrauterine growth was normal, with the exception of macrocephaly caused by hydrocephaly. Development was profoundly delayed.

Cognitive Function. Profound failure of development.

Heterozygote Expression. None

Imaging. Numerous abnormalities were present on brain imaging: marked hydrocephaly, callosal dysgenesis, cortical heterotopias and cysts, cerebellar vermis agenesis, or hypoplasia.

Comment. This entity is suggestive of Joubert syndrome, an autosomal recessive disorder. The family on which this report is based was composed of three brothers, the third being conceived by artificial donor insemination. A sister had intellectual disability of unknown cause. A number of XLID syndromes have cerebellar hypoplasia, but none of the composite of colobomas, cerebellar hypoplasia, and cortical abnormalities.

REFERENCE

Kroes HY, Nievelstein R-JAJ, Barth PG, et al.: Cerebral, cerebellar, and colobomatous anomalies in three related males: sex-linked inheritance in a newly recognized syndrome with features overlapping with Joubert syndrome. Am J Med Genet 135A:297, 2005.

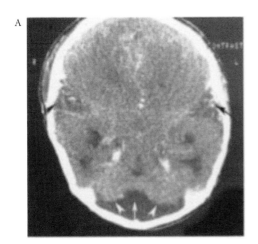 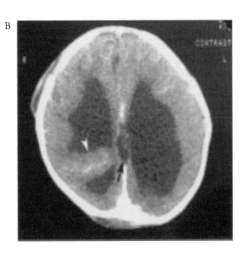

Cerebro-Cerebello-Coloboma Syndrome. CT scan showing hypoplasia of vermis *(white arrow)* and cerebellar hemispheres *(white arrowheads)* and widening of sylvian fissures *(dark arrows)* in a neonate **(A)**. Enlarged ventricles, interhemispheric cyst *(dark arrow)* and band of cortical gray matter *(white arrowhead)* in same infant **(B)**.

DIFFERENTIAL MATRIX

Syndrome	Vision or Ocular Abnormalities	Cerebellar Anomalies	Seizures	Comments
Cerebro-Cerebello-Coloboma	+	+	+	Hydrocephaly, cerebellar vermis hypoplasia, retinal coloboma, hypotonia, abnormal respiratory pattern
Bertini	+	+	+	Developmental delays and regression, postnatal growth impairment, macular degeneration, ataxia, hypotonia
Gustavson	+	+	+	Microcephaly, short stature, optic atrophy with blindness, large ears, deafness, joint contractures, rockerbottom feet, brain undergrowth, hydrocephaly, spasticity
Paine	+	+	+	Microcephaly, short stature, optic atrophy, deafness, spasticity
Christianson	+	+	O	Short stature, microcephaly, general asthenia, contractures, seizures, ophthalmoplegia, absent speech, ambulation and continence, truncal ataxia, cerebellar and brain stem hypoplasia
Schimke	+	+	O	Microcephaly, sunken eyes, downslanting palpebral fissures, narrow nose, wide spacing of teeth, cupped ears, hypotonia, choreoathetosis, contractures, impaired hearing, abducens palsy, spasticity or ataxia
Armfield	+	O	+	Short stature, cataracts or glaucoma, dental anomalies, small hands and feet, hydrocephaly, joint stiffness, facial clefting
Wittwer	+	O	+	Microcephaly, short stature, microphthalmia, hypertelorism, hypotonia, hearing loss, genitourinary anomalies
Hydrocephaly-Cerebellar Agenesis	O	+	+	Absent cerebellar hemispheres, hypotonia, hydrocephaly
Pettigrew	O	+	+	Dandy-Walker malformation, microcephaly or hydrocephaly, long face with macrostomia, small testes, contractures, choreoathetosis, spastic paraplegia, iron deposits or calcification of basal ganglia

CEREBRO-OCULO-GENITAL SYNDROME
(SIBER MICROPHTHALMIA, DUKER MICROPHTHALMIA, SIBER-DUKER MICROPHTHALMIA)

Definition. XLID with microcephaly, short stature, microphthalmia, agenesis of the corpus callosum, hypospadias or other genital anomalies, and spastic quadriplegia. The gene has not been localized.

Somatic Features. Blepharoptosis, corneal clouding with fibrovascular and dysgenesis of the stroma, pannus, uveal hypoplasia, cataracts, retinal dysplasia, and optic nerve hypoplasia accompany the microphthalmia. Aniridia has been described. The eyes move through the full range and have nystagmus. Agenesis of the corpus callosum may be demonstrated on cranial imaging. Microcephaly is constant, and low-set ears and micrognathia may be present. Small penis, hypospadias, undescended testes, fifth finger clinodactyly, joint limitation, and club foot complete the somatic phenotype.

Growth and Development. Weight is normal at birth but microcephaly or hydrocephaly is present in all cases.

Cognitive Function. Severe impairment

Neurological Findings. Spastic quadriplegia

Heterozygote Expression. No cognitive impairment and no ocular or other somatic manifestations have been described.

Imaging. Absence of corpus callosum

Neuropathology. Based on two cases: One case showed extremely small brain with cerebral cyst that communicated with the ventricle system, absent corpus callosum, and small optic nerves. The other case showed severe hydrocephalus with aqueductal stenosis; hypoplasia of cerebral hemispheres, cerebellum, midbrain, pons and basal ganglia; absence of the olfactory, optic, and oculomotor nerves; and macrogyria.

Comment. Ocular disorders of a great variety are caused by genes distributed along the entirety of the X-chromosome. These genes alter visual acuity by influencing structural development of the eyes, interference with ocular movement, obstruction of the visual medium, and disturbance of the reception and transmission of images to the occipital cortex. They are distributed from distal Xp (Aicardi, Bertini, Goltz, MIDAS, Nance-Horan, and Wittwer syndromes) to distal Xq (Graham syndrome) with a number of important loci in between (Norrie Dysplasia–Xp11.3, XLID-Choroideremia–Xq21, Mohr-Tranebjaerg syndrome–Xq22, Arts syndrome–Xq22.3, Lowe syndrome–Xq26). Other syndromes with vision loss have yet to be mapped (XLID-Retinitis Pigmentosa, Schimke syndrome). The nature of the ocular anomaly, the presence of nonocular manifestations, and the gene localizations are helpful in differentiating the XLID entities with ocular abnormalities.

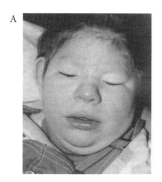
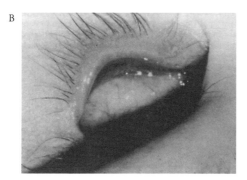
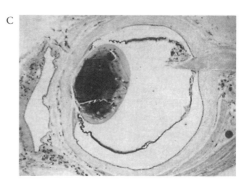

Cerebro-Oculo-Genital Syndrome. Five-year-old with microcephaly, blepharophimosis, and microphthalmia **(A)**. Microphthalmia with cornea obscured by fibrovascular membrane **(B)**; cross-section of fetal cornea showing absent Bowman's layer and Descemet's membrane **(C)**.   Courtesy of Dr. Frederick Bieber, Brigham and Women's Hospital and Massachusetts General Hospital, Boston.

REFERENCES

Duker JS, Weiss JS, Siber M, et al.: Ocular findings in a new heritable syndrome of brain, eye, and urogenital abnormalities. Am J Ophthalmol 99:51, 1985.

Siber M: X-linked recessive microencephaly, microphthalmia with corneal opacities, spastic quadriplegia, hypospadias and cryptorchidism. Clin Genet 26:453, 1984.

DIFFERENTIAL MATRIX

Syndrome	Microcephaly	Ocular Anomaly	Genitourinary Anomaly	Comments
Cerebro-Oculo-Genital	+	+	+	Hydrocephaly, short stature, agenesis of corpus callosum, microphthalmia, ptosis, hypospadias, cryptorchidism, clubfoot, spasticity
Lenz Microphthalmia	+	+	+	Malformed ears, cleft lip/palate, cardiac anomalies, thumb duplication or hypoplasia, narrow shoulders
Wittwer	+	+	+	Short stature, hearing loss, vision loss, hypertelorism, hypotonia, seizures
MIDAS	+	+	0	Dermal aplasia, dysgenesis of corpus callosum, cardiac defects, cardiomyopathy
Roifman	+	+	0	Short stature, spondyloepiphyseal dysplasia, retinal pigmentary deposits, antibody deficiency, eczema, hypotonia
XLID-Microcephaly-Testicular Failure	+	0	+	Short stature, prominent supraorbital ridges, high nasal bridge, prominent nose, macrostomia, hypogonadism
Goltz	0	+	+	Linear areas of dermal aplasia, cutaneous adipose herniations, dystrophic nails, abnormal teeth and hair, vertebral anomalies, limb reduction defects
Lowe	0	+	+	Short stature, hypotonia, aminoaciduria, progressive renal disease

CEREBRO-PALATO-CARDIAC SYNDROME (*SEE ALSO RENPENNING SYNDROME*)

(HAMEL SYNDROME, XLID-CLEFT PALATE-CARDIAC DEFECT SYNDROME, *PQBP1*-ASSOCIATED XLID)

OMIM 309500

Xp11.23

PQBP1

Definition. XLID with microcephaly, short stature, cupped ears, bulbous nose, highly arched or cleft palate, short philtrum, tented upper lip, malar hypoplasia, cardiac defect, and slender hands and feet. A mutation was found in *PQBP1*, hence the condition is allelic to Renpenning, Sutherland-Haan, Golabi-Ito-Hall, and Porteous syndromes.

Somatic Features. Microcephaly, broad nasal bridge, bulbous nose, malar hypoplasia, dysplastic cupped ears, short philtrum, tented upper lip, and small mouth contribute to a distinctive craniofacial appearance. The initially oval facial configuration elongates with age. Highly arched or cleft palate occurs consistently. Complex cardiac defects, tetralogy of Fallot in one case, atrial and ventricular septal defects and overriding aorta in another, and undiagnosed defects in two others are symptomatic in all cases. Only minor skeletal anomalies occur, including long slender hands and feet,

fifth finger clinodactyly, and contractures at the elbows and knees. Hypospadias was present in one case.

Growth and Development. All parameters of growth are retarded prenatally and postnatally. Delay of developmental milestones becomes obvious in infancy.

Neurological Findings. Hypertonicity was noted in one case.

Heterozygote Expression. The carrier mother of two affected males had an atrial septal defect but no other manifestation.

Imaging. Small brain without structural malformation was found in the single case so studied.

Comment. The Cerebro-Palato-Cardiac syndrome seems to be an exception to the generalization that XLID syndromes do not have lethal malformations. In three of the four cases described in the original family, death occurred during infancy or childhood, their cardiac defect being the principal contributor. This does not appear to be the case with Renpenning syndrome nor other allelic conditions.

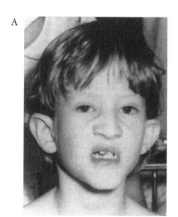 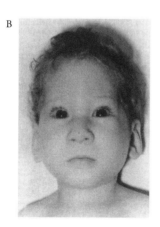 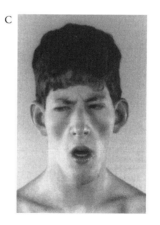 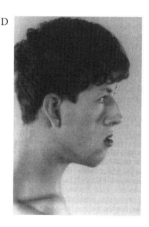

Cerebro-Palato-Cardiac Syndrome. Long narrow face, broad nasal bridge, bulbous nose, prominent mandible, cupped ears and short philtrum at age 8 years (**A**); long narrow face, broad nasal bridge, bulbous nose, malar hypoplasia, cupped ears, and small mouth in brother at ages 7 months (**B**) and 20 years (**C, D**). Courtesy of Dr. Ben Hamel, University Hospital, Nijmegen, The Netherlands and the *American Journal of Medical Genetics*, Copyright 1994, Wiley-Liss, Inc.

REFERENCES

Hamel BCJ, Mariman ECM, van Beersum SEC, et al.: Mental retardation, congenital heart defect, cleft palate, short stature, and facial anomalies: A new X-linked multiple congenital anomalies/mental retardation syndrome: Clinical description and molecular studies. Am J Med Genet 51:591, 1994.

Kalscheuer VM, Freude K, Musante L, et al.: Mutations in the polyglutamine binding protein 1 gene cause X-linked mental retardation. Nat Genet 35:313, 2003.

Lenski C, Abidi F, Meindl A, et al.: Novel truncating mutations in the polyglutamine tract binding protein 1 gene (PQBP1) cause Renpenning syndrome and X-linked mental retardation in another family with microcephaly. Am J Hum Genet 74:777, 2004.

Lubs H, Abidi FE, Echeverri R, et al.: Golabi-Ito-Hall syndrome results from a missense mutation in the WW domain of the PQBP1 gene. J Med Genet 43:e30, 2006.

Stevenson RE, Bennett CW, Abidi F, et al.: Renpenning syndrome comes into focus. Am J Med Genet A 134:415, 2005.

DIFFERENTIAL MATRIX

Syndrome	Cardiac Defect	Facial Clefting	Distinctive Facial Features	Comments
Cerebro-Palato-Cardiac (Renpenning)	+	+	+	Microcephaly, short stature, cleft palate, cupped ears, bulbous nose, short philtrum, tented upper lip, childhood death
Lenz Microphthalmia	+	+	+	Microcephaly, microphthalmia, ocular dysgenesis, malformed ears, cleft lip/palate, cardiac and genitourinary anomalies, thumb duplication or hypoplasia, narrow shoulders
Simpson-Golabi-Behmel	+	+	+	Somatic overgrowth, supernumerary nipples, polydactyly
Telecanthus-Hypospadias	+	+	+	High broad nasal root, dysplastic ears, cleft lip/palate, abnormal cranial contour or symmetry
Hereditary Bullous Dystrophy, X-linked	+	0	+	Microcephaly, short stature, upslanting palpebral fissures, protruding ears, short and tapered digits, bullous dystrophy, small testes, early death from pulmonary infection
FLNA-Associated XLID	0	+	+	Short stature, prominent brow or forehead, hypertelorism, downslanting palpebral fissures, blunting of distal phalanges, irregular spacing of digits, limited/subluxed/dislocated joints, hypoplastic fibulas, periventricular nodular heterotopias
Oral-Facial-Digital I	0	+	+	Sparse scalp hair, dystopia canthorum, flat midface, hypoplastic alae nasi, hypertrophic and aberrant oral frenuli, intraoral clefts and pseudoclefts, lingual hamartomas, brachydactyly, syndactyly, clinodactyly, structural brain anomalies, polycystic kidneys
Pallister W	0	+	+	Short stature, prominent forehead, wide nasal tip, incomplete cleft lip/palate, spasticity, contractures

CHARCOT-MARIE-TOOTH NEUROPATHY, COWCHOCK VARIANT

(XLID-MOTOR-SENSORY NEUROPATHY-DEAFNESS, COWCHOCK SYNDROME, CMTX4)

OMIM 310490

Xq25-q26

Definition. XLID associated with infancy-onset peripheral motor and sensory neuropathy and deafness. The gene has not been identified but is linked to markers in Xq25-q26.

Somatic Features. Affected males are profoundly weak and areflexic from birth. Pes cavus and hammer toes become obvious with age. Malformations or craniofacial manifestations do not occur.

Growth and Development. Growth impairment has not been described. Global developmental delay occurs, although delay of motor milestones may be more notable.

Cognitive Function. Impairment of cognitive function is inconsistent, being present in less than half of cases.

Neurological Findings. From birth, infants are areflexic and weak, so much so as to be considered affected by spinal muscular atrophy. Slow motor development may be attributed in part to muscle weakness but is too severe to be explained by this alone. Affected males eventually walk alone. Weakness appears most notable in the distal muscles of the lower limbs but is demonstrably generalized in adults. Fasciculations of the tongue and deltoid muscles may be seen in some cases. Sensorineural hearing loss has been found in most cases.

Heterozygote Expression. Clinical abnormalities have not been reported in obligate carrier females, although prolongation in sural nerve latency was documented in two.

Laboratory. Electromyography shows denervation and occasional fibrillation; median motor nerve conduction velocity is moderately slowed in some patients; sensory conduction is markedly slowed in median and sural nerves; nerve biopsy shows a paucity of myelinated nerve fibers and an increase in connective tissue; muscle biopsy shows muscle atrophy of neurogenic type.

Comment. Peripheral neuropathies constitute a heterogenous group of genetic disorders with both autosomal (17p and 1q) and X-chromosome gene loci. Only the X-linked Cowchock and Ionasescu variants have associated intellectual disability, and the mental impairment does not affect all patients. Cowchock variant may be distinguished clinically by sensorineural hearing loss and by gene localization in Xq25-q26. Both variants have onset in infancy.

REFERENCES

Cowchock FS, Duckett SW, Streletz LJ, et al.: X-linked motor-sensory neuropathy type-II with deafness and mental retardation: a new disorder. Am J Med Genet 20:307, 1985.

Fischbeck KH, ar-Rushdi N, Pericak-Vance M, et al.: X-linked neuropathy: gene localization with DNA probes. Ann Neurol 20:527, 1986.

Priest JM, Fischbeck KH, Nouri N, et al.: A locus for axonal motor-sensory neuropathy with deafness and mental retardation maps to Xq24-q26. Genomics 29:409, 1995.

DIFFERENTIAL MATRIX

Syndrome	Peripheral Motor-Sensory Neuropathy	Areflexia	Distal Leg Muscle Atrophy/ Hypoplasia	Comments
Charcot-Marie-Tooth Neuropathy, Ionasescu variant	+	+	+	Wasting of intrinsic hand muscles, enlarged ulnar nerves, pes cavus, weakness
Charcot-Marie-Tooth Neuropathy, Cowchock variant	+	+	+	Deafness, pes cavus, weakness

CHARCOT-MARIE-TOOTH NEUROPATHY, IONASESCU VARIANT

(XLID-CHARCOT-MARIE-TOOTH NEUROPATHY, X-LINKED RECESSIVE
CHARCOT-MARIE-TOOTH DISEASE TYPE 2, CMTX2)

OMIM 302801

Xp22.2

Definition. XLID associated with onset of peripheral motor and sensory neuropathy in infancy. Linkage of the disease locus with markers DXS16-DXS43 in Xp22.2 (maximal multipoint lod score 3.48) provides the basis for separation from other X-linked and autosomal forms of Charcot-Marie-Tooth neuropathy.

Somatic Features. Musculoskeletal findings are secondary to the peripheral neuropathy and include atrophy of distal leg muscles and pes cavus. Malformations and distinctive craniofacial manifestations do not occur.

Growth and Development. Growth abnormalities have not been described.

Cognitive Function. Impairment of cognitive function is found in less than half of cases.

Neurological Findings. Areflexia and weakness of the distal leg muscles are present from birth or early infancy. Foot drop or steppage gait result from atrophy of the tibialis anterior and peroneal muscles. Wasting of the intrinsic muscles of the hands and mild to moderate sensory loss in the distal limbs may also be demonstrated. Typically the ulnar nerve is enlarged and pes cavus becomes progressively more notable.

Heterozygote Expression. Carrier females do not have muscle weakness or other clinical signs of the disorder. Electromyography and nerve conduction velocity are normal, although muscle biopsy may show evidence of mild neurogenic muscle atrophy.

Laboratory. Nerve conduction is decreased, indicating demyelination, and electromyography suggests axonal involvement.

Comment. In addition to gene loci for CMT neuropathy in 1q and 17p, at least four gene loci may be present on the X chromosome (Xp22.2, Xq13.1, Xq25-q26, Xq26). Intellectual disability occurs only in the Ionasescu and Cowchock variants and in these variants is not found in all males with peripheral neuropathy. The Ionasescu and Cowchock variants both have onset in infancy and lack clinically significant carrier manifestations but may be distinguished by the presence of deafness in the Cowchock variant and by gene localization (Xp22.2 in Ionasescu variant; Xq25-q26 in Cowchock variant).

REFERENCE

Ionasescu VV, Trofatter J, Haines JL, et al.: Heterogeneity in X-linked recessive Charcot-Marie-Tooth neuropathy. Am J Hum Genet 48:1075, 1991.

DIFFERENTIAL MATRIX

Syndrome	Peripheral Motor-Sensory Neuropathy	Hearing Loss	Areflexia	Comments
Charcot-Marie-Tooth Neuropathy, Cowchock variant	+	+	+	Pes cavus, weakness
Charcot-Marie-Tooth Neuropathy, Ionasescu variant	+	0	+	Wasting of intrinsic hand muscles, enlarged ulnar nerves, pes cavus, weakness

CHASSAING-LACOMBE CHONDRODYSPLASIA

Xp11.23

HDAC6

Definition. Spondylometaphyseal dysplasia, hydrocephaly, and microphthalmia in males, and spondylometaphyseal dysplasia with rhizomelic shortening of limbs and learning disability in females.

Somatic Features. Males have a lethal spondylometaphyseal dysplasia with associated hydrocephaly and microphthalmia. Chondroosseous findings include poor mineralization of the skull; severe platyspondyly; 11 ribs; hypoplastic iliac wings; poorly ossified pubis; metaphyseal flaring of the phalanges, metacarpals, and metatarsals; hypoplastic calcaneus; and widened metaphyses of the long bones. Frontal bossing, large fontanelles, microphthalmia without coloboma, short palpebral fissures, short flat nose, low-set ears, short philtrum, and macrostomia comprise the facial features.

Females have short stature, mild body asymmetry, flat nasal bridge, retrognathia, rhizomelic limb shortening, and mild intellectual disability. The vertebral bodies show irregular articulation surfaces, short metacarpals, absence of styloid process of ulna, and short middle phalanges on toes III and IV.

Growth and Development. Variable linear and cranial growth prenatally in males. Females show intrauterine and postnatal growth retardation.

Cognitive Function. Carrier females have mild intellectual disability.

Neurological Findings. No survival in males to assess.

Comment. This lethal chondrodysplasia in males and milder chondroosseous changes, short stature, and learning disability in females is distinctive in its clinical (microphthalmia and hydrocephaly) and radiographic (platyspondyly, absent ossification of vertebrae and public bones, and metaphyseal changes in the small bones of the hands and feet) presentation. The responsible gene, *HDAC6*, is a histone deacetylase (Lacombe D, Arveiler B, personal communication).

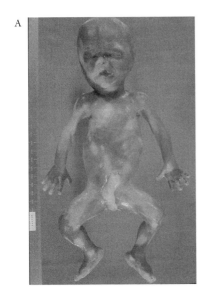
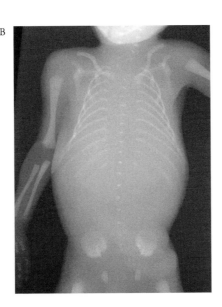
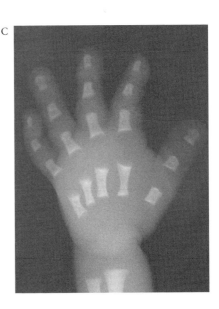

Chassaing-Lacombe Chondrodysplasia. Fetus with brachydactyly, hydrocephaly, and microphthalmia **(A)**. Radiograph of fetus showing thin ribs, platyspondyly, and underossification of vertebral bodies, hypoplasia of iliac wings, and absence of ossification of pubic bones **(B)**. Radiograph of hand showing brachydactyly and short cupped metaphyses **(C)**.

REFERENCE

Chassaing N, Siani V, Carles D, et al.: X-linked dominant chondrodysplasia with platyspondyly, distinctive brachydactyly, hydrocephaly, and microphthalmia. Am J Med Genet 136A:307, 2005.

DIFFERENTIAL MATRIX

Syndrome	Ocular Abnormality	Hydrocephaly	Skeletal Dysplasia	Comments
Chassaing-Lacombe Chondrodysplasia	+	+	+	Spondylometaphyseal dysplasia, microphthalmia in males. Spondylometaphyseal dysplasia with rhizomelic shortening of limbs and learning disability in females
Cerebro-Cerebello-Coloboma	+	+	0	Cerebellar vermis hypoplasia, retinal coloboma, hypotonia, seizures, abnormal respiratory pattern
Roifman	+	0	+	Microcephaly, short stature, spondyloepiphyseal dysplasia, retinal pigmentary deposits, antibody deficiency, eczema, hypotonia

CHRISTIAN SYNDROME
(X-LINKED SKELETAL DYSPLASIA-INTELLECTUAL DISABILITY)

OMIM 309620

Xq28

Definition. XLID with short stature, metopic ridge, vertebral anomalies, abducens palsy, and glucose intolerance. The gene has not been identified.

Somatic Features. Multiple abnormalities occur in the axial skeleton, including occipitalization of the atlas, odontoid hypoplasia, fusion of the bodies and neural arches of other cervical vertebrae, thoracic hemivertebrae with scoliosis, and hypoplasia of the sacrum. Appendicular anomalies are limited to general shortening of the bones and clinodactyly of the fifth finger. The cranium has normal circumference, typically has a prominent metopic ridge, and may have asymmetry and slight platybasia. The interorbital measurement is reduced, the palpebral fissures slant downward, and epicanthus and abducens palsy are present. Flattening of the superior helices or cupped ear may recur. All hand bones are short, the middle phalanges tending to be shorter than the others. Imperforate anus occurred in one case and constipation in another. Glucose intolerance is manifested by melituria and excessive increase in blood glucose after oral loading.

Growth and Development. Intrauterine growth appears normal. Postnatally, head growth continues to be normal, but linear growth is impaired, resulting in short stature.

Cognitive Function. Borderline normal to mild impairment

Heterozygote Expression. Carrier females may have fusion of the cervical vertebrae, short middle phalanges, and diabetes mellituria or intolerance to oral glucose loading but have normal cognitive function.

Imaging. Pneumoencephalogram was performed on one child, showing dilation of the lateral and third ventricle.

Comment. Only two other XLID syndromes (Christianson syndrome, Schimke syndrome) have abducens palsy as a manifestation. Christian syndrome and Christianson syndrome

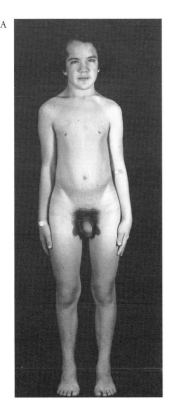

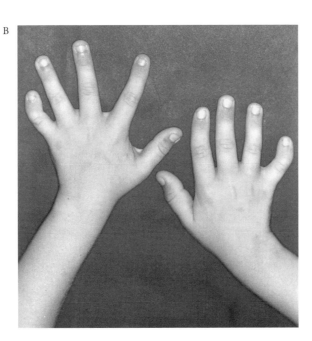

Christian Syndrome. Sixteen-year-old male with short stature **(A)**. Clinodactyly of fifth fingers **(B)**.   Courtesy of Dr. Joe C. Christian, Indiana University School of Medicine, Indianapolis.

have overlapping linkage limits but are phenotypically different. Schimke syndrome has not been mapped. Mutations in *SLC9A6* have been reported in Christianson syndrome.

REFERENCES

Christian JC, DeMeyer W, Franken EA, et al.: X-linked skeletal dysplasia with mental retardation. Clin Genet 11:128, 1977.

Dlouhy SR, Christian JC, Haines JL, et al.: Localization of the gene for a syndrome of X-linked skeletal dysplasia and mental retardation to Xq27-qter. Hum Genet 75:136, 1987.

Gilfillan GD, Selmer KK, Roxrud I, et al.: SLC9A6 mutations cause X-linked mental retardation, microcephaly, epilepsy, and ataxia, a phenotype mimicking Angelman syndrome. Am J Hum Genet 82:1003, 2008.

DIFFERENTIAL MATRIX

Syndrome	Short Stature	Abducens Palsy	Vertebral Anomalies	Comments
Christian	+	+	+	Metopic ridge
Christianson	+	+	O	Microcephaly, general asthenia, contractures, seizures, ophthalmoplegia
Schimke	+	+	O	Microcephaly, sunken eyes, downslanting palpebral fissures, narrow nose, wide spacing of teeth, cupped ears, hypotonia, hearing loss, vision loss, spasticity, choreoathetosis, contractures
Aarskog	+	O	+	Hypertelorism, downslanting palpebral fissures, ptosis, cupped ears, anteverted nares, brachydactyly, horizontal palmar crease, midfoot varus, joint laxity, shawl scrotum, cryptorchidism, inguinal hernias
Craniofacioskeletal	+	O	+	Mild cognitive impairment, microcephaly, craniofacial distinctiveness, small hands and feet, excessive fingerprint arches in females. Males die in early infancy with craniofacial, cardiac, skeletal, and genital abnormalities
Goltz	+	O	+	Cataracts, ocular dysgenesis, linear areas of dermal aplasia, cutaneous adipose herniations, dystrophic nails, abnormal teeth and hair, vertebral anomalies, limb reduction defects, genitourinary anomalies
Otopalatodigital I (*FLNA*-Associated XLID)	+	O	+	Conductive hearing impairment, prominent brow, broad nasal root, apparent ocular hypertelorism, downslanting palpebral fissures, cleft palate, blunted distal phalanges, irregular curvature and spacing of digits, limitation of elbow movement
Roifman	+	O	+	Microcephaly, spondyloepiphyseal dysplasia, retinal pigmentary deposits, antibody deficiency, eczema, hypotonia
Stoccos dos Santos	+	O	+	Heavy eyebrows, strabismus, short palpebral fissures, short philtrum, thin upper lip, prominent nasal tip, hip dislocation, hirsutism, kyphosis, precocious puberty, recurrent respiratory infections

CHRISTIANSON SYNDROME

(X-LINKED ANGELMAN-LIKE SYNDROME)

OMIM 300243

Xq26.3

SLC9A6

Definition. XLID with short stature, microcephaly, long narrow face, large ears, long straight nose, open mouth, prominent mandible, general asthenia, narrow chest, elbow flexion, long thin digits, adducted thumbs, contractures, seizures, autistic features, truncal ataxia, ophthalmoplegia, mutism, incontinence, and hypoplasia of the cerebellum and brainstem. The responsible gene encodes the sodium-hydrogen exchanger protein, NHE6.

Somatic Features. Profound disability with absence of speech, failure or loss of ambulation, incontinence, seizures, and cognitive deficiency is paralleled by somatic frailty with general asthenia, microcephaly and short stature, narrow chest, long thin digits, and contractures. There is a tendency to hold the elbows in flexed position. The long narrow face is further defined by large ears, straight thin nose, squint, open mouth, and prominent square mandible. Major malformations do not occur. Genitalia, including testicular volume, are normal.

Growth and Development. Birth weight is normal, but during childhood weight falls below the 3rd centile. Head circumference and height measure in the lower centiles or slightly below.

Cognitive Function. Profound impairment is the rule with inability to speak and assist in the rudiments of self-care.

Neurological Findings. Affected males never achieve basic skills for self-care. They never develop speech, although hearing appears intact. Incontinence of bowel and bladder persists throughout life. Ophthalmoplegia, resulting from abducens nerve dysfunction, contributes to strabismus. Muscle tone appears normal. Deep tendon reflexes are usually normal, although brisk reflexes at the knees and Babinski signs or equivocal plantar responses were noted in several patients. Clonus has rarely been described. Truncal ataxia occurs even in childhood. Generalized seizures begin in infancy or early childhood. EMG and nerve conduction are normal.

Heterozygote Expression. Carrier females may have learning impairments or mild intellectual disability and exhibit behavior problems and aggressiveness during childhood.

Neuropathology. The brain is undergrown generally, but with hypoplasia or atrophy of the cerebellar vermis and brainstem particularly. Cerebellar morphology is characterized by loss of neurons in the granular and Purkinje cell layers, microcystic changes in the molecular layer, and depletion of myelin.

Imaging. MRI shows progressive atrophy of the cerebellum and brainstem in the company of prominent cerebellar cisterns and fourth ventricle. The lateral ventricles are usually normal. Increased glutamate/glutamine peaks may be present on the MR spectroscopy.

Comment. Christianson syndrome maps to Xq23-q27, an area least populated with genes that cause X-linked intellectual disability. There are many features – profound developmental failure, microcephaly, flexed elbows, absent speech, absent or unsteady ambulation, incontinence, truncal ataxia, contractures, and generally happy demeanor – in common with Angelman syndrome. As such, Christianson syndrome joins a growing list of conditions, mostly autosomal, which mimic the Angelman phenotype. One candidate for allelism, Gustavson syndrome, has overlapping linkage limits, cerebellar hypoplasia, microcephaly, short stature, profound developmental failure, blindness, deafness, and seizures. Severe impairments are obvious from birth, and death occurs in infancy or early childhood. Other XLID syndromes with overlapping mapping limits include Arts, Miles-Carpenter, Hamel, Börjeson-Forssman-Lehmann, Hereditary Bullous Dystrophy, and XLID-Hypogammaglobulinemia syndromes, none of which is similar in phenotype with Christianson syndrome. Schimke syndrome, as yet not mapped, should be considered in the differential because of microcephaly, short stature, abducens palsy, and progressive basal ganglia dysfunction.

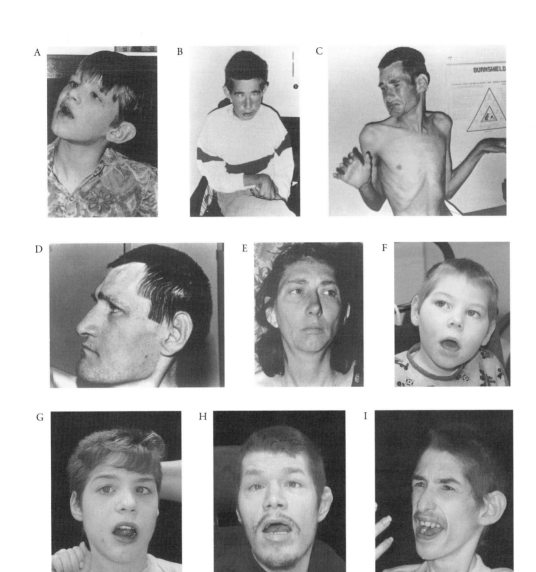

Christianson Syndrome. Ten-year-old male with incompletely folded helices, strabismus, long straight nose, and square jaw (A); 19-year-old cousin with long narrow face, bushy eyebrows, strabismus, long straight nose, large ears, and square jaw (B); 24-year-old cousin with bushy eyebrows, long straight nose, square jaw, and decreased muscle mass (C); profile of maternal uncle showing deeply-set eyes, long straight nose, prominent jaw, and large ears (D); 35-year-old carrier female with large ears and long straight nose (E). Isolated case at age 6 years with microcephaly, frontal upsweep, and hypotonic face (F). Fifteen-year-old with microcephaly and hypotonic face (G); an uncle at age 35 years with frontal upsweep, strabismus, open mouth and prominent jaw (H); and 28-year-old uncle with microcephaly, upsweep of frontal hair, gaunt face, low nasal septum, open mouth, and prominent ears (I). Illustrations A–E Courtesy of Professor Arnold Christianson, Department of Human Genetics and Developmental Biology, University of Pretoria, Republic of South Africa.

REFERENCES

Christianson AL, Stevenson RE, van der Mayden CH, et al. X linked mental retardation, mild craniofacial dysmorphology, epilepsy, ophthalmoplegia, and cerebellar atrophy in a large South African kindred. J Med Genet 36:759, 1999.

Gilfillan GD, Selmer KK, Roxrud I, et al.: SLC9A6 mutations cause X-linked mental retardation, microcephaly, epilepsy, and ataxia, a phenotype mimicking Angelman syndrome. Am J Hum Genet 82:1003, 2008.

Gustavson K-H, Annerén G, Malmgren H, et al.: New X-linked syndrome with severe mental retardation, severely impaired vision, severe hearing defect, epileptic seizures, spasticity, restricted joint mobility, and early death. Am J Med Genet 45:654, 1993.

Schroer RJ, Holden KR, Tarpey PS, et al.: Natural history of Christianson syndrome. Am J Med Genet A 152A:2775, 2010.

DIFFERENTIAL MATRIX

Syndrome	Absent Speech, Ambulation and Continence	Truncal Ataxia	Cerebellar and Brainstem Hypoplasia	Comments
Christianson	+	+	+	Short stature, microcephaly, general asthenia, contractures, seizures, ophthalmoplegia
Pelizaeus-Merzbacher	+	+	+	Optic atrophy, hypotonia, dystonia, CNS dysmyelination, ataxia, spastic paraplegia, nystagmus
Bertini	+	+	+	Macular degeneration, hypotonia, seizures, childhood death, developmental delays and regression, postnatal growth impairment
Gustavson	+	+	+	Microcephaly, short stature, optic atrophy with blindness, large ears, deafness, joint contractures, rockerbottom feet, brain undergrowth, hydrocephaly, spasticity, seizures
Schimke	+	+	+	Microcephaly, sunken eyes, downslanting palpebral fissures, narrow nose, wide spacing of teeth, cupped ears, hypotonia, abducens palsy, hearing loss, vision loss, spasticity, choreoathetosis, contractures
Paine	+	0	+	Microcephaly, short stature, optic atrophy, vision and hearing loss, spasticity, seizures
Pettigrew	0	+	+	Dandy-Walker malformation, spasticity, microcephaly or hydrocephaly, long face with macrostomia and prognathism, small testes, contractures, myoglobinuria, hemolytic anemia, seizures

CHUDLEY-LOWRY SYNDROME (*SEE ALSO ATRX*-ASSOCIATED XLID)

(XLID-HYPOTONIA-HYPOGONADISM)

OMIM 309580

Xq21.1

ATRX (XNP, XH2)

Definition. XLID with short stature, hypotonic facies, obesity, and hypogenitalism. A mutation in *ATRX* has been identified in Chudley-Lowry syndrome, making it one of a number of named XLID syndromes that are allelic to Alpha-Thalassemia Intellectual Disability.

Somatic Features. Narrow bitemporal diameter, almond-shaped eyes, depressed nasal bridge, large open mouth with arched upper lip, short philtrum, and high palate contribute to a facial appearance that suggests intrauterine and early developmental hypotonia. Only in one case, however, was hypotonia specifically noted. Skeletal manifestations include short neck, mild brachydactyly, tapering of the digits, fifth-finger camptodactyly, and genu valgum. An excess number of arch fingerprints and low total ridge count were documented. Although the testes were small or incompletely descended, sex hormone levels and secondary sexual characteristics were normal.

Growth and Development. Growth discordance, possibly postnatal in origin, results in head circumference and stature in the lower centiles and weight in the upper centiles. Global delay of developmental milestones is obvious from infancy.

Cognitive Function. Moderate to severe impairment

Behavior. Short attention span, hyperactivity, and poor adaptive function were described in two cases – one of preschool age, the other adult.

Neurological Findings. None

Heterozygote Expression. None

Imaging. CT of the brain in one case was normal.

Comment. Two groups of syndromes are called to mind by the clinical manifestations in Chudley-Lowry Syndrome. The first group is constituted of syndromes that share hypotonia, hypogonadism, and obesity as prominent findings. Notable among these are Prader-Willi, Bardet-Biedl, Börjeson-Forssman-Lehmann, Wilson-Turner, and Vasquez syndromes. The second group contains syndromes with hypotonic facies, minor skeletal abnormalities, and genital anomalies. Alpha-Thalassemia Intellectual Disability is the prototype syndrome of this latter group and the finding of an *ATRX* mutation in Chudley-Lowry syndrome confirms that these two syndromes are allelic.

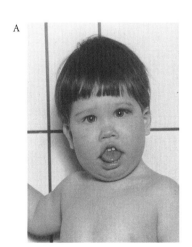 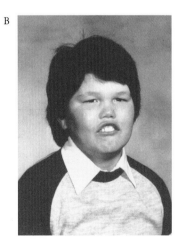 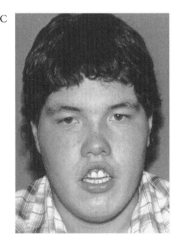

Chudley-Lowry Syndrome. Depressed nasal bridge, short philtrum, tented upper lip, and almond-shaped palpebral fissures in a 30-month-old male **(A)** and his two maternal uncles ages 19 years and 20 years **(B, C).**   Courtesy of Dr. Albert E. Chudley, Children's Hospital, Winnipeg, Manitoba.

REFERENCES

Abidi FE, Cardoso C, Lossi AM, et al.: Mutation in the 5' alternatively spliced region of the XNP/ATR-X gene causes Chudley-Lowry syndrome. Eur J Hum Genet 13:176, 2005.

Chudley AE, Lowry RB, Hoar DI: Mental retardation, distinct facial changes, short stature, obesity, and hypogonadism. A new X-linked mental retardation syndrome. Am J Med Genet 31:741, 1988.

DIFFERENTIAL MATRIX

Syndrome	Obesity	Hypotonia	Hypogenitalism	Comments
Chudley-Lowry (*ATRX*-Associated XLID)	+	+	+	Short stature, bitemporal narrowing, almond-shaped eyes, depressed nasal bridge, tented upper lip, open mouth
Börjeson-Forssman-Lehmann	+	+	+	Short stature, microcephaly, coarse face, large ears, gynecomastia, narrow sloped shoulders, visual impairment, tapered digits
Vasquez	+	+	+	Microcephaly, short stature, gynecomastia
Wilson-Turner	+	+	+	Normal growth, small hands and feet, tapered digits, gynecomastia, emotional lability
Ahmad	+	0	+	Hypogonadism, short stature, tapered fingers
Urban	+	0	+	Short stature, small hands and feet, digital contractures, osteoporosis
XLID-Hypogonadism-Tremor	+	0	+	Short stature, prominent lower lip, muscle wasting of legs, abnormal gait, hypogonadism, seizures, tremor
Young-Hughes	+	0	+	Short stature, small palpebral fissures, cupped ears, ichthyosiform scaling
Pettigrew	0	+	+	Dandy-Walker malformation, spasticity, microcephaly or hydrocephaly, long face with macrostomia and prognathism, contractures, choreoathetosis, iron deposits in basal ganglia, seizures
Prieto	0	+	+	Ventricular enlargement, facial asymmetry, hypertelorism, prominent eyes, ptosis, long narrow nose, micrognathia, inguinal hernia, cryptorchidism

CK SYNDROME

OMIM 300831

Xq28

NSDHL

Definition. XLID with microcephaly, asthenic build, distinctive facial appearance, neuronal migration disturbance, seizures, and behavioral problems. The gene is the same as mutated in CHILD Syndrome.

Somatic Features. The CK syndrome was initially reported in a single family with seven males affected in five generations (du Souich et al., 2009). The face appears hypotonic and is long and thin with upslanted palpebrae, almond-shaped eyes with epicanthus, open mouth, and micrognathia. The palate is high-arched, the teeth crowded, and the ears posteriorly rotated. Strabismus is common. The limbs are relatively long, although overall height is in the lower centiles. The joints are hyperextensible. Curvature of the spine may be present. The brain shows evidence that neuronal migration is disturbed, resulting in pachygyria and polymicrogyria. One male had aortic valve stenosis. Most exhibit abnormal behavior in a form of autistic mannerisms, excessive irritability, aggression, or attention deficit hyperactivity. A second family with a frame shift mutation in *NSDHL* was identified (McLarren et al., 2010). The second family had similar clinical findings.

Growth and Development. Intrauterine growth is impaired and continues postnatally. Microcephaly is usual and stature measures in the lower centiles. Overall asthenia with long limbs and digits is typical. Developmental milestones are globally delayed, usually to severe degree, with speech being more severely affected.

Cognitive Function. Cognitive function is severely impaired in most, but not all, cases.

Behavior. Behavioral disturbance in the form of attention deficit hyperactivity, excessive irritability, aggressiveness, or autism are universal.

Neurological Findings. All individuals develop seizures, usually in infancy. Seizures may be focal or generalized and in some cases become intractable. Brain imaging shows disturbed neuronal migration with pachygyria and polymicrogyria.

Heterozygote Expression. Carriers have normal intelligence and physical appearance.

Comment. This XLID syndrome shares somatic features with Lujan, Snyder-Robinson, and *ZDHHC9*-Associated syndromes but has more severe cognitive impairment and brain imaging evidence of abnormal neuronal migration.

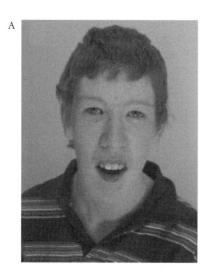 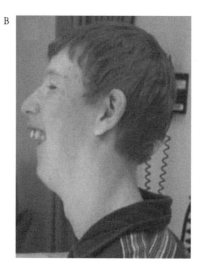 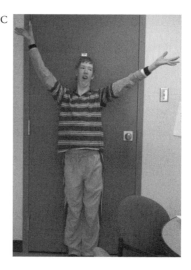

CK Syndrome. Seventeen-year-old with microcephaly; long, thin face; epicanthal folds; overbite; retracted mandible; and asthenic build **(A–C)**.
Courtesy of Drs. Christèle du Souich and Cornelius Boerkoel, University of British Columbia, Vancouver.

Mutations in different genes are responsible for these different syndromes and their similar clinical findings are not known to be caused by any similarity of gene function. *NSDHL* encodes NAD(P)H Steroid Dehydrogenase-Like protein, which functions in the cholesterol biosynthesis pathway. The mouse homologs cause "bare patches" and "striated" phenotypes.

REFERENCES

du Souich C, Chou A, Yin J, et al.: Characterization of a new X-linked mental retardation syndrome with microcephaly, cortical malformation, and thin habitus. Am J Med Genet A 149A:2469, 2009.

McLarren KW, Severson TM, du Souich C, et al.: Hypomorphic temperature-sensitive alleles of NSDHL cause CK syndrome. Am J Hum Genet 87:905, 2010.

DIFFERENTIAL MATRIX

Syndrome	Microcephaly	Neuronal Migration Disturbance	Seizures	Comments
CK	+	+	+	Asthenic build, hypotonia, long thin face, scoliosis, behavior problems
ARX-Associated XLID	+	+	+	Hydranencephaly, lissencephaly, agenesis of corpus callosum, abnormal genitalia, dystonia, ataxia, spasticity, dysarthria
Lissencephaly, X-linked	+	+	+	Defect in neuronal migration resulting in frontal pachygyria in males and subcortical band heterotopia in carrier females, hypotonia, spasticity, genital hypoplasia, dysgenesis of corpus callosum, lissencephaly, or cerebral heterotopia
Kang	+	+	0	Frontal prominence, telecanthus, small nose, short hands, seizures, downslanted mouth, brachydactyly, microcephaly, dysgenesis of corpus callosum, spastic paraplegia
Börjeson-Forssman-Lehmann	+	0	+	Short stature, coarse face, large ears, gynecomastia, narrow sloped shoulders, visual impairment, tapered digits, hypotonia, hypogonadism, obesity
Gustavson	+	0	+	Short stature, optic atrophy with blindness, large ears, deafness, joint contractures, rockerbottom feet, brain undergrowth, hydrocephaly, cerebellar hypoplasia, spasticity
Pyruvate Dehydrogenase Deficiency	+	0	+	Ataxia, dysarthria, structural brain anomalies, hypotonia, lactic acidosis
Rett	+	0	+	Truncal ataxia, autistic features, developmental regression, repetitive stereotypical hand movements
XLID-Blindness-Seizures-Spasticity	+	0	+	Poor growth, postnatal microcephaly, clubfoot, contractures, scoliosis, hypomyelination, optic atrophy or blindness, spastic paraplegia
FLNA-Associated XLID	0	+	+	Short stature, prominent brow or forehead, hypertelorism, downslanting palpebral fissures, blunting of distal phalanges, irregular spacing of digits, limited/subluxed/dislocated joints, hypoplastic fibulas, periventricular nodular heterotopias

CLARK-BARAITSER SYNDROME
(BARAITSER SYNDROME)

OMIM 300602

Definition. XLID with macrocephaly, prominent forehead and large ears, broad nasal tip, thick lower lip, supraorbital ridges, small lateral maxillary incisors, obesity, and macroorchidism. The gene has not been localized.

Somatic Features. Major malformations do not occur. Overall large stature, craniofacial manifestations, and macroorchidism define the phenotype. Macrocephaly with square forehead and prominent supraorbital ridges, large ears, broad nasal tip, thick lower lips, and small lateral maxillary incisors are the dominant facial characteristics. A central maxillary diastema may also be present. Generalized obesity adds to the fullness of the face.

Growth and Development. Details of early growth and development are not available. As adults, affected males have macrocephaly, tall stature, and obesity.

Cognitive Function. Moderate impairment

Heterozygote Expression. The mother of the two affected brothers reported by Clark and Baraitser (1987) had mild mental retardation and facial features similar to her sons.

Comment. The phenotype is based on a single family with two affected brothers and their mildly affected mother. Initially, the authors were persuaded that the condition was the same as Atkin-Flaitz syndrome. In a subsequent publication, Baraitser et al. (1995) described another family in which two male first-cousins had excessive overall growth, macrocephaly, prominence of the lower lip, obesity, and behavioral problems.

REFERENCES

Atkin JF, Flaitz K, Patil S, et al.: A new X-linked mental retardation syndrome. Am J Med Genet 21:697, 1985.

Baraitser M, Reardon W, Vijeratnam S: Nonspecific X-linked mental retardation with macrocephaly and obesity: A further family. Am J Med Genet 57:280, 1995.

Clark RD, Baraitser M: Letter to the Editor: A new X-linked mental retardation syndrome. Am J Med Genet 26:13, 1987.

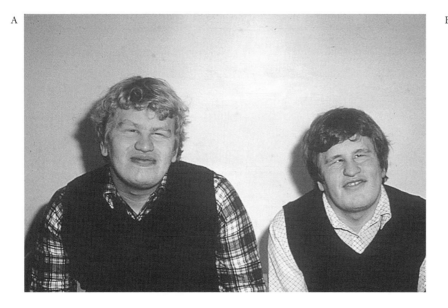
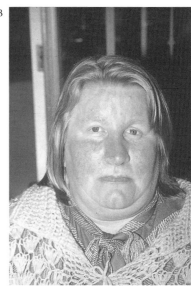

Clark-Baraitser Syndrome. Macrocephaly, prominent forehead, broad nasal tip, thick lower lip in brothers ages 21 and 22 years **(A)** and mother age 46 years **(B)**.   Courtesy of Dr. Michael Baraitser, Institute of Child Health, London.

DIFFERENTIAL MATRIX

Syndrome	Macrocephaly	Obesity	Macroorchidism	Comments
Clark-Baraitser	+	+	+	Large stature, dental abnormalities, broad nasal tip, thick lower lip
Atkin-Flaitz	+	+	+	Short stature, hypertelorism, downslanting palpebral fissures, broad nasal tip, thick lower lip, brachydactyly, seizures
XLID-Macrocephaly-Macroorchidism	+	+	+	Elongated face, prominent mandible, clumsiness, repetitive movements
XLID-Macrocephaly	+	+	0	Downslanting palpebral fissures, elbow limitation
Fragile X	+	0	+	Normal or excessive growth, prominent forehead, long face, midface hypoplasia, large ears, prominent mandible
Lujan	+	0	+	Marfanoid habitus, asthenic build, long face, prominent forehead, high palate, micrognathia, long digits, pectus excavatum, joint hyperextensibility, seizures, hyperactivity

COFFIN-LOWRY SYNDROME

(COFFIN SYNDROME, LOWRY SYNDROME)

OMIM 303600

Xp22.12

RPS6KA3 (RSK2)

Definition. XLID with short stature, distinctive facies, large and soft hands, hypotonia and joint hyperextensibility, and skeletal changes. *RPS6KA3* encodes a growth-related serine threonine kinase.

Somatic Features. Facial features evolve, becoming characteristic late in childhood or adolescence. In infancy, prominent forehead, hypertelorism, anteverted nares, cupped ears, tented upper lip, high narrow palate, hypodontia, peg-shaped incisors, and hypotonia may be notable. As years pass, the head and stature grow slowly, the face elongates and coarsens, the ears become notably large, lips and nasal structures thicken, and the mouth is kept open, showing crowding of the teeth. Mitral incompetence occurs in a minority of patients and can be associated with a dilated cardiomyopathy.

Musculoskeletal manifestations include large soft hands with tapering of the distal phalanges, pectus carinatum, bent knee habitus, flat feet, and generalized joint hyperextensibility. X-rays show delayed maturation, drumstick terminal phalanges with distal tufting and constriction of the adjacent shaft, short ulnas with angulation of the ulnar and radial epiphyses, short sternum with failure of longitudinal fusion of the paired sternal segments, pectus carinatum, notches in the anterior-superior margin of the lumbar vertebrae, narrow intervertebral spaces, mild kyphosis or scoliosis, and accentuation of lumbar lordosis.

Growth and Development. Intrauterine growth is often slow and postnatal growth notable by continued microcephaly and short stature.

Cognitive Function. Developmental milestones lag from the outset, and ultimate cognitive function is profoundly impaired.

Neurological Findings. Drop attacks and generalized seizures occur in about one-fourth of patients and sensorineural hearing loss in an equal number.

Heterozygote Expression. Carrier females consistently show a phenotype milder than males, consisting of short stature, coarse face with prominent brow, hypertelorism, thick nasal tissues, prominent lips, soft fleshy hands with thick fingers tapering distally, and variable radiographic findings similar to those in males. Cognitive function may be mildly impaired or normal.

Comment. Recognition that the entities reported by Coffin et al. in 1966 and Lowry et al. in 1971 represented one condition was made by Temtamy et al. in 1975. The condition is represented in most large facilities for the intellectually disabled. Diagnostic confusion most often results with Alpha-Thalassemia Intellectual Disability and Williams syndrome. Neither of these conditions has the large soft hands and radiographic changes found in Coffin-Lowry syndrome. Certain distinction can be achieved in cases that remain enigmatic through mutational analysis of the *RPS6KA3* gene (Coffin-Lowry) and *ATRX* gene (Alpha-Thalassemia Intellectual Disability) and through FISH studies of the elastin gene (Williams syndrome).

REFERENCES

Coffin GS, Siris E, Wegienka LC: Mental retardation with osteocartilaginous anomalies. Am J Dis Child 112:205, 1966.

Hanauer A, Alembik T, Gilgenkrantz S, et al.: Probable localisation of the Coffin-Lowry locus in Xp22.2-p22.1 by multipoint linkage analysis. Am J Med Genet 30:523, 1988.

Lowry B, Miller JR: A new dominant gene mental retardation syndrome. Am J Dis Child 121:496, 1971.

Massin MM, Radermecker MA, Verloes A, et al.: Cardiac involvement in Coffin-Lowry syndrome. Acta Paediatr 88:468, 1999.

Marques Pereira P, Schneider A, Pannetier S, et al.: Coffin-Lowry syndrome. Eur J Hum Genet. 18:627, 2010.

Temtamy SA, Miller JD, Hussels-Maumenee I: The Coffin-Lowry syndrome: An inherited faciodigital mental retardation syndrome. Pediatrics 86:724, 1975.

Trivier E, De Cesare D, Jacquot S, et al.: Mutations in the kinase Rsk-2 associated with Coffin-Lowry syndrome. Nature 384:567, 1996.

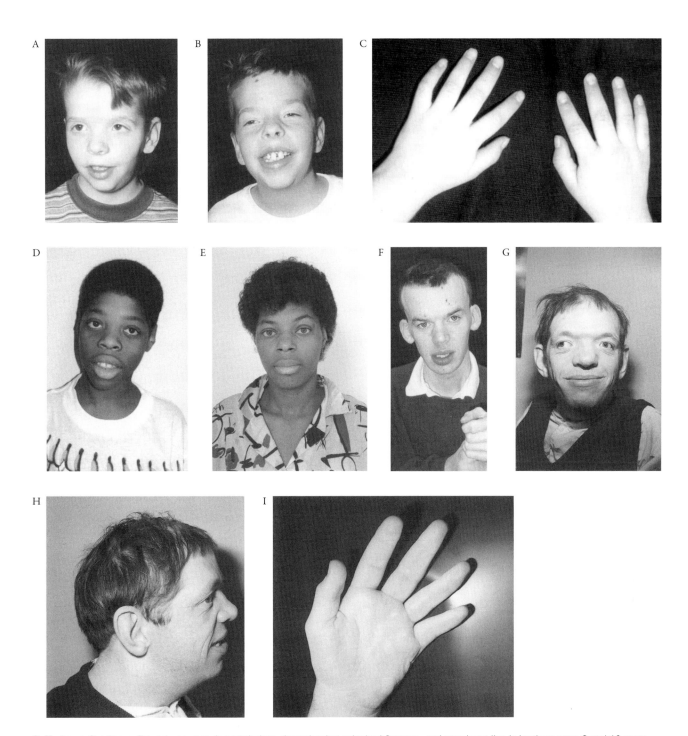

Coffin-Lowry Syndrome. Frontal upsweep, hypertelorism, downslanting palpebral fissures, and prominent lips in brothers ages 8 and 10 years (**A, B**). Fleshy tapered fingers in 8-year-old male (**C**). Hypertelorism, prominent lips and open mouth in 11-year-old male (**D**); mother of patient in **D**, showing hypertelorism and prominence of lips (**E**); cupped ears and prominent lips in 29-year-old male (**F**); microcephaly, hypertelorism, exotropia, large mouth, prominent lips, and thickened tapered digits in 44-year-old male (**G–I**).

DIFFERENTIAL MATRIX

Syndrome	Hypotonic Facies	Hypertelorism	Arch Fingerprints/ Low Ridge Count	Comments
Coffin-Lowry	+	+	+	Microcephaly, short stature, anteverted nares, tented upper lip, prominent lips and large mouth, large ears, soft hands with tapered digits, pectus carinatum
ATRX-Associated XLID	+	+	+	Microcephaly, short stature, telecanthus, small triangular nose, tented upper lip, open mouth, wide spacing of teeth, genital anomalies, musculoskeletal anomalies, hemoglobin H inclusions in erythrocytes
Prieto	+	+	+	Ventricular enlargement, facial asymmetry, prominent eyes, ptosis, long narrow face, micrognathia, inguinal hernia, cryptorchidism
Wilson-Turner	+	+	0	Normal growth, small hands and feet, obesity, hypogonadism, emotional lability
Martin-Probst	0	+	+	Microcephaly, hearing loss, short stature

ATLAS OF X-LINKED INTELLECTUAL DISABILITY SYNDROMES

CORNELIA DE LANGE SYNDROME, X-LINKED

OMIM 300590, 300269

Xp11.2

SMC1A (SMC1L1)

Definition. XLID with short stature, microcephaly, arched eyebrows, synophrys, long philtrum, thin lips, cutis marmorata, small hands and feet, hirsutism, and enlarged cerebral ventricles. Mutations in a gene in the cohesin pathway are responsible.

Somatic Features. All of the craniofacial findings of typical Cornelia de Lange syndrome may occur but are generally milder. Arched eyebrows, synophrys, long eyelashes, anteverted nostrils, long philtrum, thin lips, downturned corners of the mouth, and micrognathia are present in more than half of cases; low anterior hairline, ptosis, lacrimal duct stenosis, and cleft palate in less than half. The hands and feet are small, the thumbs may be proximally placed, and elbow limitation and fifth finger clinodactyly are usually present. There is generalized hirsutism and cutis marmorata. Males and females are both affected, although features in females may be more subtle. Major malformations do not occur.

Growth and Development. Intrauterine growth may be globally impaired, but there are examples of normal prenatal growth. Postnatally, all growth parameters slow, with childhood head circumference and height generally below the 3rd centile.

Cognitive Function. Developmental milestones are globally delayed, with ultimate cognitive achievement in the mildly disabled range.

Neurological Findings. Seizures are reported in less than half of patients.

Imaging. Structural anomalies of the brain are uncommon. Increased ventricular volume has been noted.

Comment. Only a minority of cases (about 5%) with Cornelia de Lange syndrome are X-linked. A still smaller percentage (~1%) is caused by mutations in *SMC3*, located in 10q25. About 60% of cases result from mutations in *NIPBL*, an autosomal gene. Whereas mutations in *NIPBL* may be missense or protein-truncating, all mutations found to date in *SMC1A* and *SMC3* have been frame-preserving (either missense or in frame deletions), presumably leading to mutant proteins exerting a dominant-negative effect. Although there is marked variation in expression in patients with *NIPBL* and *SMC1A*, the latter are generally milder and lack major reduction malformations of the limbs.

The genes that cause Cornelia de Lange syndrome are either regulators or structural components of the cohesion complex, which has the primary role of controlling sister chromatid segregation during meiosis and mitosis. *SMC1A* and *SMC3* encode two of the four core structural subunits, and *NIPBL* encodes a key regulatory protein.

Deardorff et al. (2011) have recently reported loss of function mutations in the X-linked histone deacetylase gene, *HDAC8*, in patients with facial features consistent with Cornelia de Lange Syndrome, but without major limb malformations.

REFERENCES

Deardorff MA, Bando M, Saitoh K, et al.: HDAC8 mutations in Cornelia de Lange syndrome. 2011 David W. Smith Workshop on Malformations and Morphogenesis, Lake Arrowhead, CA, September 9–14, 2011.

Deardorff MA, Kaur M, Yaeger D, et al.: Mutations in cohesion complex members SMC3 and SMC1A cause a mild variant of Cornelia de Lange syndrome with predominant mental retardation. Am J Hum Genet 80:485, 2007.

Egemen A, Ulger Z, Ozkinay F, et al.: A de novo t(X;8)(p11.2; q24.3) demonstrating Cornelia de Lange syndrome phenotype. Genet Couns 16:27, 2005.

Liu J, Krantz ID: Cornelia de Lange syndrome, cohesion, and beyond. Clin Genet 76:303, 2009.

Musio A, Selicorni A, Focarelli ML, et al.: X-linked Cornelia de Lange syndrome owing to SMC1L1 mutations. Nat Genet 38:528, 2006.

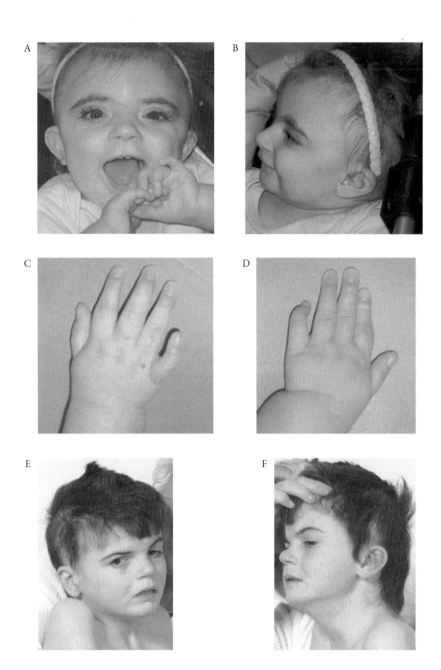

Cornelia de Lange Syndrome, X-Linked. One-year-old girl with microcephaly, arched eyebrows, cupped retroverted ears, thin upper lip, small hands with small thumbs and fifth finger clinodactyly (A–D). Fifteen-year-old girl with microcephaly, thin arched eyebrows, thin upper lip, downturned corners of the mouth, and retroverted ears (E, F).   Courtesy of Dr. Ian Krantz, Children's Hospital of Philadelphia.

DIFFERENTIAL MATRIX

Syndrome	Microcephaly	Distinctive Facies	Small Hands and Feet	Comments
Cornelia de Lange Syndrome, X-linked	+	+	+	Arched eyebrows, synophrys, long philtrum, thin lips, cutis marmorata, hirsutism, enlarged cerebral ventricles, proximal thumbs, elbow restriction, short stature, small testes
ATRX-Associated XLID	+	+	+	Short stature, telecanthus/hypertelorism, small triangular nose, tented upper lip, open mouth, wide spacing of teeth, abnormal genitalia, minor musculoskeletal anomalies, hypotonia, erythrocyte HbH inclusions in some
Craniofacioskeletal	+	+	+	Mild cognitive impairment, short stature, craniofacial distinctiveness, excessive fingerprint arches in females. Males die in early infancy with craniofacial, cardiac, skeletal, and genital abnormalities
XLID-Microcephaly-Testicular Failure	+	+	+	Short stature, prominent supraorbital ridges, high nasal bridge, prominent nose, macrostomia, hypogonadism
Hereditary Bullous Dystrophy, X-linked	+	O	+	Short stature, upslanting palpebral fissures, protruding ears, digits short and tapered, bullous dystrophy, small testes, early death from pulmonary infection, cutaneous lesions, cardiac defects
Otopalatodigital I (*FLNA*-Associated XLID)	O	+	+	Short stature, prominent brow, broad nasal root, apparent ocular hypertelorism, downslanting palpebral fissures, blunted distal phalanges, irregular curvature and spacing of digits, limitation of elbow movement, cleft palate, hearing impairment, digital anomalies
Otopalatodigital II (*FLNA*-Associated XLID)	O	+	+	Short stature, prominent forehead, flat/broad nasal bridge, ocular hypertelorism, downslanting palpebral fissures, flat midface, blunted flexed overlapping fingers, rockerbottom feet, hypoplastic fibulae, subluxed/dislocated joints, cleft palate, hearing impairment, digital anomalies

CRANIOFACIOSKELETAL SYNDROME

OMIM 300712

Xq26-q27

Definition. X-linked dominant disorder with mild cognitive impairment, short stature, microcephaly, craniofacial distinctiveness, small hands and feet, and excessive fingerprint arches in females. Affected males die in early infancy with craniofacial, cardiac, skeletal, and genital abnormalities. Suggestive linkage has been found to Xq26-q27.

Somatic Features. Affected females have microcephaly, short stature, small ears, short philtrum, overhanging columella, thin upper lip, small mandible, small hands and feet, short fifth fingers, clinodactyly of toes IV and V, flat feet, and excessive fingerprint arches. Cleft palate has been present in one instance. On radiographs, the frontal sinuses were underdeveloped, absent, or asymmetrically developed with one side being short. The vertebral bodies appeared foreshortened, the iliac wings full and narrow, and all long bones had cortical thickening with reduced marrow cavity.

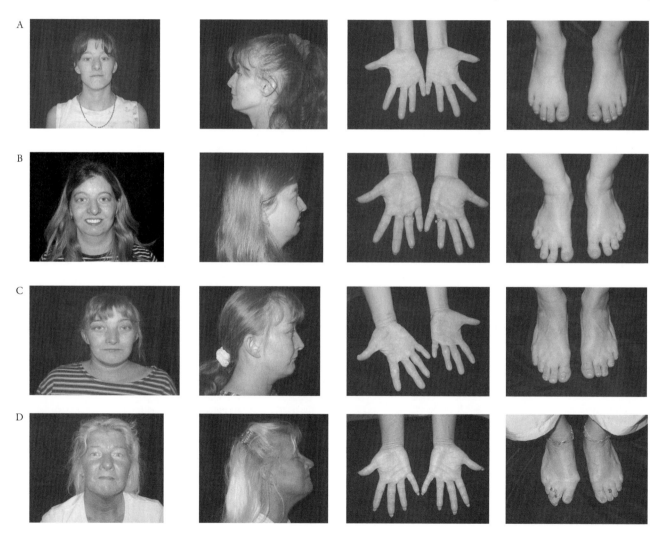

Craniofacioskeletal Syndrome. Twenty-six-year-old woman with microcephaly, hypotelorism, narrow alae nasi, retroverted ears, thin lips, short fifth fingers, and normal feet (A). Twenty-eight-year-old sister with microcephaly, retroverted ears, overhanging columella, short philtrum (repaired cleft lip), small jaw, wide forefoot with spacing of toes and bulbous distal toes (B). Thirty-year-old sister with microcephaly, overhanging columella, thin upper lip, short hands, single crease on fifth fingers, short fourth toes, and syndactyly of second and third toes (C). Forty-nine-year-old mother of these three sisters with microcephaly, widow's peak, overhanging columella, retroverted ears, short philtrum, thin upper lip, and lateral deviation of toes of right foot (D).

Two affected males had prenatal growth impairment and multiple malformations and died in the early postnatal months. One had broad cranium with wide sutures, prominent eyes, short palpebral fissures, small nose, micrognathia, hypospadias, undescended testes, short fingers with single flexion creases, and low calcium. Autopsy showed hydrocephaly, cerebellar hypoplasia, interrupted aortic arch, atrial septal defect, and hydronephrosis. The second male showed broad cranium with wide sutures, downslanting palpebral fissures, small ears, short nose, short fingers and nails, and small penis. Also, he had choanal atresia, distal tracheal stenosis, VSD, hydronephrosis, and low serum calcium.

Growth and Development. Slow growth prenatally continues postnatally and is reflected in head size, height, and weight.

Neurological Findings. No overt neurological signs occur in females. Brain imaging showed small brain with an extra gyrus of the superior temporal region.

Cognitive Function. Cognitive function in females is mildly impaired with IQ measurements between 65 and 85.

Behavior. No behavioral abnormalities occur.

Comment. This X-linked condition with expression in females and lethality in males can be clearly distinguished on clinical findings from the other X-linked dominant conditions. Description as an XLID syndrome is based on female expression, greater severity with lethality in males, the near complete skewing of X-inactivation in females, and suggestive linkage to Xq26–27.

The skeletal changes in females and the low serum calcium in the affected males suggest that calcium-phosphorous metabolism may be disturbed in this condition. An X chromosome locus for hypoparathyroidism has been found in Xq27, but the gene has not been identified.

REFERENCE

Stevenson RE, Brasington CK, Skinner C, et al.: Craniofacioskeletal syndrome: An X-linked dominant disorder with early lethality in males. Am J Med Genet A 143A:2321, 2007.

DIFFERENTIAL MATRIX

Syndrome	Microcephaly	Short Stature	Distinctive Facies	Comments
Craniofacioskeletal	+	+	+	Mild cognitive impairment, craniofacial distinctiveness, small hands and feet, excessive fingerprint arches in females. Males die in early infancy with craniofacial, cardiac, skeletal, and genital abnormalities
ATRX-Associated XLID	+	+	+	Telecanthus/hypertelorism, small triangular nose, tented upper lip, open mouth, wide spacing of teeth, abnormal genitalia, minor musculoskeletal anomalies, hypotonia, erythrocyte HbH inclusions in some
Börjeson-Forssman-Lehmann	+	+	+	Coarse face, large ears, gynecomastia, narrow sloped shoulders, visual impairment, tapered digits, hypotonia, hypogonadism, obesity
Coffin-Lowry	+	+	+	Anteverted nares, tented upper lip, prominent lips and large mouth, large ears, soft hands with tapered digits, pectus carinatum, hypotonic facies, hypertelorism, arch fingerprints/low ridge count
Miles-Carpenter	+	+	+	Ptosis, small palpebral fissures, open mouth, pectus excavatum, scoliosis, long hands, camptodactyly, rockerbottom feet, arch fingerprints, unsteady gait, skeletal abnormality, spasticity
Pettigrew	+	+	+	Dandy-Walker malformation, hydrocephaly, long face with macrostomia, small testes, contractures, choreoathetosis, cerebellar hypoplasia, spastic paraplegia, iron deposits or calcification of basal ganglia, seizures
XLID-Microcephaly-Testicular Failure	+	+	+	Prominent supraorbital ridges, high nasal bridge, prominent nose, macrostomia, hypogonadism
Hereditary Bullous Dystrophy, X-linked	+	+	0	Upslanting palpebral fissures, protruding ears, digits short and tapered, bullous dystrophy, small testes, early death from pulmonary infection, cutaneous lesions, cardiac defects

CREATINE TRANSPORTER DEFICIENCY

OMIM 300036

Xq28

SLC6A8

Definition. XLID caused by cerebral creatine deficiency with decreased muscle mass, hypotonia, expressive language impairment, seizures, and aberrant behavior. Mutations in the solute transporter *SLC6A8* are the cause and may represent one of the most common causes of XLID (1–3%).

Somatic Features. Malformations do not occur in creatine transporter deficiency. Decreased muscle mass occurs and may be associated with hypotonia and decreased strength. Hypotonic face with lax soft tissues, ptosis, and flatness of the midface have been described as related findings. Cardiac involvement in the form of mild cardiomyopathy or arrhythmias has been noted in a few cases. Soft skin and hyperextensible joints have also been noted in a minority.

Growth and Development. Prenatal growth is usually normal, but thereafter growth slows. Stature ultimately falls below the 3rd centile in about half of affected males. Head circumference usually remains in the normal percentiles, although some males with microcephaly have been described.

Cognitive Function. A wide range of cognitive function has been described. Milder impairment has been noted in the younger patients suggesting the possibility that the disorder is progressive. Speech and language function appears distinctly more severely impaired than motor function.

Behavior. Most patients manifest some type of behavioral disturbance. These include hyperactivity, anxiety, autism, and psychosis.

Neurological Findings. Hypotonia is noted frequently, but appears less prominent with age. Seizures occur in about half of patients. Seizures are varied in type and in some cases are recalcitrant to anticonvulsant therapy. Spasticity, dystonia or ataxia have also been noted in half of cases.

Heterozygote Expression. Carrier females commonly have manifestations in the form of learning disability and aberrant behavior.

Imaging. No consistent structural anomalies have been noted on brain imaging. Markedly decreased creatine and phosphocreatine signal is typical on magnetic resonance spectroscopy.

Laboratory. Urine creatine:creatinine ratio and plasma creatine are increased and serve as a useful screening test.

Comment. The manifestations in this condition are so varied and inconsistent that some observers prefer to classify it as nonsyndromal. It is included here as a syndrome because of frequent seizures and behavioral manifestations and because of the metabolic disturbance. Creatine has been

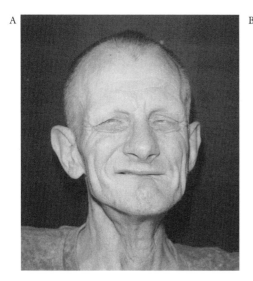
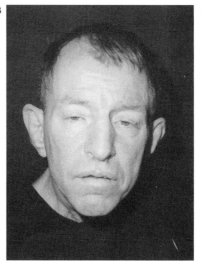
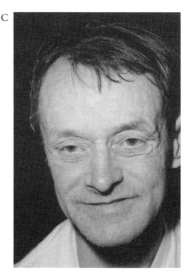

Creatine Transporter Deficiency. Sixty-four-year-old with narrow palpebral fissures and lax soft tissues of the face (**A**); 65-year-old brother with ptosis, narrow palpebral fissures and expressionless face (**B**); and 66-year-old brother with prominent forehead and lax skin around the eyes (**C**).

supplemented orally in a number of cases. Some improvement in muscle mass and strength has been reported in several cases, but no improvement has been noted in cognitive function or behavior.

REFERENCES

Anselm IM, Alkuraya FS, Salomons GS, et al.: X-linked creatine transporter defects: A report on two unrelated boys with a severe clinical phenotype. J Inherit Metab Dis 29:214, 2006.

Hahn, KA, Salomons GS, Tackels-Horne D, et al: X-linked mental retardation with seizures and carrier manifestations is caused by a mutation in the creatine-transporter gene (SLC6A8) located in Xq28. Am J Hum Genet 70:2349, 2002.

Kleefstra T, Rosenberg EH, Salomons GS, et al.: Progressive intestinal, neurological and psychiatric problems in two adult males with cerebral creatine deficiency caused by an SLC6A8 mutation. Clin Genet 68:379, 2005.

Longo N, Ardon O, Vanzo R, et al.: Disorders of creatine transport and metabolism. Am J Med Genet C Semin Med Genet 157:72, 2011.

Mancardi MM, Caruso U, Schiaffino MC, et al.: Severe epilepsy in X-linked creatine transporter defect (CRTR-D). Epilepsia 48:1211, 2007.

Marco EJ, Skuse DH: Autism-lessons from the X chromosome. SCAN 1:183, 2006.

Póo-Argüelles P, Arias A, Vilaseca MA, et al.: X-linked creatine transporter deficiency in two patients with severe mental retardation and autism. J Inherit Metab Dis 29:220, 2006.

Raymond FL: X-linked mental retardation: a clinical guide. J Med Genet 43:193, 2006.

Rosenberg EH, Almeida LS, Kleefstra T, et al.: High prevalence of SLC6A8 deficiency in X-linked mental retardation. Am J Hum Genet 75:97, 2004.

Salomons GS, van Dooren SJ, Verhoeven NM, et al.: X-linked creatine-transporter gene (SLC6A8) defect: a new creatine deficiency syndrome. Am J Hum Genet 68:1497, 2001.

Valayannopoulos V, Boddaert N, Chabli A, et al.: Treatment by oral creatine, L-arginine and L-glycine in six severely affected patients with creatine transporter defect. J Inherit Metab Dis [epub ahead of print June 10, 2011].

Van de Kamp JM, Mancini GMS, Pouwels PJW, et al.: Clinical features of X-inactive in females heterozygous for creatine transporter defects. Clin Genet 79:264, 2011.

DUCHENNE MUSCULAR DYSTROPHY

(PSEUDOHYPERTROPHIC MUSCULAR DYSTROPHY)

OMIM 310200

Xp21.2

DMD

Definition. XLID associated with pseudohypertrophic muscular dystrophy. Duchenne Muscular Dystrophy and the milder Becker Muscular Dystrophy are allelic disorders caused by mutation in dystrophin, a large gene occupying most of Xp21.2.

Somatic Features. Major malformations or distinctive craniofacial manifestations do not occur. Hypertrophy of muscles – particularly those of the calf – provide an early diagnostic clue, even before weakness is evident. Muscle destruction persists and progresses relentlessly, leading to loss of ambulation in the teen years and death in early adult life. In the final stage, widespread muscle wasting, weakness, and contractures are present.

Cognitive Function. A wide range of cognitive function can be found. Most cases have normal intelligence, but the average IQ measures 80 to 85, and about 20% will have IQ measures below 70. Three percent have severe mental retardation. Verbal abilities test lower than performance abilities. Affected brothers tend to have comparable cognitive function. An adequate explanation for the cognitive impairment has not been established but is presumed to be a pleiotropic effect of abnormal dystrophin on brain development. Cardiomyopathy may become symptomatic by the midteen years.

Neurological Findings. Neuromuscular findings generally follow a predictable and relentlessly progressive pattern. Weakness of the lower limbs and pelvic girdle initially manifest as clumsiness and inability to climb stairs. Hypertrophy of the calf muscles may give parents a false sense that the muscles are strong. Toe-walking leads to pelvic tilt and compensatory hyperlordosis of the lumbar spine, both evident during the preschool years and accompanied by loss of deep tendon reflexes.

Heterozygote Expression. Although carriers usually have normal muscle strength and intellectual function, 5% to

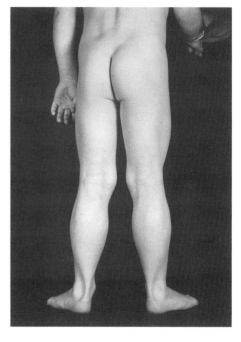

Duchenne Muscular Dystrophy. Five-year-old male showing hypertrophy of the calf muscles.

10% may have slight muscle weakness, and a lesser number may have cognitive impairment. Carrier manifestations have been attributed to preferential inactivation of the normal X-chromosome. Carriers frequently have high normal or elevated creatine kinase levels. Muscle biopsy may show centralization of nuclei and variability in size of muscle fibers.

REFERENCES

Beggs AH, Kunkel LM: Improved diagnosis of Duchenne/Becker muscular dystrophy. J Clin Invest 85:613, 1990.

Duchenne GBA: Recherches sur la paralysie musculaire pseudo-hypertrophique, ou paralysie myosclérosique. Générales de Médecine 11:5, 1868. Translation in Arch Neurol 19:629, 1968.

Mendell JR, Kissel JT, Amato AA, et al.: Myoblast transfer in the treatment of Duchenne's muscular dystrophy. New Eng J Med 333:832, 1995.

Mostacciuolo ML, Lombardi A, Cambissa V, et al.: Population data on benign and severe forms of X-linked muscular dystrophy. Hum Genet 75:217, 1987.

Rosman NP, Kakulas BA: Mental deficiency associated with muscular dystrophy – a neurological study. Brain 89:769, 1966.

DIFFERENTIAL MATRIX

Syndrome	Muscle Hypertrophy	Weakness	Areflexia	Comments
Duchenne Muscular Dystrophy	+	+	+	Hypertrophy of calf muscles, elevated muscle enzymes, muscle wasting, contractures
Arts	0	+	+	Growth deficiency, hypotonia, ataxia, deafness, vision loss, seizures, childhood death
Charcot-Marie-Tooth Neuropathy, Cowchock variant	0	+	+	Peripheral motor and sensory neuropathy, deafness, pes cavus
Charcot-Marie-Tooth Neuropathy, Ionasescu variant	0	+	+	Peripheral motor and sensory neuropathy, wasting of intrinsic hand muscles, enlarged ulnar nerves, pes cavus
Myotubular Myopathy	0	+	+	Hypotonic facies, open mouth, tented upper lip, hydrocephaly, long digits, cryptorchidism, hypotonia
Phosphoglycerate Kinase Deficiency	0	+	+	Expressionless face, seizures, myoglobinuria, hemolytic anemia

DYSKERATOSIS CONGENITA

(ZINSSER-ENGMANN-COLE SYNDROME)

OMIM 305000

Xq28

DKC1

Definition. XLID associated with dyskeratosis, hyperpigmentation, leukoplakia, alopecia, pancytopenia, hypersplenomegaly, and predisposition to malignancy. About one-fourth of all patients with dyskeratosis congenita have the X-linked form.

Somatic Features. The major cutaneous manifestation is reticulate hyperpigmentation with predisposition for the neck, upper chest, and arm. The lesions may be telangiectatic and have interspersed areas of hypopigmented atrophic skin. The palms and soles have hyperkeratosis, and alopecia and hyperhidrosis are common. Bullae may follow minimal trauma. The nails develop longitudinal ridging or splitting as well as friability and may decrease in size or may be completely lost. Fingernail changes precede toenail changes. Leukoplakia forms on the oral mucosa but may affect other mucosal linings as well. When the epithelium of the lacrimal ducts is involved, blepharitis, conjunctivitis, and epiphora may result. Excessive cavities or tooth loss may be a part of the condition. In some cases, the face appears pinched secondary to loss of subcutaneous tissue. Small penis and testes have been described, but hypogonadism appears quite rare.

Pancytopenia occurs in about half of cases, heralded by thrombocytopenia or anemia. Squamous cell carcinoma may occur in areas of cutaneous lesions or mucosal leukoplakia. Esophageal and pancreatic carcinomas and Hodgkin's lymphoma occur in a small minority of cases.

Growth and Development. Usually normal, with occasional cases having short stature

Cognitive Function. Normal cognitive function is the rule, but with mild impairment in about one-third of cases.

Natural History. Only rarely are any cutaneous manifestations present at birth. Usually they make their appearance between ages 5 and 12 years. Mucous membrane lesions appear slightly later, and hematologic abnormalities occur in the midteen years with malignancy in young adult life.

Heterozygote Expression. None. The cases of female involvement likely represent autosomal inheritance.

Laboratory. Excessive chromatid breakage, both spontaneous and radiation-induced, has been reported in fibroblast cultures.

Comment. Cognitive impairment is neither prerequisite for nor a common feature of dyskeratosis congenita. An autosomal form, Hoyeraal-Hreidarsson syndrome, has significant developmental delay, immunological abnormalities, and cerebellar hypoplasia. The autosomal and X-linked forms of dyskeratosis congenita are unified by the finding of short telomeres.

REFERENCES

Arngrimsson R, Dokal I, Luzzatto L, et al.: Dyskeratosis congenita: three additional families show linkage to a locus in Xq28. J Med Genet 30:618, 1993.

Connor JM, Gatherer D, Gray FC, et al.: Assignment of the gene for dyskeratosis congenita to Xq28. Hum Genet 72:348, 1986.

Davidson HR, Connor JM: Dyskeratosis congenita. J Med Genet 25:843, 1988.

DeBauche DM, Pai GS, Stanley WS: Enhanced G$_2$ chromatid radiosensitivity in dyskeratosis congenita fibroblasts. Am J Hum Genet 46:350, 1990.

Heiss NS, Knight SW, Vulliamy TJ, et al.: X-linked dyskeratosis congenita is caused by mutations in a highly conserved gene with putative nucleolar functions. Nat Genet 19:32, 1998.

Savage SA, Bertuch AA: The genetics and clinical manifestations of telomere biology disorders. Genet Med 12:753, 2010.

Sirinavin C, Trowbridge AA: Dyskeratosis congenita: clinical features; and genetic aspects. J Med Genet 12:339, 1975.

Vulliamy TJ, Marrone A, Knight SW, et al.: Mutations in dyskeratosis congenita: their impact on telomere length and the diversity of clinical presentation. Blood 107:2680, 2006.

Zinsser F: Atrophia cutis reticularis cum pigmentatione, dystrophia unguim et leukoplakia oris. Ikonographia Dermatologica 5:219, 1910.

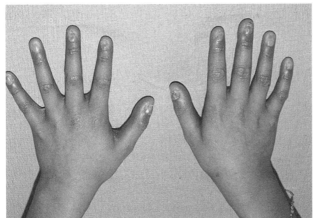

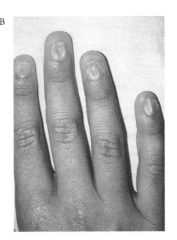

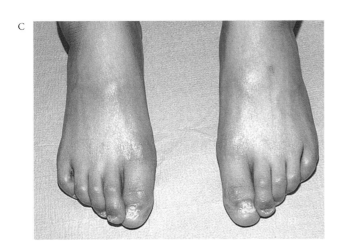

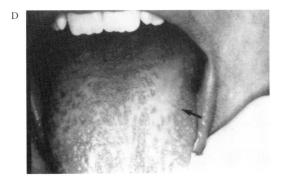

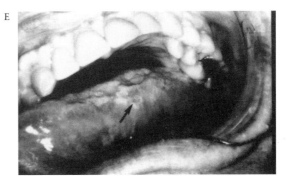

Dyskeratosis Congenita. Dystrophic nails of hands and feet (A–C); white plaques **(arrows)** of the tongue **(D, E)**.   Courtesy of Dr. Shashidhar Pai, Medical University of South Carolina, Charleston.

DIFFERENTIAL MATRIX

Syndrome	Ectodermal Manifestations	Short Stature	Malignancy Predisposition	Comments
Dyskeratosis Congenita	+	+	+	Alopecia, hyperpigmented lesions, palmar and plantar hyperkeratosis, mucosal leukoplakia, pancytopenia
Cantu	+	+	0	Microcephaly, follicular keratosis, cortical atrophy, alopecia, seizures
Hereditary Bullous Dystrophy, X-linked	+	+	0	Microcephaly, upslanting palpebral fissures, protruding ears, short and tapered digits, cardiac defects, small testes, early death from pulmonary infection

EPILEPSY-INTELLECTUAL DISABILITY IN FEMALES (EIDF)

OMIM 300088

Xq22.1

PCDH19

Definition. XLID with epilepsy in females. The gene encodes a protocadherin protein.

Somatic Features. Malformations or distinctive craniofacial features do not appear to be a component of this syndrome. Individual cases have had cataracts, microcephaly, syndactyly, or strabismus – perhaps unrelated findings. Neurological manifestations begin during infancy (age 4–18 months) with the onset of generalized or partial seizures. Seizures increase in frequency for a period of time but decrease by age 2 to 3 years. Coincident with the seizures is developmental regression. Ultimately, the deterioration results in marked cognitive impairment in some individuals, but less severe impairment in others. The more severely impaired showed stereotyped movements, hand-wringing, hand-flapping, and some loss of fine motor skills.

Growth and Development. Details of intrauterine and postnatal growth have not been reported. Only one girl has had microcephaly. Developmental milestones appear normal until the onset of seizures.

Cognitive Function. A range of impairment exists from profound to mild.

Neurological Findings. Generalized tonic-clonic, myoclonic, tonic, atonic, or absence seizures predominate, but partial and focal seizures have been described. The onset is usually in infancy and may be precipitated by fever. During or following a period of developmental and cognitive regression, patients may develop hyper-reflexia and stereotypic repetitive activities such as hand-wringing or hand-flapping.

Heterozygote Expression. Only carrier females have seizures and mental regression. Hemizygous males manifest no seizures or symptoms.

Comment. Males who carry the gene do not experience seizures or developmental regression and appear normally fertile. This sparing of males in an apparently X-linked dominant disorder is unique and is as yet not explained.

REFERENCES

Dibbens LM, Tarpey PS, Hynes K, et al.: X-linked protocadherin 19 mutations cause female-limited epilepsy and cognitive impairment. Nat Genet 40:776, 2008.

Fabisiak K, Erickson R: A familial form of convulsive disorder with or without mental retardation limited to females: extension of a pedigree limits possible genetic mechanisms. Clin Genet 38:353, 1990.

Hynes K, Tarpey P, Dibbens LM, et al.: Epilepsy and mental retardation limited to females with PCDH19 mutations can present de novo or in single generation families. J Med Genet 47:211, 2010.

Juberg RC, Hellman CD: A new familial form of convulsive disorder and mental retardation limited to females. J Pediatr 79:726, 1971.

Page DC: Save the Males! Nat Genet 17:3, 1997.

Ryan SG, Chance PF, Zou C-H, et al.: Epilepsy and mental retardation limited to females: an X-linked dominant disorder with male sparing. Nat Genet 17:92, 1997.

Scheffer IE, Turner SJ, Dibbens LM, et al.: Epilepsy and mental retardation limited to females: an under-recognized disorder. Brain 131:918, 2008.

FITZSIMMONS SYNDROME

(XLID-SPASTIC PARAPLEGIA-PALMOPLANTAR HYPERKERATOSIS)

OMIM 309560

Definition. XLID with lower limb spasticity, pes cavus, and hyperkeratosis of the palms and soles. The gene has not been localized.

Somatic Features. Lower limb spasticity with pes cavus, clawing of the toes, wasting of the distal legs and ankles, and shuffling gait become apparent at about age 2 years. The upper limbs remain normal. Hyperkeratosis of the palms and soles becomes apparent later, in mid-childhood. The soles are more severely affected and erosions may occur over pressure points. The nails are thickened and fissured. Teeth and sweat production appear normal. A facial phenotype with high forehead, prominent nose, frontal balding, and sparse hair was noted in the index family. Hyperextensibility of the digits has been seen and in one case resulted in spontaneous thumb dislocation.

Growth and Development. Prenatal and postnatal growth appears normal. Development lags from the outset and is obvious prior to age 1 year.

Cognitive Function. Mild impairment

Neurological Findings. Hyperreflexia and spasticity begin by age 2 years and appear to become static during adulthood.

Heterozygote Expression. Females may show evidence of cutaneous and neurological involvement but have normal intelligence. Although quite mild in comparison to the manifestations in males, fissuring and erythema of the palms, thickening of the soles, and thickened and fissured nails have been described in females. Deep tendon reflexes in the lower limbs are increased and the toes may show some clawing.

Comment. Ectodermal manifestations occur in only a few XLID syndromes.

REFERENCES

Armour CM, Humphreys P, Hennekam RC, Boycott KM. Fitzsimmons syndrome: spastic paraplegia, brachydactyly and cognitive impairment. Am J Med Genet A 149A:2254, 2009.

Fitzsimmons JS, Fitzsimmons EM, McLachlan JI, et al.: Four brothers with mental retardation, spastic paraplegia and palmoplantar hyperkeratosis. A new syndrome? Clin Genet 23:329, 1983.

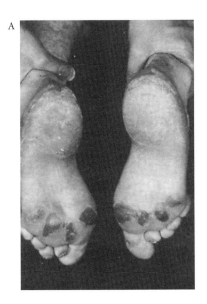
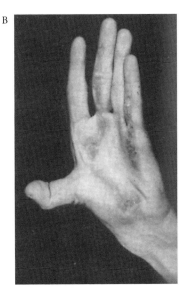
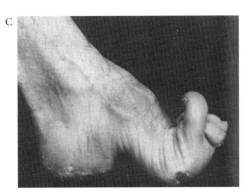

Fitzsimmons Syndrome. Hyperkeratotis of the soles **(A)**; hyperkeratosis of the palms and dislocated thumb **(B)**; pes cavus with dorsiflexion of the halux and clawing of the toes **(C)**.   Courtesy of *Clinical Genetics*, Copyright 1983, Munksgaard, Copenhagen.

DIFFERENTIAL MATRIX

Syndrome	Alopecia/Sparse Hair	Cutaneous Manifestations	Spastic Paraplegia	Comments
Fitzsimmons	+	+	+	Pes cavus, hyperkeratosis of palms and soles, dystrophic nails
Cantu	+	+	0	Microcephaly, short stature, follicular keratosis, cortical atrophy, seizures
Dykeratosis Congenita	+	+	0	Short stature, hyperpigmented lesions, palmar and plantar hyperkeratosis, mucosal leukoplakia, nail ridging or splitting, pancytopenia, skin and mucosal lesions premalignant
Hereditary Bullous Dystrophy, X-linked	+	+	0	Microcephaly, short stature, upslanting palpebral fissures, protruding ears, digits short and tapered, cardiac defects, small testes, early death from pulmonary infection

FLNA-ASSOCIATED XLID

(*FLNA* SPECTRUM, OTOPALATODIGITAL SPECTRUM, OTOPALATODIGITAL SYNDROME I, OTOPALATODIGITAL SYNDROME II, PERIVENTRICULAR NODULAR HETEROTOPIA, CRANIOORODIGITAL SYNDROME)

OMIM 300077

Xq28

FLNA (FLN1)

Definition. A number of disparate XLID syndromes are subsumed in *FLNA*-Associated XLID. Because of the marked phenotypic difference, each syndrome has a separate entry in this Atlas and a brief summary here.

Otopalatodigital Syndrome I is a well-established X-linked syndrome with short stature, distinctive craniofacial features, and mild intellectual disability. Frontal bossing with prominent supraorbital ridges and depressed nasal bridge, hypertelorism, downslanting palpebral fissures, small mouth, cleft palate, micrognathia, and prominent occiput are notable craniofacial features. The digits are irregularly curved with blunted or bulbous tips and short nails. Thumbs and great toes are short and broad. Shortening of the trunk, pectus excavatum, restricted elbow movement, and abnormal modeling or bowing of the long bones attest to the global involvement of the skeleton. Among an array of radiographic findings, abnormal configuration and coalitions of the carpals and tarsals and accessory proximal ossification centers of the metacarpals and metatarsals are most helpful. Carrier females may have mild expression of the craniofacial and skeletal features. Mutations are typically missense and most often found in the actin-binding domain.

Otopalatodigital Syndrome II (Cranioorodigital Syndrome) has similar facial manifestations as otopalatodigital syndrome I but more severe skeletal anomalies and intellectual disability. Prominence of the frontal area with wide sutures and delayed fontanelle closure, flat nasal bridge, hypertelorism, downslanted palpebral fissures, small mouth, low-set retroverted ears, cleft palate, and micrognathia are typical. Skeletal manifestations are widespread: short stature, narrow thorax, pectus excavatum, small or absent fibulas, short and blunted thumbs and great toes, overlapping flexed and blunted fingers, rockerbottom feet, and, in some cases, postaxial polydactyly, absent thumbs, syndactyly, and clinodactyly. On radiographs, the calvarium is underossified, but the base of the skull, supraorbital ridges and long bones are dense. The sinuses are absent or poorly aerated. The phalanges are short and may not be ossified. The halluces and first metatarsals may be absent. The clavicles are thin and irregular, vertebrae flat, and ribs narrow proximally, but widened distally. Carrier females may have similar but milder facial, digital, and radiographic findings. Missense mutations of *FLNA* are usual.

Periventricular Nodular Heterotopias generally occur in females and are accompanied by multiple types of seizures. Although male lethality is suggested in some pedigrees, this is not universal, with some males having similar MRI finding as females. Truncating mutations in *FLNA* are typical.

Frontometaphyseal Dysplasia is a skeletal dysplasia with major impact on the craniofacies, long bones, and digits. Although reduced cognitive skills have been reported, they likely result from impaired hearing.

Melnick-Needles Syndrome is a generalized skeletal dysplasia in females with more severe and lethal expression in males. Females have normal intelligence.

Other Reports. Unger et al. (2007) reported a missense mutation in a male with broad forehead, frontal hair upsweep, chronic constipation, and mild delay in language acquisition. They considered the boy to represent a variant of Optiz FG syndrome (the so-called "FGS locus 2"). We believe this to be incorrect, with the patient having craniofacial findings unlike Opitz FG syndrome and the chronic constipation resulting from intestinal hypomobility rather than anorectal maldevelopment.

REFERENCES

Fitch N, Jequier S, Gorlin R: The oto-palato-digital syndrome, proposed type II. Am J Med Genet 15:655, 1983.

Fox JW, Lamperti ED, Eksioglu YZ, et al.: Mutations in filamin 1 prevent migration of cerebral cortical neurons in human periventricular heterotopia. Neuron 21:1315, 1998.

Gorlin RJ, Cohen MM Jr: Frontometaphyseal dysplasia. A new syndrome. Am J Dis Child 118:487, 1969.

Robertson SP: Filamin A: phenotypic diversity. Curr Opin Genet Dev 15:301, 2005.

Robertson SP, Twigg SRF, Sutherland-Smith AJ, et al.: Localized mutations in the gene encoding the cytoskeletal protein filamin A cause diverse malformations in human. Nat Genet 33:487, 2003.

Robertson SP, Walsh S, Oldridge M, et al.: Linkage of otopalatodigital syndrome type 2 (OPD2) to distal Xq28: evidence for allelism with OPD1. Am J Hum Genet 69:223, 2001.

Sheen VL, Dixon PH, Fox JW, et al.: Mutations in the X-linked filamin 1 gene cause periventricular nodular heterotopia in males as well as in females. Hum Mol Genet 10:1775, 2001.

Unger S, Mainberger A, Spitz C, et al.: Filamin A mutation is one cause of FG syndrome. Am J Med Genet A 143A:1876, 2007.

Verloes A, Lesenfants S, Barr M, et al.: Fronto-otopalatodigital osteo-dysplasia: clinical evidence for a single entity encompassing Melnick-Needles syndrome, otopalatodigital syndrome types 1 and 2, and frontometaphyseal dysplasia. Am J Med Genet 90:407, 2000.

DIFFERENTIAL MATRIX

Syndrome	Neuronal Migration Disturbance	Distinctive Facies	Skeletal Abnormalities	Comments
FLNA-Associated XLID	+	+	+	Short stature, prominent brow or forehead, hypertelorism, downslanting palpebral fissures, blunting of distal phalanges, irregular spacing of digits, limited/subluxed/dislocated joints, hypoplastic fibulas
Coffin-Lowry	0	+	+	Microcephaly, short stature, anteverted nares, tented upper lip, prominent lips and large mouth, large ears, soft hands with tapered digits, pectus carinatum, hypotonic facies, hypertelorism, arch fingerprints/low ridge count
Mucopolysaccharidosis IIA	0	+	+	Hepatosplenomegaly, hernias, joint stiffness, thick skin, hirsutism, behavioral disturbance, short stature, coarse facies, macrocephaly
Pallister W	0	+	+	Prominent forehead, wide nasal tip, incomplete cleft lip/palate, spasticity, short stature, facial clefting, seizures
XLID-Spondyloepimetaphyseal Dysplasia	0	+	+	Coarse facies, chest deformation, small corpus callosum, cerebral atrophy

FRAGILE X SYNDROME

(MARKER X SYNDROME, FRAXA SYNDROME, MARTIN-BELL SYNDROME)

OMIM 300624

Xq27.3

FMR1

Definition. XLID with prominent forehead, long face, recessed midface, large ears, prominent mandible, and macro-orchidism. Greater than 99% of the mutations in *FMR1* described are expansions of an unstable CGG repeat in the 5'-untranslated region of the gene. The number of CGG repeats in this region are divided into three categories: repeats of less than 55 are considered normal, repeats of 55 through 200 are unstable and termed *premutations*, and repeats of more than 200 are termed *full mutations* and cause the Fragile X syndrome.

Somatic Features. A characteristic facial appearance – prominent forehead, elongation of the face, large ears with incompletely folded helices, hypoplasia of the midface, pale irides, and prominent mandible – evolves during the childhood and teenage years. In early childhood, the facial elongation and prominence of the mandible may be less notable. The palate may be high and the teeth crowded. There is a tendency to joint laxity, manifest as excessive hyperextensibility of digits, flat feet, and, less commonly, scoliosis and mitral valve prolapse. Testicular enlargement may be detected by measurement at any age. In adulthood,

testicular volume usually exceeds 25 milliliters. Major malformations do not occur.

Growth and Development. Prenatal and early postnatal growth is robust with head circumference, length, and weight exceeding the average for age. Motor milestones lag from the outset, usually requiring twice the time for achievement of sitting alone, pulling up, and walking. Language development may be even further delayed.

Behavior. Perhaps the most formidable management issue in the Fragile X syndrome is the difficult temperament. Children exhibit hyperactivity, attention deficit, tantrums, perseverative speech, shyness, social anxiety, aggressive outbursts, and autistic behaviors, including tactile defensiveness, hand-flapping, hand-biting, and gaze avoidance. Most of these behaviors persist into adult life.

Neurological Findings. Childhood hypotonia and generalized seizures commonly resolve by adulthood. An adult-onset disorder characterized by ataxia, dementia, and tremor has been described in males with premutation size (55–200 CGG repeats) *FMR1* expansions.

Heterozygote Expression. About half of females with full mutations will have mental retardation, usually of less severe degree than males with full mutations. The adult-onset disorder with ataxia, dementia, and tremor associated with

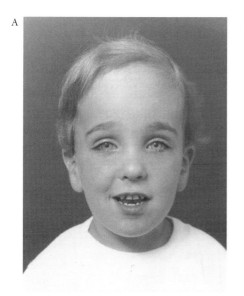

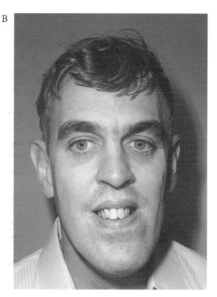

Fragile X Syndrome. Macrocephaly and prominent forehead at age 3 years (A); typical adult facial appearance with long face, large ears, and prominent jaw (B).

premutation-sized *FMR1* expansions occurs less commonly and with lesser severity in female carriers.

Imaging. Many children have had CNS imaging because of developmental delay and macrocephaly. The brain in Fragile X syndrome appears overgrown, with an increase in ventricular volume and a decrease in size of the cerebellar vermis.

Comment. Fragile X syndrome is caused by expansions of greater than 200 CGGs in a CGG repeat region in the 5'-untranslated region of the *FMR1* gene. It is the most commonly diagnosed XLID syndrome. In the general population, males have a prevalence of about 1 in 4000. Fragile X syndrome accounts for about 2% of males and about 0.3% of females with intellectual disability.

Males with premutations with 55 through 200 CGG repeats in 5'-untranslated region of the *FMR1* gene may develop a progressive syndrome of ataxia, tremor, and cognitive decline, generally after age 50 years. Females with similar premutations appear to be affected less often and with less severity.

REFERENCES

Berry-Kravis E, Goetz CG, Leehey MA, et al.: Neuropathic features in fragile X premutation carriers. Am J Med Genet A 143:19–26, 2007.

de Vries BBA, Halley DJJ, Oostra BA, Niermeijer MF: The fragile X syndrome. J Med Genet 35:579–589, 1998.

Lubs H: A marker X chromosome. Am J Hum Genet 21:231, 1969.

Martin JP, Bell J: A pedigree of mental defect showing sex-linkage. J Neurol Psychiatry 6:154, 1943.

Oberle I, Rousseau F, Heitz D, et al.: Instability of a 550-base pair DNA segment and abnormal methylation in fragile X syndrome. Science 252:1097, 1991.

DIFFERENTIAL MATRIX

Syndrome	Macrocephaly	Macroorchidism	Behavioral Aberrations	Comments
Fragile X	+	+	+	Normal or excessive growth, prominent forehead, long face, midface hypoplasia, large ears, prominent mandible
Atkin-Flaitz	+	+	0	Short stature, hypertelorism, downslanting palpebral fissures, broad nasal tip, thick lower lip, brachydactyly, seizures
Clark-Baraitser	+	+	0	Large stature, obesity, dental abnormalities, broad nasal tip, thick lower lip
XLID-Macrocephaly-Macroorchidism	+	+	0	Elongated face, prominent mandible, clumsiness, repetitive movements
Lujan	+	0	+	Asthenic build, long face, prominent forehead, high palate, micrognathia, long digits, pectus excavatum, joint hyperextensibility, hyperactivity, marfanoid habitus, seizures
Mucopolysaccharidosis IIA	+	0	+	Short stature, coarse facies, hepatosplenomegaly, hernias, joint stiffness, thick skin, hirsutism
Opitz FG	+	0	+	High forehead, downslanted palpebral fissures, everted lower lip, dysgenesis of corpus callosum, cardiac defects, imperforate anus, constipation, broad flat thumbs and great toes, digital anomalies, hypotonia
Waisman-Laxova	+	0	+	Spasticity, strabismus
PPM-X	0	+	+	Spastic paraplegia, psychosis, parkinsonian features

GIUFFRÈ-TSUKAHARA SYNDROME

(XLID-MICROCEPHALY-RADIOULNAR SYNOSTOSIS, TSUKAHARA SYNDROME)

OMIM 603438

Definition. XLID with microcephaly and radioulnar synostosis. Assignment to the X-chromosome is tentative, based on males being affected intellectually and skewed X-inactivation in one mother.

Somatic Features. Microcephaly apparent from birth is found in males and females. Bilateral radioulnar synostosis has been noted at birth, but may escape notice until early childhood. Various minor facial characteristics have been described but appear different from family to family. Fifth-finger clinodactyly and scoliosis may be manifestations of the syndrome.

Cognitive Function. Males may have intellectual impairment, mild in nature. Girls, even those with microcephaly and radioulnar synostosis, are intellectually normal.

Comment. The evidence for X-linkage is not conclusive. Giuffrè et al. (1994) considered their two families to represent autosomal dominant inheritance. Tsukahara et al. (1995) reported an isolated case in a male with similarities to the cases of Udler at al. (1998) and Selicorni et al. (2005).

Gaspar et al. (2008) reported a boy with microcephaly, facial dysmorphism, radioulnar synostosis, and delayed development whose mother had radioulnar synostosis and an IQ of 72. They conclude these cases all represent the same heritable entity with apparent X-linked semi-dominant inheritance.

REFERENCES

Gaspar H, Albermann K, Baumer A, et al.: Clinical delineation of Giuffré-Tsukahara syndrome: Another case with microcephaly and radio-ulnar synostosis with apparent X-linked semi-dominant inheritance. Am J Med Genet A 146A:1453, 2008.

Giuffrè L, Corsello G, Giuffrè M, et al.: New syndrome: Autosomal dominant microcephaly and radio-ulnar synostosis. Am J Med Genet 51:266, 1994.

Selicorni A, Ferrarini A, Cagnoli G, et al.: Additional case of Tsukahara's syndrome or new syndrome: Further delineation of the association of microcephaly and radio-ulnar synostosis. Am J Med Genet 132A:189, 2005.

Tsukahara M, Matsuo K, Furukawa S: Radio-ulnar synostosis, short stature, microcephaly, scoliosis, and mental retardation. Am J Med Genet 58:159, 1995.

Udler Y, Halpern GJ, Shohat M, et al.: Tsukahara syndrome of radio-ulnar synostosis, short stature, microcephaly, scoliosis, and mental retardation. Am J Med Genet 80:526, 1998.

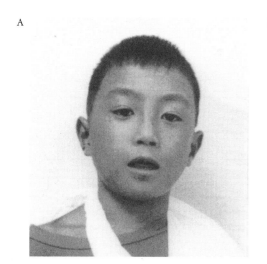
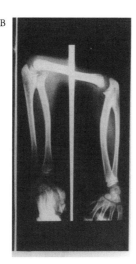

Giufré-Tsukahara Syndrome. Nine-year-old boy with microcephaly, bushy eyebrows, epicanthal folds, and simple philtrum with thin upper lip **(A)**. Radiograph showing synostosis of the proximal radius and ulna **(B)**.
Courtesy of the *American Journal of Medical Genetics*. Copyright 1995. Wiley Liss, Inc.

GLYCEROL KINASE DEFICIENCY

(XLID-HYPERGLYCEROLEMIA)

OMIM 307030

Xp21.3

GKD

Definition. XLID and slow growth, hypogonadism, spasticity, muscular dystrophy, and osteoporosis associated with hyperglycerolemia, glyceroluria, and glycerol kinase deficiency. The full syndrome is seen only where glycerol kinase deficiency is a component of the contiguous gene syndrome involving adjacent genes for gonadotropin deficiency, adrenal hypoplasia, and Duchenne Muscular Dystrophy. Isolated glycerol kinase deficiency may be asymptomatic or may cause recurrent episodes of lethargy, hypothermia, vomiting, and acidemia.

Somatic Features. No somatic manifestations should be anticipated in isolated glycerol kinase deficiency. Short stature, hypogonadotropic hypogonadism, osteoporosis with fractures, muscular weakness with pseudohypertrophy, spasticity, seizures, esotropia, and developmental impairment may occur when adjacent genes are deleted as part of the complex glycerol kinase deficiency contiguous gene syndrome.

Growth and Development. Postnatal growth deficiency and delayed development occur only when genes adjacent to glycerol kinase are deleted as part of a contiguous gene syndrome.

Neurological Findings. Recurrent episodes of lethargy, hypothermia, vomiting, acidemia, and stupor have occurred in children with isolated glycerol kinase deficiency. These symptoms resolved with institution of a low-fat diet. Muscle weakness and spasticity may occur in patients with large deletions involving adjacent genes.

Heterozygote Expression. Female carriers of isolated glycerol kinase deficiency do not show clinical manifestations, nor do those females with deletions of adjacent genes as part of the complex glycerol kinase deficiency contiguous gene syndrome.

Comment. Most patients with glycerol kinase deficiency have had deletions of this gene that extended to involve adjacent genes. The gene order appears to be Xpter-*GTD-AHC-GK-DMD-OTC*-Xcen. It is not clear that glycerol kinase deficiency alone may cause intellectual disability. Certainly there exist adult forms of glycerol kinase deficiency that have no clinical manifestations. Grier et al. (1989) has reported a case of presumed isolated glycerol kinase deficiency in a male infant with recurrent hypothermia and lethargy. Ginns et al. (1982) and Eriksson et al. (1983) reported children with recurrent episodes of vomiting, acidemia, and stupor. A low-fat diet resulted in clinical and developmental improvement in these cases. Developmental impairment might result from these recurrent episodes. Perhaps more likely, mental retardation may result from involvement of a separate gene. There appears to be one such gene distal to the adrenal hypoplasia gene. Alternatively, mental impairment may result from deletions that extend into the 3' end of the *DMD* gene.

REFERENCES

Bartley JA, Patil S, Davenport S, et al.: Duchenne muscular dystrophy, glycerol kinase deficiency, and adrenal insufficiency associated with Xp21 interstitial deletion. J Pediatr 108, 189, 1986.

Eriksson A, Lindstedt S, Ransnas L, et al.: Deficiency of glycerol kinase (EC2.7.1.30). Clin Chem 29:718, 1983.

Ginns EI, Barranger JA, McClean SW, et al.: Hyperglycerolemia secondary to glycerol kinase deficiency in a child without neurological deficits. Pediatr Res 16:191A, 1982.

Grier RE, Howell RR, Wu D, et al.: Isolated glycerol kinase deficiency: nutritional and molecular genetic studies. Am J Hum Genet 45(suppl):A6, 1989.

McCabe ERB, Fennessey PV, Guggenheim MA, et al.: Human glycerol kinase deficiency with hyperglycerolemia and glyceroluria. Biochem Biophys Res Commun 78:1327, 1977.

McCabe ERB, Guggenheim MA, Fennessey PV, et al.: Glyceroluria, psychomotor retardation, spasticity dystrophic myopathy, and osteoporosis in a sibship. Pediatr Res 11:527, 1977.

Matsumoto T, Kondoh T, Yoshimoto M, et al.: Complex glycerol kinase deficiency: molecular-genetic, cytogenetic, and clinical studies of five Japanese patients. Am J Med Genet 31:603, 1988.

Walker AP, Muscatelli F, Monaco AP: Isolation of the human Xp21 glycerol kinase gene by positional cloning. Hum Mol Genet 2:107, 1993.

Willard HF: Cloning of the X-linked glycerol kinase gene. Hum Mol Genet 2:95, 1993.

DIFFERENTIAL MATRIX

Syndrome	Hypothermia	Lethargy	Recurrent Vomiting	Comments
Glycerol Kinase Deficiency	+	+	+	Short stature, hypogonadotrophic hypogonadism, osteoporosis, fractures, muscle weakness, spasticity, and seizures when a part of GKD contiguous gene syndrome. Isolated GKD may be asymptomatic
Menkes	+	+	0	Growth deficiency, sparse kinky hair, pallor, limited movement, hypertonicity, seizures, metaphyseal widening and spurs, arterial tortuosity, childhood death
Ornithine Transcarbamoylase Deficiency	0	+	+	Chronic or intermittent hyperammonemia, microcephaly, protein-induced vomiting and lethargy, ataxia, seizures
Pyruvate Dehydrogenase Deficiency	0	+	+	Microcephaly, ataxia, dysarthria, structural brain anomalies, hypotonia, lactic acidosis

GOLABI-ITO-HALL SYNDROME: (*SEE ALSO* RENPENNING SYNDROME)

OMIM 300463

Xp11.23

PQBP1

Definition. XLID with short stature, microcephaly, narrow or triangular face, telecanthus, epicanthus, upslanting palpebral fissures, cupped ears, and ectodermal manifestations. A missense mutation in *PQBP1* has been demonstrated, making Golabi-Ito-Hall syndrome allelic to Renpenning, Hamel Cerebro-Palato-Cardiac, Sutherland-Haan, and Porteous syndromes.

Somatic Features. Characteristic manifestations are found in each of the craniofacial segments. The cranium is small and the triangular facial configuration present in childhood elongates during the teen years. The upper face is perhaps most distinctive because of the narrow forehead with prominence of the glabella or metopic ridging, telecanthus, epicanthus, and upslanting palpebral fissures. A long nose with high nasal root and cupped ears are the major midfacial manifestations. The lower facial segment shows a thin upper lip, prominent maxillary central incisors, narrow palate with wide palatine ridges, and – at least in early childhood – a small mandible. A variety of ectodermal manifestations, including dry brittle scalp hair, nail hypoplasia, cutis marmorata, and large maxillary central incisors, have been described. Chest asymmetry was noted in two cases and atrial septal defect in two cases.

Growth and Development. Birth weight and head circumference are normal but in the lower percentiles. Postnatally, all growth parameters lag leading to microcephaly and short stature. Global developmental delay becomes obvious during infancy and early childhood.

Cognitive Function. The degree of cognitive impairment was not reported. An IQ of 23 was found in one affected male who also had neonatal complications.

Neurological Findings. Abnormal neurological findings – lower limb hyper-reflexia, Babinski signs, petit mal seizures, and mild sensorineural hearing loss – were described in only one case, who required resuscitation at birth.

Heterozygote Expression. None reported

Laboratory. Chronic hematuria of unknown cause occurred in one case.

Comment. Only a single family has been reported. The presence of chronic hematuria and sensorineural hearing loss in one affected male suggests Alport syndrome, an X-linked entity that does not have intellectual disability.

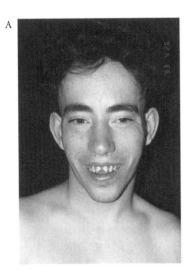 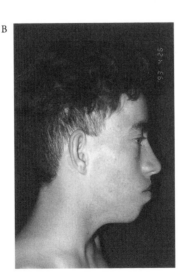 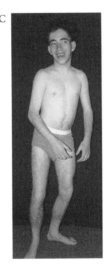 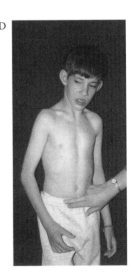

Golabi-Ito-Hall Syndrome. Affected male at age 21 years showing short stature, microcephaly, triangular face, cupped ears, upslanted palpebral fissures, long nose, thin upper lip, and small mandible (**A–C**); affected cousin at age 13 years (**D**).

REFERENCES

Golabi M, Ito M, Hall BD: A new X-linked multiple congenital anomalies/mental retardation syndrome. Am J Med Genet 17:367, 1984.

Kalscheuer VM, Freude K, Musante L, et al.: Mutations in the polyglutamine binding protein 1 gene cause X-linked mental retardation. Nat Genet 35:313, 2003.

Lenski C, Abidi F, Meindl A, et al.: Novel truncating mutations in the polyglutamine tract binding protein 1 gene (PQBP1) cause Renpenning syndrome and X-linked mental retardation in another family with microcephaly. Am J Hum Genet 74:777, 2004.

Lubs H, Abidi FE, Echeverri R, et al.: Golabi-Ito-Hall syndrome results from a missense mutation in the WW domain of the PQBP1 gene. J Med Genet 43:e30, 2006.

Stevenson RE, Bennett CW, Abidi F, et al.: Renpenning syndrome comes into focus. Am J Med Genet A 134A:415, 2005.

DIFFERENTIAL MATRIX

Syndrome	Distinctive Craniofacial Findings	Cardiac Malformation	Ectodermal Manifestation	Comments
Golabi-Ito-Hall (Renpenning)	+	+	+	Microcephaly, short stature, telecanthus, high nasal root, cupped ears, thoracic asymmetry, sacral dimple, dry/brittle/sparse hair, cutis marmorata, nail hypoplasia
Hereditary Bullous Dystrophy, X-linked	+	+	+	Microcephaly, short stature, upslanting palpebral fissures, protruding ears, short and tapered digits, bullous dystrophy, small testes, early death from pulmonary infection
MIDAS	+	+	+	Microphthalmia, ocular dysgenesis, corneal opacification, dermal aplasia, dysgenesis of corpus callosum
ATRX-Associated XLID	+	+	0	Microcephaly, short stature, small testes, telecanthus, small triangular nose, tented upper lip, open mouth, wide spacing of teeth, genital anomalies, musculoskeletal anomalies, hemoglobin H inclusions in erythrocytes
Lenz Microphthalmia	+	+	0	Microcephaly, microphthalmia, ocular dysgenesis, malformed ears, cleft lip/palate, cardiac and genitourinary anomalies, thumb duplication or hypoplasia, narrow shoulders
Opitz FG	+	+	0	Macrocephaly, broad forehead, downslanted palpebral fissures, everted lower lip, dysgenesis of corpus callosum, imperforate anus, constipation, flat thumbs and great toes, hypotonia
Simpson-Golabi-Behmel	+	+	0	Somatic overgrowth, supernumerary nipples, polydactyly
Telecanthus-Hypospadias	+	+	0	High broad nasal root, dysplastic ears, cleft lip/palate, abnormal cranial contour or symmetry
Oral-Facial-Digital I	+	0	+	Sparse scalp hair, dystopia canthorum, flat midface, hypoplastic alae nasi, hypertrophic and aberrant oral frenuli, intraoral clefts and pseudoclefts, lingual hamartomas, brachydactyly, syndactyly, clinodactyly, structural brain anomalies, polycystic kidneys

GOLDBLATT SPASTIC PARAPLEGIA SYNDROME

OMIM 312920

Xp21.3

Definition. XLID with nystagmus, optic atrophy, muscle hypoplasia, contractures, ataxia, and spasticity. The gene has not been identified.

Somatic Features. Malformations or facial abnormalities do not occur. Optic atrophy with nystagmus and exotropia are present. The leg muscles are underdeveloped, and signs of spasticity and ataxia present.

Growth and Development. Not known

Cognitive Function. Mildly impaired

Neurological Findings. Nystagmus and in some cases exotropia have been reported. Spastic paraplegia with increased deep tendon reflexes and Babinski signs are present from infancy. Ataxia, dysarthria, dysmetria and dysdiadochokinesia may be present as well. Independent ambulation is not achieved, but muscle power of the arms and continence of bowel and bladder are normal.

Heterozygote Expression. None

Comment. Although more clinically severe, the neuromuscular and ocular findings suggest that this syndrome may be a variant of Pelizaeus-Merzbacher syndrome, the gene for which (*PLP1*) has been localized to Xq21.1. To date, mutational analysis has not been reported.

REFERENCE

Goldblatt J, Ballo R, Sachs B, et al.: X-linked spastic paraplegia: evidence for homogeneity with a variable phenotype. Clin Genet 35:116, 1989.

DIFFERENTIAL MATRIX

Syndrome	Ataxia	Spastic Paraplegia	Muscle Hypoplasia	Comments
Goldblatt Spastic Paraplegia	+	+	+	Optic atrophy, exotropia, nystagmus, dysarthria, contractures
Allan-Herndon-Dudley	+	+	+	Childhood hypotonia, dysarthria, athetosis, large ears with cupping or abnormal architecture, contractures
Apak Ataxia-Spastic Diplegia	+	+	+	Short stature, clubfoot
XLID-Spastic Paraplegia-Athetosis	+	+	+	Nystagmus, weakness, dysarthria, contractures
Mohr-Tranebjaerg	+	+	0	Neurologic deterioration with childhood onset, dystonia
Pelizaeus-Merzbacher	+	+	0	Optic atrophy, nystagmus, hypotonia, dystonia, CNS dysmyelination
Pettigrew	+	+	0	Microcephaly or hydrocephaly, long face with macrostomia and prognathism, Dandy-Walker malformation, small testes, contractures, choreoathetosis, iron deposits in basal ganglia, seizures
XLID-Spastic Paraplegia, type 7	+	+	0	Nystagmus, reduced vision, absent speech and ambulation, bowel and bladder dysfunction
XLID-Hypogonadism-Tremor	+	0	+	Short stature, prominent lower lip, muscle wasting of legs, abnormal gait, hypogonadism, obesity, seizures, tremor

GOLTZ SYNDROME
(FOCAL DERMAL HYPOPLASIA, GOLTZ-GORLIN SYNDROME)

OMIM 305600

Xp11.23

PORCN

Definition. XLID in females associated with linear areas of thin or absent skin, herniated cutaneous papules of adipose tissue, dystrophic nails, abnormal teeth and hair, cataracts, and reduction defects of the limbs.

Somatic Features. Focal areas of dermal hypoplasia or aplasia date from birth, occur on all skin surfaces except the palms and soles, vary considerably in size, and tend to be linear when on the limbs. Affected areas of skin are thin and depressed, forming irregular plaques that may be darker or lighter than adjacent normal skin. Histologically, the connective tissue of the corium is replaced completely or partially by adipose tissue. Yellowish saccular herniations of fat encased in the thinnest covering of epidermis occur, perhaps with a predilection in body folds and in the perioral and perianal areas, and are considered a pathognomonic finding.

Other ectodermal tissues have involvement as well. The hair is generally sparse and in localized areas of the scalp and pubic area may be totally absent. Dystrophic or absent nails occur, particularly when adjacent skin is involved. Oligodontia, hypoplastic teeth, notched incisors, malocclusion or irregular spacing, and delayed eruption can be found in nearly half of cases.

Ocular defects, often unilateral or asymmetric, include epiphora, strabismus, microphthalmia, iris colobomas, cataracts, optic atrophy, and retinal colobomas.

In addition to contributions from the ocular, dental, and cutaneous abnormalities, the facies may be otherwise distinctive with facial asymmetry, simply formed and

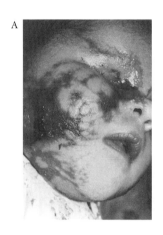
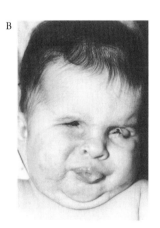
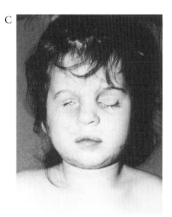
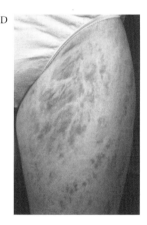

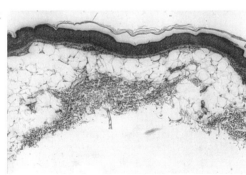
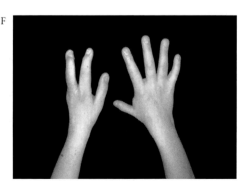

Goltz Syndrome. Oculocutaneous manifestations involving the face showing microphthalmia, small palpebral fissures, and hypoplastic or aplastic areas of skin at ages 2 weeks, 3 months, and 2 years (A-C); thinning of skin of the proximal thigh with herniations of adipose tissue (D). Replacement of connective tissue of the corium with adipose tissue (E); upper limb malformation with absence of the ulnar rays of the left hand and thumb hypoplasia of the right hand (F). Illustrations **A-C** courtesy of Dr. Arthur S. Aylsworth, University of North Carolina School of Medicine, Chapel Hill. Illustrations **D-F** courtesy of Dr. Robert Gorlin, University of Minnesota, Minneapolis.

cupped ears, broad nasal tip, and, in some cases, notching of the alae nasi. Cleft lip, cleft palate, cleft tongue, and notching of the alveolar ridge may also occur.

Most cases have malformation of the hands and feet, typically reduction defects with the missing rays being central, medial, or lateral. Limb asymmetry, syndactyly, hemivertebrae, and clavicular anomalies occur as well. Longitudinal striations in the metaphyses of the long bones have been demonstrated in about 20% of cases.

Other anomalies may include omphalocele, inguinal hernia, hiatal hernia, and unusually placed hernias at the sites of dermal hypoplasia. Renal dysplasia and horseshoe kidney have also been reported.

Growth and Development. Growth is globally impaired, beginning prior to birth and often resulting in microcephaly and short stature. Asymmetry commonly affects the face, limbs, and trunk. Most achieve developmental milestones at the normal time; others are variably delayed.

Cognitive Function. In most cases, cognitive function is normal. The minority of cases with impaired function (perhaps 15%), are represented primarily among those with microcephaly and severe ocular malformation.

Imaging. CNS structures are usually normal. Rarely noted abnormalities include hydrocephalus and agenesis of the corpus callosum.

Comment. The degree of somatic involvement may incorrectly predict the measure of visual and cognitive disability. Most cases are sporadic, although in some instances female relatives have had mild evidence of ectodermal involvement. As with other female limited disorders, gestational lethality in males has been proposed. Several mildly affected males have been reported, their involvement being limited to the skin and so mild as to preclude diagnosis until they fathered daughters with typical manifestations. These males likely represent mosaics with only a minority of somatic cells affected.

REFERENCES

Burgdorf WHC, Dick GF, Soderberg MD, et al.: Focal dermal hypoplasia in a father and daughter. Am Acad Dermatol 4:273, 1981.

Goltz RW: Focal dermal hypoplasia syndrome. An Update. Arch Dermatol 128:1108, 1992.

Goltz RW, Peterson WC, Gorlin RJ, et al.: Focal dermal hypoplasia. Arch Dermatol 86:52, 1962.

Grzeschik KH, Bornholdt D, Oeffner F, et al.: Deficiency of PORCN, a regulator of Wnt signaling, is associated with focal dermal hypoplasia. Nat Genet 39:833, 2007.

Maas SM, Lombardi MP, van Essen AJ, et al.: Phenotype and genotype in 17 patients with Goltz-Gorlin syndrome. J Med Genet 46:716, 2009.

Temple IK, MacDowall P, Baraitser M, et al.: Focal dermal hypoplasia (Goltz syndrome). J Med Genet 27:180, 1990.

Wang X, Reid Sutton V, Omar Peraza-Llanes J, et al.: Mutations in X-linked PORCN, a putative regulator of Wnt signaling, cause focal dermal hypoplasia. Nat Genet 39:836, 2007.

DIFFERENTIAL MATRIX

Syndrome	Ocular Abnormality	Urogenital Anomalies	Cutaneous Manifestations	Comments
Goltz	+	+	+	Linear areas of dermal aplasia, dystrophic nails, abnormal teeth and hair, vertebral anomalies, limb reduction defects
Lenz Microphthalmia	+	+	+	Short stature, microcephaly, microphthalmia, cupped or dysplastic ears, thumb anomalies, cleft lip/palate, sloped shoulders, clavicular hypoplasia, barrel chest, kyphoscoliosis
Cerebro-Oculo-Genital	+	+	0	Microcephaly, hydrocephaly, short stature, agenesis of corpus callosum, microphthalmia, ptosis, hypospadias, cryptorchidism, clubfoot, spasticity
Lowe	+	+	0	Short stature, hypotonia, aminoaciduria, progressive renal disease
Wittwer	+	+	0	Microcephaly, short stature, microphthalmia, hearing loss, vision loss, hypertelorism, hypotonia, seizures
MIDAS	+	0	+	Corneal opacification, dermal aplasia, dysgenesis of corpus callosum, cardiac defects, cardiomyopathy

GRAHAM ANOPHTHALMIA SYNDROME

(GRAHAM SYNDROME, X-LINKED ANOPHTHALMIA)

OMIM 301590

Xq27-q28

Definition. XLID with anophthalmia and ankyloblepharon. The gene has not been identified, but it may be localized to Xq27-q28.

Somatic Features. Clinical anophthalmia, ankyloblepharon, shallow orbits, and short eyebrows and eyelids make up the facial phenotype. Other common characteristics have not been described. One male had preauricular tags and cleft soft palate.

Cognitive Function. Severe impairment.

Growth and Development. Unknown

Heterozygote Expression. None

Comment. Only a single family with seven affected males in two generations has been reported. Limitation of the clinical manifestations to the ocular and periocular region makes possible differentiation from other microphthalmia-intellectual disability syndromes.

REFERENCE

Graham CA, Redmond RM, Nevin NC: X-linked clinical anophthalmos: Localization of the gene to Xq27-Xq28. Ophthalmic Pediatr Genet 12:43, 1991.

A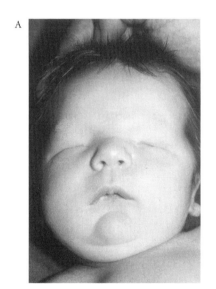
B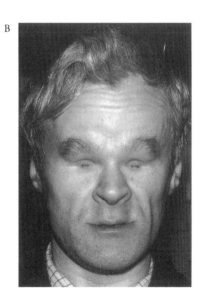

Graham Anophthalmia Syndrome. Affected males in infancy and adulthood showing bilateral anophthalmia and ankyloblepharon.   Courtesy of Dr. Norman Nevin, Northern Ireland Regional Genetic Center, Belfast.

DIFFERENTIAL MATRIX

Syndrome	Ocular Dysgenesis	Short or Fused Palpebral Fissures	Comments
Graham Anophthalmia	+	+	Microphthalmia, shallow orbits, short eyebrows
Aicardi	+	+	Lacunar retinopathy, costovertebral anomalies, agenesis of corpus callosum, seizures
Goltz	+	+	Cataracts, linear areas of dermal aplasia, cutaneous adipose herniations, dystrophic nails, abnormal teeth and hair, vertebral anomalies, limb reduction defects, genitourinary anomalies
MIDAS	+	+	Microphthalmia, corneal opacification, dermal aplasia, dysgenesis of corpus callosum, cardiac defects, cardiomyopathy
Lenz Microphthalmia	+	+	Short stature, microcephaly, cupped or dyplastic ears, thumb anomalies, urogenital anomalies, cleft lip/palate, sloped shoulders, clavicular hypoplasia, barrel chest, kyphoscoliosis
Cerebro-Oculo-Genital	+	+	Microcephaly, hydrocephaly, short stature, agenesis of corpus callosum, microphthalmia, ptosis, hypospadias, cryptorchidism, clubfoot, spasticity
Wittwer	+	0	Microcephaly, short stature, hearing loss, vision loss, hypertelorism, genitourinary anomalies, hypotonia, seizures

GUSTAVSON SYNDROME
(XLID-OPTIC ATROPHY-DEAFNESS-SEIZURES)

OMIM 309555

Xq23-q27.3

Definition. XLID with microcephaly, short stature, blindness, deafness, seizures, spasticity, and early death. The responsible gene has not been identified but localized to the large region flanked by DXS424 (Xq23) and DXS297 (Xq27.3).

Somatic Features. Microcephaly, optic atrophy, large ears, marked short stature, and contractures of the large joints give a distinctive, if not specific, presentation. The fontanelles are quite small, if palpable at all. Vertical talus gives the foot a rockerbottom or calcaneovalgus configuration. Ultrasound and CT imaging have demonstrated marked undergrowth of the brain, enlarged cerebral ventricles, cerebellar hypoplasia, and, in one case, Dandy-Walker malformation.

Growth and Development. Marked intrauterine growth impairment occurs with decreased head circumference, length, and weight. Length appears to be more severely reduced than other growth parameters. Growth impairment continues postnatally. No meaningful developmental progress is made, and death occurs in infancy or early childhood.

A
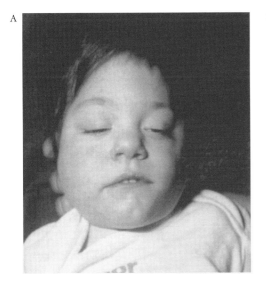

B
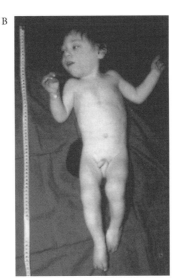

C
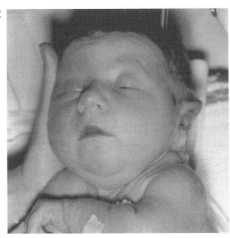

D
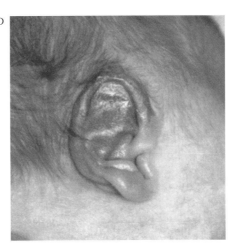

Gustavon Syndrome. Affected male at age 14 months showing short broad nose, large ears, and spastic positioning **(A, B)**; 3-day-old male cousin with receding chin and large dysplastic ears **(C, D).**   Courtesy of Dr. Karl-Henrik Gustavson, University of Uppsala, Sweden and *The American Journal of Medical Genetics*, Copyright 1993 Wiley-Liss, Inc.

Cognitive Function. No apparent cognitive skills develop prior to death.

Neurological Findings. From birth, these infants are severely impaired, with increased muscle tone and hyperreflexia. They do not respond to visual or auditory stimulation. Seizures and apneic episodes recur. Contractures of the large joints and equinovarus, calcaneovalgus, or rockerbottom feet are present at birth.

Heterozygote Expression. Carrier females typically show no manifestations. One infant girl, however, was severely and typically affected, a circumstance possibly explained by preferential inactivation of her normal X chromosome.

Imaging. Brain undergrowth, especially affecting the cerebellum, with enlarged cerebral ventricles and Dandy-Walker malformation (one case) has been demonstrated by ultrasound and cranial tomography.

Comment. A similar phenotype (microcephaly, short stature, impaired vision and hearing, spasticity and contractures) and course (profound developmental failure, seizures, and early death) are shared by a number of conditions in which severe intrauterine brain injury has been sustained. Prenatal infections with herpes virus, cytomegalovirus, rubella, and toxoplasma gondii constitute environmental causes that may be distinguished by serological testing, intracranial calcifications, and evidence of continuing postnatal infection of various tissues. Reardon et al. (1994) have reviewed a number of genocopies, some possibly X-linked, which may in some cases be distinguished by the presence of intracranial calcification and thrombocytopenia. Other entities with cerebellar hypoplasia and spastic paraplegia that map to the same region are allelic to Pelizaeus-Merzbacher disease (mutations in *PLP1*) and Christianson syndrome (mutations in *SLC9A6*).

REFERENCES

Arena JF, Schwartz C, Stevenson R, et al.: Spastic paraplegia with iron deposits in the basal ganglia: a new X-linked mental retardation syndrome. Am J Med Genet 43:479, 1992.

Christianson AL, Stevenson RE, van der Meyden CH, et al.: X linked severe mental retardation, craniofacial dysmorphology, epilepsy, ophthalmoplegia, and cerebellar atrophy in a large South African kindred is localised to Xq24-q27. J Med Genet 36:759, 1999.

Gilfillan GD, Selmer KK, Roxrud I, et al.: SLC9A6 mutations cause X-linked mental retardation, microcephaly, epilepsy, and ataxia, a phenotype mimicking Angelman syndrome. Am J Hum Genet 82:1003, 2008.

Gustavson K-H, Annerén G, Malmgren H, et al.: New X-linked syndrome with severe mental retardation, severely impaired vision, severe hearing defect, epileptic seizures, spasticity, restricted joint mobility, and early death. Am J Med Genet 45:654, 1993.

Malmgren H, Sundvall M, Dahl N, et al.: Linkage mapping of a severe X-linked mental retardation syndrome. Am J Hum Genet 52:1046, 1993.

Reardon W, Hockey A, Silberstein P, et al.: Autosomal recessive congenital intrauterine infection-like syndrome of microcephaly, intracranial calcification, and CNS disease. Am J Med Genet 52:58, 1994.

Stevenson RE, Tarpey P, May MM, et al.: Arena syndrome is caused by a missense mutation in PLP1. Am J Med Genet A 149A:1081, 2009.

DIFFERENTIAL MATRIX

Syndrome	Cerebellar Hypoplasia	Seizures	Spasticity	Comments
Gustavson	+	+	+	Microcephaly, short stature, optic atrophy with blindness, large ears, deafness, joint contractures, rockerbottom feet, brain undergrowth, hydrocephaly
Paine	+	+	+	Microcephaly, short stature, optic atrophy, vision and hearing loss
Pelizaeus-Merzbacher	+	+	+	Optic atrophy, nystagmus, hypotonia, ataxia, dystonia, CNS dysmyelination
Pettigrew	+	+	+	Dandy-Walker malformation, microcephaly or hydrocephaly, long face with macrostomia and prognathism, small testes, contractures, myoglobinuria, hemolytic anemia
Schimke	+	+	+	Microcephaly, sunken eyes, downslanting palpebral fissures, narrow nose, wide spacing of teeth, cupped ears, hypotonia, abducens palsy, hearing loss, vision loss, choreoathetosis, contractures
Bertini	+	+	0	Macular degeneration, hypotonia, childhood death, developmental delays and regression, postnatal growth impairment
Cerebro-Cerebello-Coloboma	+	+	0	Hydrocephaly, cerebellar vermis hypoplasia, retinal coloboma, hypotonia, abnormal respiratory pattern
Christianson	+	+	0	Short stature, microcephaly, general asthenia, contractures, ophthalmoplegia

HALL OROFACIAL SYNDROME

Hall and Robl (1999) reported two brothers and a maternal first-cousin with moderate intellectual disability, normal growth, upslanted and short palpebral fissures, and prominent nasal tip. Two had hypertelorism, high nasal bridge, low-set ears, short fifth fingers, and inguinal hernias. One had cleft lip, and one had cleft palate. Postnatal growth deficiency, ear pit, kyphosis, cubitus valgus, small thumbs, clubfoot, multicystic kidney, and undescended testes were each noted once in the three males. The condition has not been mapped nor is there other evidence of X-linkage.

REFERENCE

Hall BD, Robl JM: New x-linked MR/MCA syndrome associated with cleft lip/palate, upslanted/short palpebral fissures, high nasal bridge, prominent nasal tip, inguinal hernia and minor digital defects. Am J Hum Genet 65:A151, 1999.

HEREDITARY BULLOUS DYSTROPHY, X-LINKED

(MACULAR TYPE BULLOUS DYSTROPHY)

OMIM 302000

Xq27.3-qter

Definition. XLID with short stature, microcephaly, alopecia, macular bullous dystrophy, tapered fingers, and hypogenitalism. The gene has not been identified.

Somatic Features. Microcephaly, scalp alopecia, upslanting palpebral fissures, and protruding ears give the face its characteristic appearance. The corneas may be cloudy. Alopecia begins before birth or during the first year of life. Bullous lesions usually make their appearance during the first year as well. The lesions consist of macules or papules on skin-exposed areas, particularly the face and dorsal surface of the hands and lips. Some lesions are vesicular and leave hypopigmented or hyperpigmented areas upon resolution. Cutaneous cancer has been noted in at least one case. Cataracts may develop in adult life. The teeth are normal and nail dystrophy has been noted in only one case. The fingers are short and tapered and may show acrocyanosis. The testes may be small or undescended. Incompletely characterized heart defects appear to be common. One case had pulmonary valve stenosis and a right-sided conduction defect. Death in childhood or early adult life from pulmonary infections is not unusual.

Growth and Development. Markedly slow growth is evident at birth and catch-up growth thereafter does not occur. All growth parameters are affected.

Cognitive Function. Most cases appear to have mental retardation, although the severity has not been reported.

Heterozygote Expression. None

Imaging. With the exception of its small size, brain structure is normal.

Comment. Although a defect in the immune system has been suspected as an underlying factor in the respiratory infections that lead to death in childhood or early adult life, no such defect has been demonstrated.

REFERENCES

Lungarotti MS, Martello C, Barboni G, et al.: X-linked mental retardation, microcephaly, and growth delay associated with hereditary bullous dystrophy macular type: Report of a second family. Am J Med Genet 51:598, 1994.

Mendes da Costa S, Van der Valk JW: Typus maculatus der bullosen hereditären dystrophie. Arch Derm Syph 91:1, 1908.

Wijker M, Ligtenberg JL, Schoute F, et al.: The gene for hereditary bullous dystrophy, X-linked macular type, maps to the Xq27.3-qter region. Am J Hum Genet 56:1096, 1995.

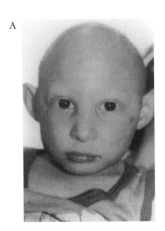
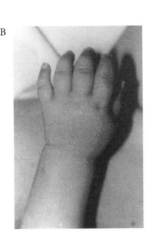
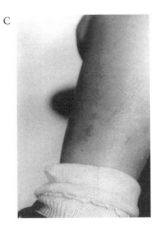
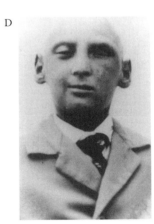

Hereditary Bullous Dystrophy, X-Linked. Microcephaly, alopecia, protruding ears, upslanting palpebral fissures, tapered fingers, and macular, papular, and vesicular lesions on the forearm and legs (A-C); microcephaly and alopecia in a maternal uncle (D).   Courtesy of Dr. Serena Lungarotti, University of Perugia, Perugia, Italy.

DIFFERENTIAL MATRIX

Syndrome	Microcephaly	Cutaneous Lesions	Cardiac Defects	Comments
Hereditary Bullous Dystrophy, X-linked	+	+	+	Short stature, upslanting palpebral fissures, protruding ears, digits short and tapered, bullous dystrophy, small testes, early death from pulmonary infection
Cantu	+	+	O	Short stature, alopecia, follicular keratosis, cortical atrophy, seizures
Cornelia de Lange Syndrome, X-linked	+	+	O	Short stature, arched eyebrows, synophrys, long philtrum, thin lips, cutis marmorata, small hands and feet, hirsutism, enlarged cerebral ventricles, proximal thumbs, elbow restriction
Goltz	+	+	O	Cataracts, ocular dysgenesis, linear areas of dermal aplasia, cutaneous adipose herniations, dystrophic nails, abnormal teeth and hair, vertebral anomalies, limb reduction defects, genitourinary anomalies
Roifman	+	+	O	Short stature, spondyloepiphyseal dysplasia, retinal pigmentary deposits, antibody deficiency, eczema, hypotonia
Renpenning	+	O	+	Short stature, small testes
Fitzsimmons	O	+	+	Pes cavus, hyperkeratosis of palms and soles, dystrophic nails, spastic paraplegia
MIDAS	O	+	+	Microphthalmia, ocular dysgenesis, corneal opacification, dermal aplasia, dysgenesis of corpus callosum, cardiomyopathy

HOLMES-GANG SYNDROME (*SEE ALSO ATRX*-ASSOCIATED XLID)
(*ATRX* SPECTRUM)

OMIM 309580

Xq21.1

ATRX (XNP, XH2)

Definition. XLID with microcephaly, large fontanelle, hypotonic facies with short nose and anteverted nares, and club foot. A mutation has been found in *ATRX*, confirming allelism with Alpha-Thalassemia Intellectual Disability).

Somatic Features. Microcephaly, large anterior fontanelle, apparent hypertelorism, epicanthus, short nose with flat nasal bridge and anteverted nares, and tented upper lip with short philtrum comprise the craniofacial phenotype. The feet are clubbed. In one case, renal hypoplasia/dysplasia, thyroglossal duct cyst and incomplete lung lobation were found at autopsy.

Growth and Development. Intrauterine growth is slow and growth delay persists postnatally. Developmental progress is severely delayed, with death in infancy or early childhood.

Heterozygote Expression. None

Neuropathology. Markedly small brain with hypoplasia of cerebral white matter and indistinct temporal gyri.

A
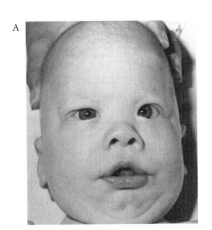

B
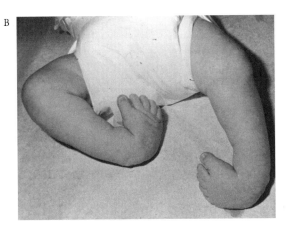

C
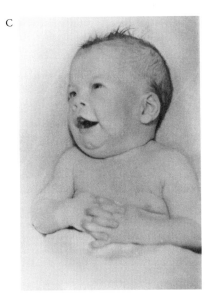

Holmes-Gang Syndrome. Five-month-old with microcephaly, epicanthal folds, flat nasal bridge, short triangular nose, anteverted nares, tented upper lip, and club feet (**A, B**); maternal uncle with similar facial features at age 5 months (**C**). Courtesy of Dr. Lewis B. Holmes, Massachusetts General Hospital, Boston.

Comment. This syndrome is based on observations in a single family. Similarity of the craniofacial findings, largely caused by hypotonia, with those in Alpha-Thalassemia Intellectual Disability has led to the identification of a mutation in the *ATRX* gene in Xq13.3.

REFERENCES

Holmes LB, Gang DL: Brief clinical report: An X-linked mental retardation syndrome with craniofacial abnormalities, microcephaly and club foot. Am J Med Genet 17:375, 1984.

Stevenson RE, Abidi F, Schwartz CE, et al.: Holmes-Gang syndrome is allelic with XLMR-hypotonic face syndrome. Am J Med Genet 94:383, 2000.

DIFFERENTIAL MATRIX

Syndrome	Microcephaly	Hypotonic Facies	Short Nose	Comments
Holmes-Gang (*ATRX*-Associated XLID)	+	+	+	Short stature, small testes, telecanthus, small triangular nose, tented upper lip, open mouth, wide spacing of teeth, genital anomalies, musculoskeletal anomalies, hemoglobin H inclusions in erythrocytes
Coffin-Lowry	+	+	0	Short stature, hypertelorism, anteverted nares, tented upper lip, prominent lips and large mouth, large ears, soft hands with tapered digits, pectus carinatum
Miles-Carpenter	+	+	0	Short stature, ptosis, small palpebral fissures, open mouth, pectus excavatum, scoliosis, long hands, camptodactyly, rockerbottom feet, arch fingerprints, spasticity, unsteady gait
Proud (*ARX*-Associated XLID)	+	+	0	Hearing loss, vision loss, agenesis of corpus callosum, cryptorchidism, inguinal hernias, ataxia, spasticity, seizures
Smith-Fineman-Myers	+	+	0	Ptosis, flat philtrum, scoliosis, midfoot varus, narrow feet, seizures
XLID-Psoriasis	0	+	+	Hypertelorism, open mouth, large ears, seizures, psoriasis

HOMFRAY SEIZURES-CONTRACTURES

A single family in which Homfray et al. (1995) considered a teenage male and his maternal uncle with coarse facies, generalized seizures, and nonprogressive flexion contractures of the neck, shoulders, elbows, wrists, hips, knees, ankles, and toes as representative of an XLID syndrome. The IQ measurements were 50 and 47. Another nephew possibly had intellectual disability.

REFERENCE

Homfray T, Holland T, Patton M: A new X-linked mental retardation syndrome. Clin Dysmorphol 4:289, 1995.

HYDE-FORSTER SYNDROME

OMIM 300064

Hyde-Forster reported two brothers with brachycephaly, flat occiput, plagiocephaly, "coarse features," and severe developmental delay. One brother had microcephaly, seizures, and mild cerebral atrophy on CT imaging. The younger brother had prominence of the forehead. Two maternal aunts had learning problems but no craniofacial manifestations. In the absence of additional details or other similar cases, designation of these cases as a unique XLID syndrome should be deferred.

REFERENCE

Hyde-Forster I, McCarthy G, Berry AC: A new X linked syndrome with mental retardation and craniofacial dysmorphism? J Med Genet 29:736, 1992.

HYDRANENCEPHALY WITH ABNORMAL GENITALIA (*SEE ALSO ARX*-ASSOCIATED XLID)

(X-LINKED LISSENCEPHALY, TYPE 2)

OMIM 300215

Xp21.3

ARX

Definition. XLID associated with hydranencephaly and abnormalities of the male genitalia. This disorder belongs to the *ARX*-Associated XLID spectrum.

Somatic Features. Microcephaly and hydranencephaly are present, and the genitalia show microphallus, hypospadias, cryptorchidism, or may be incompletely differentiated. The craniofacial features may be mildly dysmorphic but are nonspecific and may include a low forehead, micrognathia, and facial hypotonia.

Growth and Development. Because of the severe brain malformation, development and growth are severely impaired. Death usually occurs in infancy.

Neurological Findings. Severe hypotonia and seizures as neonates

Heterozygote Expression. Up to 35% of heterozygotes may have mild developmental disabilities. Some females have abnormalities of the corpus callosum and/or seizures.

Imaging. This disorder is separated from the other ARX-associated conditions by the finding of hydranencephaly and overlaps closely with X-linked Lissencephaly and Abnormal Genitalia (XLAG).

Neuropathology. Simplified gyral pattern with disorganized cortex and abnormal neuronal migration with the cortex only 6 to 7 millimeters thick as opposed to the thicker cortex (15–20 millimeters) seen in lissencephaly caused by mutations in *DCX*.

Comment. Hydranencephaly with abnormal genitalia and XLAG represent the most severe end of the spectrum of the *ARX*-associated disorders. Nonsense and other truncating mutations lead to loss of gene function and the severe phenotypes. A consistent genotype-phenotype correlation has been documented by Kato et al. (2004). Missense mutations are associated with a milder neurological phenotype, and expansions of the polyalanine tracts are usually associated with milder and nonmalformation phenotypes.

REFERENCES

Kato M, Das S, Petras K, et al.: Mutations of ARX are associated with striking pleiotropy and consistent genotype-phenotype correlation. Hum Mutat 23:147, 2004.

Bonneau D, Toutain A, Laquerriere A, et al.: X-linked lissencephaly with absent corpus callosum and ambiguous genitalia (XLAG): clinical, magnetic resonance imaging, and neuropathological findings. Ann Neurol 51:340, 2002.

Gécz J, Cloosterman D, Partington M: ARX: a gene for all seasons. Curr Opin Genet Dev 16:308, 2006.

Shoubridge C, Fullston T, Gécz J: ARX spectrum disorders: making inroads into the molecular pathology. Hum Mutat 31:889, 2010.

Friocourt G, Parnavelas JG: Mutations in ARX result in several defects involving GABAergic neurons. Front Cell Neurosci. 4:4, 2010.

DIFFERENTIAL MATRIX

Syndrome	Hydrocephaly or Hydranencephaly	Abnormal Genitalia	Seizures	Comments
Hydranencephaly with Abnormal Genitalia (*ARX*-Associated XLID)	+	+	+	Simple cerebral gyri, neuronal migration abnormality, hypotonia
Armfield	+	O	+	Short stature, cataracts or glaucoma, dental anomalies, small hands and feet, joint stiffness, ocular abnormality, orofacial clefting
Cerebro-Cerebello-Coloboma	+	O	+	Cerebellar vermis hypoplasia, retinal coloboma, hypotonia, abnormal respiratory pattern
CK	+	O	+	Asthenic build, hypotonia, long thin face, scoliosis, behavior problems, microcephaly, neuronal migration disturbance
Gustavson	+	O	+	Microcephaly, short stature, optic atrophy with blindness, large ears, deafness, joint contractures, rockerbottom feet, brain undergrowth, hydrocephaly, cerebellar hypoplasia, spasticity
Pettigrew	+	O	+	Dandy-Walker malformation, microcephaly, long face with macrostomia, small testes, contractures, choreoathetosis, cerebellar hypoplasia, spastic paraplegia, iron deposits or calcification of basal ganglia
Hydrocephaly-Cerebellar Agenesis	+	O	+	Absent cerebellar hemispheres, hypotonia, cerebellar anomalies
Proud (*ARX*-Associated XLID)	O	+	+	Microcephaly, cryptorchidism, inguinal hernias, ataxia, dysgenesis of corpus callosum, impaired vision and/or hearing, spasticity
Lissencephaly and Abnormal Genitalia (*ARX*-Associated XLID)	O	+	+	Neuronal migration disturbance, agenesis of corpus callosum, hypotonia, early childhood death

HYDROCEPHALY-CEREBELLAR AGENESIS SYNDROME

(XLID-HYDROCEPHALUS-CEREBELLAR AGENESIS SYNDROME)

OMIM 307010

Definition. XLID with hydrocephaly, cerebellar agenesis, hypotonia, seizures, and early death. The gene has not been localized.

Somatic Features. No craniofacial manifestation, aside from enlarged head circumference secondary to hydrocephaly, has been described. In one case, rudimentary scrotum was present. Focal glomerulosclerosis and mild hemosiderin deposits in multiple organs were noted.

Growth and Development. Prenatal growth impairment in one case. Delivery by cesarian section is required because of hydrocephalus.

Neurological Findings. Hypotonia, areflexia, hyporeflexia, and seizures manifest almost immediately, and the infants die shortly after birth.

Neuropathology. Absent cerebellar hemispheres, thinning and gliosis of the cerebral cortex, absence of the foramina of Magendie and Luschka, and dilation of the lateral ventricles, aqueduct of Sylvius, foramin of Monro, and third and fourth ventricles were found at postmortem examination.

Comment. This entry is based on one family with three affected males, one of whom had postmortem examination. A hydrocephalic female second cousin related through males was presumed to have a coincidental unrelated hydrocephalus. The early demise of the affected males makes comparison with other X-linked conditions with cerebellar anomalies and hydrocephalus problematic. Based on a case of OFD II with cerebellar hypoplasia and hydrocephalus, it has been suggested that these two X-linked conditions may be allelic.

REFERENCES

Riccardi VM, Marcus ES: Congenital hydrocephalus and cerebellar agenesis. Clin Genet 13:443, 1978.
Stratton RF, Bluestone DL: Oto-palato-digital syndrome type II with X-linked cerebellar hypoplasia/hydrocephalus. Am J Med Genet 41:169, 1991.

DIFFERENTIAL MATRIX

Syndrome	Hydrocephaly	Cerebellar Anomalies	Seizures	Comments
Hydrocephaly-Cerebellar Agenesis	+	+	+	Absent cerebellar hemispheres, hypotonia
Cerebro-Cerebello-Coloboma	+	+	+	Hypotonia, abnormal respiratory pattern
Gustavson	+	+	+	Microcephaly, short stature, optic atrophy with blindness, large ears, deafness, joint contractures, rockerbottom feet, brain undergrowth, cerebellar hypoplasia, spasticity
Pettigrew	+	+	+	Dandy-Walker malformation, spasticity, microcephaly or hydrocephaly, long face with macrostomia, small testes, contractures, choreoathetosis, iron deposits in basal ganglia
Armfield	+	0	+	Short stature, cataracts or glaucoma, dental anomalies, small hands and feet, joint stiffness
Bertini	0	+	+	Macular degeneration, hypotonia, ataxia, childhood death, hypoplasia of cerebellar vermis and corpus callosum, developmental delays and regression, postnatal growth impairment
Christianson	0	+	+	Short stature, microcephaly, general asthenia, contractures, ophthalmoplegia
Paine	0	+	+	Microcephaly, short stature, optic atrophy, vision and hearing loss, spasticity

HYDROCEPHALY-MASA SPECTRUM

(COMPLICATED SPASTIC PARAPLEGIA, SPASTIC PARAPLEGIA 1, XLID-CLASP THUMB,
INTELLECTUAL DISABILITY-APLASIA-SHUFFLING GAIT-ADDUCTED THUMBS SYNDROME,
X-LINKED HYDROCEPHALUS-STENOSIS OF AQUEDUCT OF SYLVIUS, L1 SYNDROME,
X-LINKED PARTIAL AGENESIS OF CORPUS CALLOSUM)

OMIM 303350, 304100, 307000

Xq28

L1CAM

Definition. XLID with hydrocephalus, adducted thumbs, and spastic paraplegia.

Somatic Features. Severe hydrocephalus leads to intrauterine or neonatal death in many cases. Dilation of the cerebral ventricles, present in about half of survivors, underlies the variable macrocephaly. Dysgenesis of the corpus callosum has been noted in one-third of cases. Although a wide range of craniofacial features other than the large head size have been described, none is consistently present. Clasp thumb, secondary to deficiency of the extensor pollicis muscles or abductor pollicis muscles, or hypoplasia of the thumb with underdevelopment of the thenar eminence is found in most cases.

Growth and Development. In most cases, statural growth is normal but may measure in the lower centiles. Hip and knee flexion may falsely lower the height measurement. Macrocephaly of variable degree occurs and depends at least in part on dilation of the cerebral ventricles. Motor and speech milestones are mildly to moderately delayed. Slow motor development is most notable in males with hypotonia.

Cognitive Features. Impairment of cognitive function is quite variable, with some patients functioning in the lower range of normal and others having profound intellectual disability. There appears to be a correlation between the severity of cognitive impairment and degree of hydrocephaly.

Neurological Findings. Although motor and speech development is delayed from the outset, neurological changes are delayed in some patients until later in childhood or the teen years. Hypotonia in early childhood is associated with slow

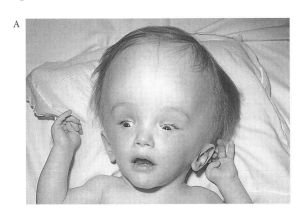
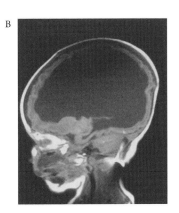
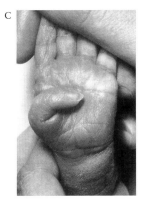
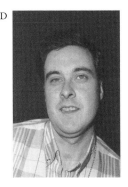
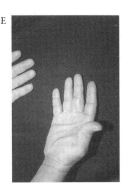
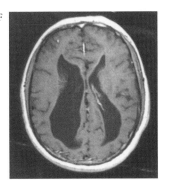
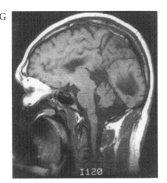

Hydrocephaly-MASA Spectrum. Infant showing massive hydrocephaly and clasp thumb (**A**); massive hydrocephaly on sagittal MRI (**B**); clasp thumb in newborn infant (**C**); 32-year-old with normal head circumference, facial asymmetry, and adducted thumbs (**D, E**); and MRI of 44-year-old uncle with hydrocephaly and agenesis of the corpus callosum (**F, G**).

motor development. Spasticity, manifested by hyperactive deep tendon reflexes, Babinski signs, and shuffling gait, and less so by increased muscle tone, usually begins in school age. The severity of intellectual disability tends to correlate with the degree of hydrocephaly and the level of spasticity.

Heterozygote Expression. Carrier females usually show no evidence of hydrocephaly, thumb anomalies, gait disturbance, spasticity, or cognitive impairment. Skewed X-inactivation has been suggested as the explanation for expression (cognitive function lower than noncarrier sisters, hydrocephalus, adducted thumbs) in a few carrier females.

Comment. Linkage analysis and mutational analysis of the *L1CAM* gene have permitted the inclusion of four entities previously considered separate (X-linked Hydrocephalus, MASA syndrome, XLID-Clasp Thumb syndrome, and Complicated Spastic Paraplegia 1) into a single spectrum. Preliminary evidence suggests that the phenotype can be correlated with the type of mutation affecting the *L1CAM* gene. Mutations that result in truncated L1CAM protein give rise to a severe phenotype. This probably results from the loss of the extracellular domain responsible for cell-cell and cell-matrix interactions. Mutations affecting the cytoplasmic domain at the carboxyl end are not as severe because only the cytoplasmic signal pathway is affected. Missense mutations in the extracellular domains produce a variety of phenotypes. The length of infant survival is associated with the location of missense mutations; those in key residues of either the immunoglobulin (Ig) or fibronectin (FN) domains result in survival of less than one year.

REFERENCES

Bertolin C, Boaretto F, Barbon G, et al.: Novel mutations in the L1CAM gene support the complexity of L1 syndrome. J Neurol Sci 294:124, 2010.

Bianchine JW, Lewis RC Jr: The MASA syndrome: a new heritable mental retardation syndrome. Clin Genet 5:298, 1974.

Bickers DA, Adams RD: Hereditary stenosis of the aqueduct of Sylvius as a cause of congenital hydrocephalus. Brain 72:246, 1949.

Boyd E, Schwartz CE, Schroer RJ, et al.: Agenesis of the corpus callosum associated with MASA syndrome. Clin Dysmorphol 2:332, 1993.

Finckh U, Schröder J, Ressler B, et al.: Spectrum and detection rate of L1CAM mutations in isolated and familial cases with clinically suspected L1-disease. Am J Med Genet 92:40, 2000.

Jouet M, Rosenthal A, MacFarlane J, et al.: A missense mutation confirms the L1 defect in X-linked hydrocephalus. Nat Genet 4:331, 1993.

Schrander-Stumpel C, Höweler C, Jones M, et al.: The spectrum of X-linked hydrocephalus (HSAS), MASA syndrome, and complicated spastic paraplegia (SPG1): clinical review with six additional families. Am J Med Genet 56:1, 1995.

Vits L, Van Camp G, Coucke P, et al.: MASA syndrome is due to mutations in the neural cell adhesion gene L1CAM. Nat Genet 7:408, 1994.

Vos YJ, de Walle HEK, Bos KK, et al.: Genotype-phenotype correlations in L1 syndrome: a guide for genetic counseling and mutation analysis. J Med Genet 47:169, 2010.

DIFFERENTIAL MATRIX

Syndrome	Hydro-cephaly	Dysgenesis of Corpus Callosum	Spasticity	Comments
Hydrocephaly-MASA Spectrum	+	+	+	Adducted thumbs
Juberg-Marsidi-Brooks	+	+	+	Microcephaly, short stature, deep-set eyes, blepharophimosis, cupped ears, bulbous nose, small mouth, thin upper lip, pectus excavatum, flexion contractures
Kang	+	+	+	Microcephaly, frontal prominence, telecanthus, small nose, short hands, seizures, downslanted mouth, brachydactyly
Proud (*ARX*-Associated XLID)	+	+	+	Microcephaly, hearing loss, vision loss, cryptorchidism, inguinal hernias, ataxia, seizures
Gustavson	+	0	+	Microcephaly, short stature, optic atrophy with blindness, large ears, deafness, joint contractures, rockerbottom feet, brain undergrowth, cerebellar hypoplasia, seizures
Pettigrew	+	0	+	Dandy-Walker malformation, microcephaly or hydrocephaly, long face with macrostomia and prognathism, small testes, contractures, choreoathetosis, iron deposits in basal ganglia, seizures
VACTERL-Hydrocephalus	+	0	+	Vertebral anomalies, radial limb defects, tracheal and esophageal anomalies, renal malformations, anal anomalies
AP1S2-Associated XLID	+	0	+	Calcifications of basal ganglia, muscle hypoplasia, sensory impairment
Pyruvate Dehydrogenase Deficiency	0	+	+	Microcephaly, ataxia, dysarthria, structural brain anomalies, hypotonia, lactic acidosis

HYPOPARATHYROIDISM, X-LINKED

OMIM 307700

Xq27.1

Definition. XLID with hypocalcemia, seizures, and cataracts secondary to hypoparathyroidism.

Somatic Features. No malformations or dysmorphism occurs. The endocrinopathy becomes apparent in the period of infancy with hypocalcemia, hyperphosphatemia, and seizures. If not treated, slow growth, delay of dental eruption, developmental failure, and cataracts ensue.

Growth and Development. With treatment, growth and development progress normally; without treatment, slowing of statural growth and development are to be expected.

Cognitive Function. Cognitive function depends on the promptness and consistency of treatment. Absent treatment, severe intellectual impairment may be expected.

Heterozygote Expression. None

Comment. Based on limited studies, the metabolic disturbance is caused by absence of parathormone which, in turn, results from absence of the parathyroid gland. Bowl et al. (2005) suggested that the hypoparathyroidism may be secondary to an interstitial deletion-insertion near the *SOX3* gene in Xq27.1.

REFERENCES

Bowl MR, Nesbit MA, Harding B, et al.: An interstitial deletion-insertion involving chromosomes 2p25.3 and Xq27.1, near SOX3, causes X-linked recessive hypoparathyroidism. J Clin Invest 115:2822, 2005.

Peden VH: True idiopathic hypoparathyroidism as a sex-linked recessive trait. Am J Hum Genet 12:323, 1960.

Thakker RV, Davies KE, Whyte MP, et al.: Mapping the gene causing X-linked recessive idiopathic hypoparathyroidism to Xq26-Xq27 by linkage studies. J Clin Invest 86:40, 1990.

Whyte MP, Weldon VV: Idiopathic hypoparathyroidism presenting with seizures during infancy: X-linked recessive inheritance in a large Missouri kindred. J Pediatr 99:608, 1981.

INCONTINENTIA PIGMENTI

(BLOCH-SULZBERGER SYNDROME)

OMIM 308310

Xq28

IKBKG (NEMO)

Definition. XLID associated with incontinentia pigmenti. The condition is caused by deletions or mutations in *IKBKG* (*NEMO*) and is one of the conditions that occur primarily in females.

Somatic Features. Pigmentary changes are required for the diagnosis. Typically, these changes are triphasic, beginning at birth or within the first 6 weeks of life as irregular crops of erythematous vesicular lesions. Within 6 to 8 weeks, these lesions become verrucous in nature and persist for several months. Irregular hyperpigmentation replaces the verrucous lesions and persist for years. The hyperpigmented skin follows the lines of Blaschko and histologically shows incontinence of pigment in the basal layer of the epidermis and phagocytosis of the dendritic processes of melanocytes. By adult life, the hyperpigmentation fades, leaving atrophic depigmented scarring.

A variety of neurological, ocular, and dental abnormalities have been reported. More than half of patients have microcephaly, mental retardation, spasticity, or seizures. Microphthalmia, strabismus, nystagmus, cataracts, optic atrophy, and blindness may occur. Oligodontia, abnormally shaped teeth, and delayed dental eruption are particularly common.

Growth and Development. Intrauterine and postnatal growth appears normal. Delay of developmental milestones occurs predominantly among cases with neurological manifestations.

Cognitive Function. Variable and dependent on involvement of the CNS. Those cases with seizures and/or spasticity are most likely to have cognitive impairment.

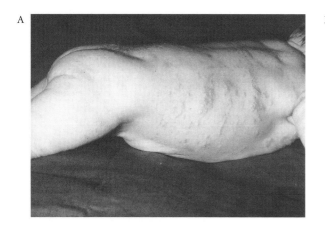
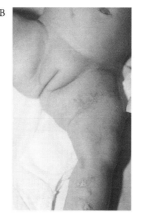
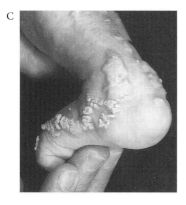
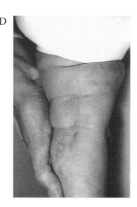
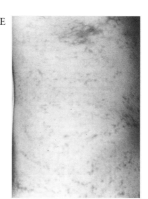

Incontinentia Pigmenti. Vesicular lesions (**A**), and verrucous lesions (**B, C**) during infancy. Residual hyperpigmented lesions during childhood (**D, E**).
Illustrations **A, C,** and **E** Courtesy of Dr. Robert G. Carney, Jr., Decatur, Illinois.

Comment. Incontinentia pigmenti usually occurs among females. Pedigrees showing a paucity of males and an increased number of spontaneous abortions lend support to the concept that it represents a dominant X-linked disorder with gestational lethality in males.

REFERENCES

Bloch B: Krankendemonstrationen aus der dermatologischen klinik Zürich. Schw Med Woch 57:404, 1926.

Carney RG: Incontinentia pigmenti. A world statistical analysis. Arch Dermatol 112:535, 1976.

Gilgenkrantz S, Tridon P, Pinel-Briquel N, et al.: Translocation (X;9) (p11;q34) in a girl with incontinentia pigmenti (IP): implications for the regional assignment of the IP locus to Xp11? Ann Genet 28:90, 1985.

Hodgson SV, Neville B, Jones RWA, et al.: Two cases of X autosome translocation in females with incontinentia pigmenti. Hum Genet 75:98, 1985.

Landy SJ, Donnai D: Incontinentia pigmenti (Block-Sulzberger syndrome). J Med Genet 30:53, 1993.

Lenz W: Half chromatid mutations may explain incontinentia pigmenti in males. Am J Hum Genet 27:690, 1975.

Sefiani A, Abel L, Heuertz S, et al.: The gene for incontinentia pigmenti is assigned to Xq28. Genomics 4:427, 1989.

Sulzberger MB: Über eine bisher nicht beschriebene congenitale Pigmentanomalie (Incontinentia pigmenti). Archiv Derm Syph 154:19, 1927.

The International Incontinentia Pigmenti (IP) Consortium: Genomic rearrangement in NEMO impairs NF-κB activation and is a cause of incontinentia pigmenti. Nature 405:466, 2000.

DIFFERENTIAL MATRIX

Syndrome	Cutaneous Changes	Ocular Anomalies	Dental Anomalies	Comments
Incontinentia Pigmenti	+	+	+	Cutaneous vesicles, verrucous lesions, and irregular hyperpigmentation, microcephaly, ocular anomalies, oligodontia, abnormally shaped teeth, spasticity, seizures
Goltz	+	+	+	Cataracts, ocular dysgenesis, linear areas of dermal aplasia, cutaneous adipose herniations, dystrophic nails, abnormal teeth and hair, vertebral anomalies, limb reduction defects, genitourinary anomalies
MIDAS	+	+	0	Microphthalmia, ocular dysgenesis, corneal opacification, dermal aplasia, dysgenesis of corpus callosum, cardiac defects, cardiomyopathy
Dyskeratosis Congenita	+	0	+	Short stature, alopecia, hyperpigmented lesions, palmar and plantar hyperkeratosis, mucosal leukoplakia, nail-ridging or splitting, pancytopenia, skin and mucosal lesions premalignant

JUBERG-MARSIDI-BROOKS SYNDROME

(SKLOWER-BROOKS SYNDROME, BROOKS-WISNIEWSKI-BROWN SYNDROME, JUBERG-MARSIDI SYNDROME)

OMIM 300612

Xp11.22

HUWE1

Definition. XLID with prenatal and postnatal undergrowth, microcephaly, bifrontal narrowing, blepharophimosis, cupped ears, bulbous nose, small mouth, flexion contractures, seizures, deafness, and hypotonia that in some cases progresses to spasticity. Mutations have been found in *HUWE1*, an E3 ubiquitin ligase gene.

Somatic Features. Abnormalities in all regions of the face contribute to the distinctive appearance. Bifrontal narrowing, deeply-set eyes, blepharophimosis or short palpebral fissures, epicanthus inversus, and, in some cases, hypotelorism characterize the upper face. A full or bulbous nose and low-set, retroverted, and cupped ears punctuate a flattened midface. An overall triangular lower face is further distinguished by a small mouth and mandible and a thin tented upper lip. The neck appears short and the posterior hairline low. Although microcephalic, the cerebral ventricles are enlarged, and dysgenesis of the corpus callosum may be noted on brain imaging. Undergrowth and decreased muscle bulk gives the appearance of generalized frailness. Pectus excavatum; contractures at the hips, elbows, and knees; and fifth-finger clinodactyly also occur.

Growth and Development. Intrauterine growth is retarded, with some infants weighing less than 2000 grams at birth. All parameters of postnatal growth are markedly slow. Development lags far behind. Speech is limited, if present at all. Some cases never achieve independent ambulation or continence.

Cognitive Function. Severe impairment

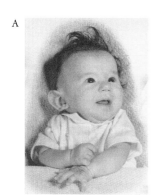
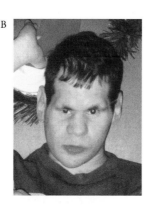
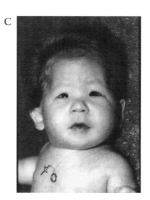
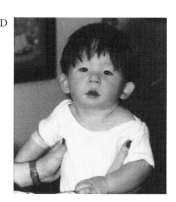
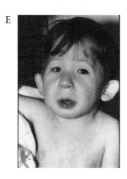
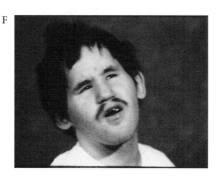

Juberg-Marsidi-Brooks Syndrome. Microcephaly, cupped ears and thin upper lip in infant and 27-year-old nephew from original family reported by Juberg and Marsidi (**A, B**). Microcephaly, blepharophimosis, deeply set eyes, depressed nasal bridge, simple cupped ears, and bulbous nasal tip in affected male at ages 4 months (**C**); 2 years (**D**); and 4 years (**E**). Affected uncle at age 14 years showing microcephaly, blepharophimosis, deeply set eyes, cupped ears (**F**). Illustrations C–F Courtesy of Dr. Susan Brooks, University of Medicine and Dentistry of New Jersey, New Brunswick.

Neurological Findings. Hypotonia is notable from infancy. Hyperreflexia and spasticity, especially of the lower limbs, become evident in infancy as well. Poor vision is associated with strabismus, nystagmus, myopia, and optic atrophy. Hearing loss occurs in some cases. Generalized seizures occasionally begin in infancy.

Heterozygote Expression. None

Imaging. Cranial CT and MRI show enlarged ventricles and dysgenesis of the corpus callosum.

Comment. Microcephaly in the presence of hydrocephaly attests to the marked underdevelopment of the brain. This is reflected in the general frailness, slow growth, and profound developmental failure in this syndrome. In these aspects and others, Juberg-Marsidi-Brooks syndrome is similar to Gustavson, Pettigrew, and Schimke syndromes.

Juberg and Marsidi (1980) reported three males with severe intellectual disability and growth impairment, cupped ears, deafness, epicanthus, strabismus, flat nasal bridge, arched upper lip, hypogenitalism, hypotonia, seizures, and deafness. Scoliosis and hip flexion became apparent in the teen years. Brain imaging was not obtained. Two of the three cases died in childhood.

The cases of Brooks et al. (1994) have quite similar facial findings, severe growth failure, hypotonia, seizures, and deafness. Both families have mutations in *HUWE1*, an E3 ubiquitin ligase gene located in Xp11.22. Duplications in *HUWE1* and adjacent genes have been associated with nonsyndromal XLID. Missense mutations have also been found in three other families including the XLID-macrocephaly syndrome reported by Turner et al. (1994), a family with moderate intellectual disability and normal facial appearance, and a family with severe intellectual disability, knee contractures, and facial characteristics in published photographs similar to Juberg-Marsidi-Brooks syndrome. A family considered to have Brooks syndrome by Morava et al. (1996) has not had molecular studies. The family considered by Mattei et al. (1983) to have Juberg-Marsidi syndrome has a mutation in *ATRX* and, hence, represents a misdiagnosis.

REFERENCES

Brooks SS, Wisniewski K, Brown WT: New X-linked mental retardation (XLMR) syndrome with distinct facial appearance and growth retardation. Am J Med Genet 51:586, 1994.

Froyen G, Corbett M, Vandewalle J, et al.: Submicroscopic duplications of the hydroxysteroid dehydrogenase HSD17B10 and the E3 ubiquitin ligase HUWE1 are associated with mental retardation. Am J Hum Genet 82:432, 2008.

Juberg RC, Marsidi I: A new form of X-linked mental retardation with growth retardation, deafness, and microgenitalism. Am J Hum Genet 32:714, 1980.

Mattéi JF, Collignon P, Ayme S, et al.: X-linked mental retardation, growth retardation, deafness and microgenitalism. A second familial report. Clin Genet 23:70, 1983.

Morava E, Storcz J, Kosztolányi G: X-linked mental retardation syndrome: Three brothers with the Brooks-Wisniewski-Brown syndrome. Am J Med Genet 64:59, 1996.

Turner G, Gedeon A, Mulley J: X-linked mental retardation with heterozygous expression and macrocephaly: pericentromeric gene localization. Am J Med Genet 51:575, 1994.

DIFFERENTIAL MATRIX

Syndrome	Microcephaly and Hydrocephaly	Spasticity	Seizures	Comments
Juberg-Marsidi-Brooks	+	+	+	Short stature, dysgenesis of corpus callosum, deep-set eyes, blepharophimosis, cupped ears, bulbous nose, small mouth, thin upper lip, pectus excavatum, flexion contractures
Gustavson	+	+	+	Short stature, optic atrophy with blindness, large ears, deafness, joint contractures, rockerbottom feet, brain undergrowth, cerebellar hypoplasia
Pettigrew	+	+	+	Dandy-Walker malformation, microcephaly or hydrocephaly, long face with macrostomia and prognathism, small testes, contractures, choreoathetosis, iron deposits in basal ganglia
Schimke	+	+	0	Sunken eyes, downslanting palpebral fissures, narrow nose, wide spacing of teeth, cupped ears, hypotonia, abducens palsy, hearing loss, vision loss, choreoathetosis, contractures
CK	+	0	+	Asthenic build, neuronal migration disturbance, hypotonia, long thin face, scoliosis, behavior problems

KANG SYNDROME
(X-LINKED AGENESIS OF CORPUS CALLOSUM)

Definition. XLID with microcephaly, frontal prominence, telecanthus, downturned mouth, short broad hands with brachydactyly, agenesis of corpus callosum, and spastic diplegia. The gene has not been localized.

Somatic Features. The face appears broad with frontal prominence, telecanthus, small nose with anteverted nares, and downturned mouth. Microcephaly or hydrocephaly occurs with malformations of the brain (agenesis of corpus callosum, interhemispheric cysts, gyral dysplasia, and lateral displacement of the ventricles). One case had unilateral cataract. The hands are short and broad, with short fingers and single flexion creases on the fifth fingers. The genitalia appear normal. Spastic diplegia ensues.

Growth and Development. Details of postnatal growth and development have not been reported. Birth weights appear normal.

Cognitive Function. Mild impairment

Neurological Findings. Spastic diplegia becomes evident during infancy.

Heterozygote Expression. None

Imaging. Ultrasound and CT show dysgenesis of the corpus callosum, interhemispheric cysts, dilation of the lateral and third ventricles, and cortical gyral dysplasia.

Comment. Although dysgenesis of the corpus callosum may be found in apparently asymptomatic individuals in the general population, this developmental anomaly occurs more commonly among individuals with intellectual disability and especially among the subgroup with metabolic errors. Other anomalies of the CNS often accompany dysgenesis of the corpus callosum and may be responsible for neurological symptoms. Complete or partial agenesis of the corpus callosum occurs inconsistently in a number of XLID syndromes: Aicardi, Cerebro-Oculo-Genital, Goltz, Lujan, MIDAS, Optiz FG and Oral-Facial-Digital I syndromes and Pyruvate Dehydrogenase Deficiency, X-Linked Hydrocephaly-MASA Spectrum and *ARX*-Associated XLID. As such, it seems a helpful but nonmandatory clue to diagnosis.

REFERENCES

Bamforth F, Bamforth S, Poskitt K, et al.: Abnormalities of corpus callosum in patients with inherited metabolic diseases. Lancet 2:451, 1988.

Fratelli N, Papageorghiou AT, Prefumo F, et al.: Outcome of prenatally diagnosed agenesis of the corpus callosum. Prenat Diagn 27:512, 2007.

Grogono JL: Children with agenesis of the corpus callosum. Dev Med Child Neurol 10:613, 1968.

Kang W-M, Huang C-C, Lin S-J: X-linked recessive inheritance of dysgenesis of corpus callosum in a Chinese Family. Am J Med Genet 44:619, 1992.

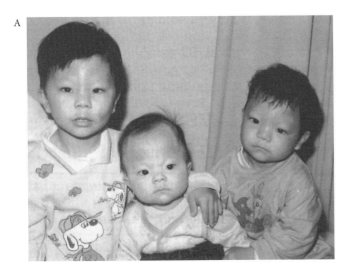
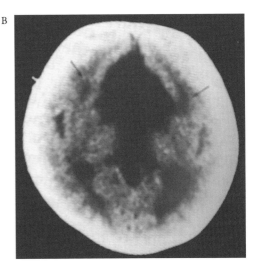

Kang Syndrome. Affected brothers at ages 8 years (*left*) and 3 years (*right*) and maternal cousin at age 8 months (*center*), showing frontal prominence, telecanthus, broad nasal root, and downturned mouth (A); cranial tomography of infant at age 8 months showing a large interhemispheric cyst and displacement of lateral ventricles [*arrows*] (B).   Courtesy of Dr. Shio-Jean Lin, National Cheng Kung University Hospital, Taiwan.

Syndrome	Microcephaly	Dysgenesis of Corpus Callosum	Spastic Paraplegia	Comments
Kang	+	+	+	Frontal prominence, telecanthus, small nose, short hands, seizures, downslanted mouth, brachydactyly
Proud (*ARX*-Associated XLID)	+	+	+	Hearing loss, vision loss, cryptorchidism, inguinal hernias, ataxia, seizures
Pyruvate Dehydrogenase Deficiency	+	+	+	Microcephaly, ataxia, dysarthria, structural brain anomalies, hypotonia, lactic acidosis
Goltz	+	+	0	Cataracts, ocular dysgenesis, linear areas of dermal aplasia, cutaneous adipose herniations, dystrophic nails, abnormal teeth and hair, vertebral anomalies, limb reduction defects, genitourinary anomalies
Paine	+	0	+	Short stature, optic atrophy, vision and hearing loss, seizures
Pettigrew	+	0	+	Dandy-Walker malformation, microcephaly or hydrocephaly, long face with macrostomia and prognathism, small testes, contractures, choreoathetosis, iron deposits in basal ganglia, seizures
Schimke	+	0	+	Sunken eyes, downslanting palpebral fissures, narrow nose, wide spacing of teeth, cupped ears, hypotonia, abducens palsy, hearing loss, vision loss, spasticity, choreoathetosis, contractures
Hydrocephaly-MASA Spectrum	0	+	+	Hydrocephaly, adducted thumbs

LENZ MICROPHTHALMIA SYNDROME

(LENZ SYNDROME)

OMIM 309800

Definition. XLID with microcephaly, microphthalmia, malformed or cupped ears, cleft lip and cleft palate, dental anomalies, urogenital anomalies, narrow shoulders, duplication of the thumbs, or other digital malformations and spinal curvature. One gene locus has been found in Xq27-q28. Mutations in *BCOR*, which is located in Xp11.4, have been reported in two families.

Somatic Features. The facies appear normal with the exception of asymmetric and often colobomatous microphthalmia, blepharoptosis, and dysplastic ears. The colobomas may extend to the optic disc, and retinal detachment, lens dislocation, and cataract may be present. The ears may be simply formed and cupped or small and dysplastic. Thumb duplication or hypoplasia is the usual hand malformation. Syndactyly, camptodactyly, and clinodactyly may affect hands and feet. A variety of urogenital anomalies have included renal agenesis, hydronephrosis, hypospadias, and cryptorchidism. Cleft lip and palate, crowding or wide spacing of the teeth, and cardiac malformations are seen in a minority of cases. Sloping shoulders, thinning of the lateral third of the clavicle, barrel chest, kyphoscoliosis, and gibbus anomaly are common.

Growth and Development. Detailed information on growth is not available. Some affected males have intrauterine growth impairment. All parameters of postnatal growth appear slow, with measurements ultimately falling below the 3rd centile. Developmental milestones are globally but variably delayed.

Cognitive Function. Some degree of cognitive impairment occurs in all cases, but considerable variation in severity has been reported.

Heterozygote Expression. Carrier females may have short stature, microcephaly, and digital anomalies.

Imaging. No intracranial malformations have been described.

Comment. Lenz Microphthalmia syndrome may be distinguished from other X-linked microphthalmia syndromes on the basis of associated manifestations. Norrie disease has congenital and bilateral blindness, retinal dysplasia, progressing to collapse of the ocular globe and hearing loss. Goltz syndrome has dermal aplasia, cutaneous herniations of fat, and dysplasia of other ectodermal tissues and is expressed in females only. MIDAS syndrome, another disorder with female limited expression, has linear areas of dermal aplasia, CNS and cardiac malformations, and cardiomyopathy.

There appears to be locus heterogeneity among the families with Lenz Microphthalmia. A mutation in *BCOR*, located in Xp11.4, was found in two families but has not been found in other families. Mutations in *BCOR* are responsible for Oculofaciocardiodental syndrome, a syndrome with overlapping somatic manifestations but with milder intellectual disability, if at all. A second gene locus in Xq27-q28 overlaps with the locus for Graham Anophthalmia, suggesting that these two XLID syndromes may be allelic.

REFERENCES

Forrester S, Kovach MJ, Reynolds NM, et al.: Manifestations in four males with and an obligate carrier of the Lenz microphthalmia syndrome. Am J Med Genet 98:92, 2001.

Glanz A, Forse A, Polomeno RC, et al.: Lenz microphthalmia: A malformation syndrome with variable expression of multiple congenital anomalies. Can J Ophthalmol 18:41, 1983.

Hilton E, Johnston J, Whalen S, et al.: BCOR analysis in patients with OFCD and Lenz microphthalmia syndromes, mental retardation with ocular anomalies, and cardiac laterality defects. Eur J Hum Genet 17:1325, 2009.

Horn D, Chyrek M, Kleier S, et al.: Novel mutations in BCOR in three patients with oculo-facio-cardio-dental syndrome, but none in Lenz microphthalmia syndrome. Eur J Hum Genet 13:563, 2005.

Lenz W: Recessiv-geschlechtsgebundene mikrophthalmie mit multiplen mißbildungen. Zeit Kinderheil 77:384, 1955. (Translation in Proc Greenwood Genet Ctr 17:5, 1998.)

Ng D, Thakker N, Corcoran CM, et al.: Oculofaciocardiodental and Lenz microphthalmia syndromes result from distinct classes of mutations in BCOR. Nat Genet 36:411, 2004.

Traboulsi EI, Lenz W, Gonzales-Ramos M, et al.: The Lenz microphthalmia syndrome. Am J Ophthalmol 105:40, 1988.

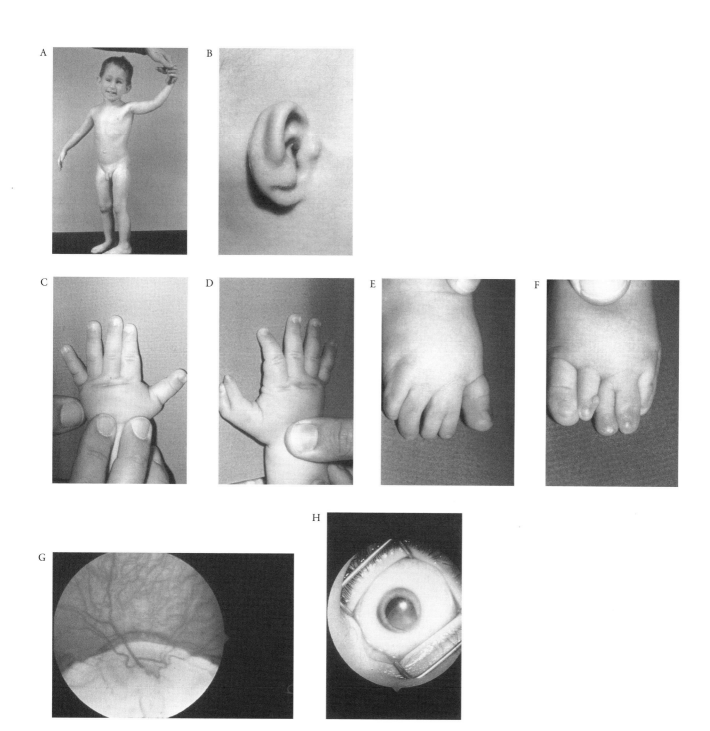

Lenz Microphthalmia Syndrome. Three-year-old male with bilateral microphthalmia, more severe on the right, short palpebral fissure on right, cupped ears, and hypoplastic thumbs (**A**); manifestations in a second patient showing dysplastic ears, preaxial polydactyly, syndactyly, choreoretinal coloboma involving the nerve head and iris coloboma with subluxed lens (**B–H**).   Courtesy of Dr. Elias Traboulsi, Cleveland Clinic, Cleveland.

DIFFERENTIAL MATRIX

Syndrome	Ocular Anomaly	Limb Anomaly	Urogenital Anomaly	Comments
Lenz Microphthalmia	+	+	+	Microcephaly, malformed ears, cleft lip/palate, cardiac anomalies, thumb duplication or hypoplasia, narrow shoulders
Goltz	+	+	+	Linear areas of dermal aplasia, cutaneous adipose herniations, dystrophic nails, abnormal teeth and hair, vertebral anomalies
Cerebro-Oculo-Genital	+	0	+	Microcephaly, hydrocephaly, short stature, agenesis of corpus callosum, microphthalmia, ptosis, hypospadias, cryptorchidism, clubfoot, spasticity
Lowe	+	0	+	Short stature, hypotonia, aminoaciduria, progressive renal disease
Wittwer	+	0	+	Microcephaly, short stature, hearing loss, hypertelorism, hypotonia, seizures

LESCH-NYHAN SYNDROME

(XLID-HYPERURICEMIA, HYPOXANTHINE GUANINE PYROPHOSPHATE RIBOSYL TRANSFERASE DEFICIENCY)

OMIM 300322

Xq26.2

HPRT

Definition. XLID with uric acid urinary stones, spasticity, choreoathetosis, seizures, and self-mutilation, associated with hyperuricemia.

Somatic Features. Malformations and developmental abnormalities of the craniofacial structures do not occur. The lips and tongue may be irregular, avulsed, or scarred secondary to biting. The digits may be similarly mutilated. Hematuria, crystalluria, and stones result from hyperuricemia.

Growth and Development. Intrauterine growth is normal. There is a tendency toward poor weight gain and general asthenia, but the head circumference and length are usually normal. Profound developmental failure accompanied by choreoathetoid and dystonic movement becomes obvious by age 6 months. In most cases, speech and independent sitting or ambulation are never achieved.

Cognitive Function. Variable cognitive impairments have been documented with IQ measurements between 40 and 65.

Behavior. Uncontrollable urge to self-mutilation by biting constitutes the most dramatic behavioral abnormality. Patients may attempt injury to their heads or limbs and appear unusually aggressive toward others in their environment.

Neurological Findings. Constant involuntary movements dominate the neurological phenotype. Choreoathetoid movement of the fingers, flailing movement of the limbs, excessive startle reactions, and opisthotonic posturing are interrupted only by sleep. Spasticity with hypertonicity, increased deep tendon reflexes, clonus, and Babinski signs dates from infancy but usually becomes notable after choreoathetosis is well-established. Most distressing is the self-mutilation of the lips and digits from biting, a clearly painful phenomenon that usually begins after age 2 years. Seizures occur in about half of cases.

Imaging. Brain malformations do not occur, but the overall brain size may be small and the ventricles mildly dilated.

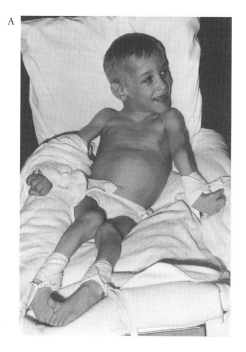
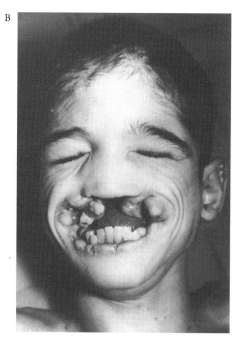

Lesch-Nyhan Syndrome. Seven-year-old boy with inability to sit without support, choreoathetoid posturing of the upper limbs, and spasticity; restraints are used to prevent mutilation **(A)**; 14-year-old boy with extreme facial mutilation from biting **(B)**.   Courtesy of Dr. William Nyhan, University of California, San Diego, La Jolla.

Laboratory. Excessive production of uric acid leads to hyperuricemia, excessive urinary excretion of uric acid, elevated urinary uric acid:creatine ratios, crystalluria, and uric acid stones. A megaloblastic anemia occurs in a minority of cases.

Comment. Although self-injury is a common phenomenon among persons with severe intellectual disability, self-mutilation by biting appears unique to individuals with Lesch-Nyhan syndrome. They do not appear to have any reduction in sensation to pain. No therapy has been successful, other than protection against self-mutilation by tooth extraction and wrapping of the hands.

REFERENCES

Ceballos-Picot I, Mockel L, Potier MC, et al.: Hypoxanthine-guanine phosphoribosyl transferase regulates early developmental programming of dopamine neurons: implications for Lesch-Nyhan disease pathogenesis. Hum Mol Genet 18:2317, 2009.

Hoefnagel D, Andrew ED, Mireault NG, et al.: Hereditary choreoathetosis, self-mutilation and hyperuricemia in young males. New Eng J Med 273:130, 1965.

Lesch M, Nyhan WL: A familial disorder of uric acid metabolism and central nervous system function. Am J Med 36:561, 1964.

DIFFERENTIAL MATRIX

Syndrome	Spasticity	Choreo-athetosis	Seizures	Comments
Lesch-Nyhan	+	+	+	Self-mutilation, hyperuricemia
Pettigrew	+	+	+	Dandy-Walker malformation, microcephaly or hydrocephaly, long face with macrostomia and prognathism, small testes, contractures, iron deposits in basal ganglia
Proud (*ARX*-Associated XLID)	+	+	+	Microcephaly, hearing loss, vision loss, agenesis of corpus callosum, cryptorchidism, inguinal hernias, ataxia
XLID-Spastic Paraplegia-Athetosis	+	+	+	Nystagmus, weakness, dysarthria, muscle wasting, contractures
Allan-Herndon-Dudley	+	+	0	Large ears with cupping or abnormal architecture, muscle hypoplasia, childhood hypotonia, contractures, dysarthria, athetosis, ataxia
Schimke	+	+	0	Microcephaly, sunken eyes, downslanting palpebral fissures, narrow nose, wide spacing of teeth, cupped ears, hypotonia, abducens palsy, hearing loss, vision loss, contractures
Goldblatt Spastic Paraplegia	+	0	+	Optic atrophy, exotropia, nystagmus, ataxia, dysarthria, muscle hypoplasia, contractures
Gustavson	+	0	+	Microcephaly, short stature, optic atrophy with blindness, large ears, deafness, joint contractures, rockerbottom feet, brain undergrowth, hydrocephaly, cerebellar hypoplasia
Paine	+	0	+	Microcephaly, short stature, optic atrophy, vision and hearing loss
Pelizaeus-Merzbacher	+	0	+	Optic atrophy, nystagmus, hypotonia, ataxia, dystonia, CNS dysmyelination
Ataxia-Deafness-Dementia, X-linked	+	0	+	Optic atrophy, vision loss, hearing loss, ataxia, hypotonia, childhood death

LISSENCEPHALY AND ABNORMAL GENITALIA, X-LINKED (*SEE ALSO ARX*-ASSOCIATED XLID)

OMIM 300215

Xp21.3

ARX

Definition. XLID associated with lissencephaly, agenesis of the corpus callosum, seizures, hypothalamic dysfunction, and abnormal genitalia.

Somatic Features. Mild craniofacial dysmorphism may be present, including low forehead and micrognathia. The genitalia show microphallus, hypospadias, cryptorchidism, or may be undifferentiated or indeterminate.

Growth and Development. Birth growth parameters are typically in the 5th to 25th centiles, but profound delays and brain anomalies lead to poor growth and microcephaly. Most affected males die by age 6 months.

Cognitive Function. Profound developmental failure. Early death may prevent adequate assessment of cognitive function.

Neurological Findings. Hypotonia and intractable seizures present in the early neonatal period.

Heterozygote Expression. Some carrier females may have absence or hypoplasia of the corpus callosum, mild intellectual disability, and seizures.

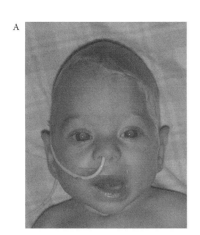
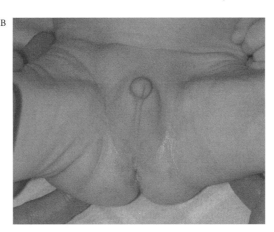
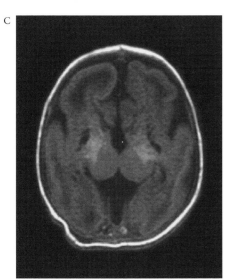
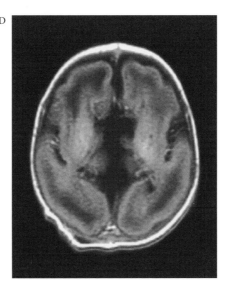

Lissencephaly and Abnormal Genitalia, X-linked. Infant with upsweep of frontal hair but otherwise normal face (**A**), and hypoplasia of the genitalia with hypospadias and thickened penoscrotal raphe (**B**). MR images showing lissencephaly with posterior agyria and frontal pachygyria, moderately thick cortex, cavitation of basal ganglia, enlarged third ventricles, and agenesis of the corpus callosum (**C, D**).   Courtesy of Dr. William Dobyns, Seattle Children's Research Institute, Seattle.

Imaging. Cranial imaging demonstrates lissencephaly with the posterior cortex more severely affected. The cortex is mildly to moderately thickened and the corpus callosum is absent. The lateral ventricles are usually enlarged.

Neuropathology. A trilayered cortex containing pyramidal neurons, neuronal migration defects, disorganized basal ganglia, and gliotic and spongy white matter is seen.

Comments. XLAG is the most severe entity of the *ARX*-Associated disorders. Deletions and nonsense mutations lead to loss of gene function and the severe phenotype. A consistent genotype-phenotype correlation has been documented. Missense mutations are usually associated with Proud Syndrome (agenesis of the corpus callosum and abnormal genitalia), and a recurrent in-frame 24-base pair duplication in a polyalanine tract in exon 2 is typically associated with a nonmalformation neurological phenotype in which intellectual disability presents with infantile spasms (West syndrome), dystonia (Partington syndrome), or autism. Isolated intellectual disability may also be seen, and mutations of *ARX* are the most common cause of intellectual disability in the reported nonsyndromal (MRX) families.

ARX, a transcriptional regulator gene, is expressed in the forebrain and testes and is important in neuronal proliferation and migration. It plays a central role in cerebral development and patterning and has a secondary role in testis development.

REFERENCES

Bhat SS, Rogers RC, Holden KR, et al.: A novel in-frame deletion in *ARX* is associated with lissencephaly with absent corpus callosum and hypoplastic genitalia. Am J Med Genet 15:70, 2005.

Bonneau D, Toutain A, Laquerriere A, et al.: X-linked lissencephaly with absent corpus callosum and ambiguous genitalia (XLAG): clinical, magnetic resonance imaging, and neuropathological findings. Ann Neurol 51:340, 2002.

Dobyns WB, Berry-Kravis E, Havernick NJ, et al.: X-linked lissencephaly with absent corpus callosum and ambiguous genitalia. Am J Med Genet 86:331, 1999.

Friocourt G, Poirier K, Rakic S, et al.: The role of ARX in cortical development. Eur J Neurosci 23:869, 2006.

Kato M, Das S, Petras K, et al.: Mutations of ARX are associated with striking pleiotropy and consistent genotype-phenotype correlation. Hum Mutat 23:147, 2004.

DIFFERENTIAL MATRIX

Syndrome	Dysgenesis of Corpus Callosum	Seizures	Neuronal Migration Disturbance	Comments
Lissencephaly and Abnormal Genitalia (*ARX*-Associated XLID)	+	+	+	Abnormal genitalia, hypotonia, early childhood death
Aicardi	+	+	+	Ocular dysgenesis, lacunar retinopathy, costovertebral anomalies
Lissencephaly, X-linked	+	+	+	Hypotonia, spasticity, genital hypoplasia, subcortical band heterotopia in carrier females
Bertini	+	+	0	Macular degeneration, hypotonia, ataxia, childhood death, hypoplasia of cerebellar vermis and corpus callosum, developmental delays and regression, postnatal growth impairment
Juberg-Marsidi-Brooks	+	+	0	Microcephaly, short stature, deep-set eyes, blepharophimosis, cupped ears, bulbous nose, small mouth, thin upper lip, pectus excavatum, flexion contractures
Kang	+	+	0	Microcephaly, frontal prominence, telecanthus, small nose, short hands, downslanted mouth, brachydactyly
Proud (*ARX*-Associated XLID)	+	+	0	Microcephaly, hearing loss, vision loss, cryptorchidism, inguinal hernias, ataxia, spasticity
Pyruvate Deyhydrogenase Deficiency	+	+	0	Microcephaly, ataxia, dysarthria, structural brain anomalies, hypotonia, lactic acidosis
CK	0	+	+	Microcephaly, long thin face, scoliosis, asthenic build, seizures, hypotonia, behavior problems

LISSENCEPHALY, X-LINKED

(X-LINKED LISSENCEPHALY-AGENESIS OF CORPUS CALLOSUM, SUBCORTICAL BAND HETEROTOPIA)

OMIM 300067

Xq22.3

DCX

Definition. XLID with microcephaly, defect in neuronal migration, hypoplastic genitalia, hypotonia, spasticity, and seizures.

Somatic Features. The craniofacial features are not distinctive and major malformations outside the central nervous system do not occur. Cranial size is small, and the brain has variable evidence of defective neural migration. In males, this is usually evident as frontal pachygyria and in females as subcortical band heterotopia. Less commonly, males have agyria, polymicrogyria, and dysgenesis of the corpus callosum. The genitalia are underdeveloped.

Growth and Development. Males have very limited development and have failure of growth including microcephaly.

Neurological Findings. Beginning soon after birth, males develop seizures of various types – tonic, tonic-clonic, myoclonic, and infantile spasms. Hypotonia, spasticity, or both (truncal hypotonia with hypertonia and hyperreflexia of the limbs) occur.

Natural History. Seizures begin soon after birth and are poorly controlled by anticonvulsants. There is little psychomotor progress, limited environmental interaction, poor growth, and death occurs the first year of life, usually in the first months.

Heterozygote Expression. Females often have mild-to-moderate intellectual disability, but some have normal intelligence and others severe intellectual disability. In childhood, there may be psychomotor delay, behavioral problems, and hyperactivity. Seizures usually begin in childhood but may not begin until young adulthood and are of various types – tonic, tonic-clonic, atonic, atypical absence, partial complex, infantile spasms, and Lennox-Gastaut.

Imaging. In males, pachygyria (particularly frontal), agyria (posterior), agenesis of corpus callosum, dilated ventricles, and cerebellar vermis hypoplasia occurs. In females, there is a layer of gray matter heterotopia between the cortex and ventricles, separated from the cortex by white matter. The thickness of this heterotopic band correlates with the severity of the cognitive impairment and of the seizures.

Neuropathology. Neuronal migration defect with agyria and pachygyria in males and subcortical band heterotopia in females.

Comment. Although some of the clinical manifestations of the X-linked disorders of neuronal migration overlap, other clinical findings and brain imaging should allow them to be differentiated. Mutation analysis of *ARX*, *DCX* and *FLNA* is available for the three most common of these disorders.

REFERENCES

Berry-Kravis E, Israel J: X-linked pachygyria and agenesis of the corpus callosum: Evidence for X chromosome lissencephaly locus. Ann Neurol 36:229, 1994.

des Portes V, Pinard JM, Billuart P, et al.: A novel CNS gene required for neuronal migration and involved in X-linked subcortical laminar heterotopia and lissencephaly syndrome. Cell 92:51, 1998.

des Portes V, Pinard JM, Smadja D, et al.: Dominant X linked subcortical laminar heterotopia and lissencephaly syndrome (XSCLH/LIS): Evidence for the occurrence of mutation in males and mapping of a potential locus in Xq22. J Med Genet 34:177, 1997.

Dobyns WB, Andermann E, Andermann F, et al.: X-linked malformations of neuronal migration. Neurology 47:321, 1996.

Gleeson JG, Allen KM, Fox JW, et al.: *Doublecortin*, a brain specific gene mutated in human X-linked lissencephaly and double cortex syndrome, encodes a putative signaling protein. Cell 92:63, 1998.

Haverfield EV, Whited AJ, Petras KS, et al,: Intragenic deletions and duplications of the LIS1 and DCX genes: a major disease-causing mechanism in lissencephaly and subcortical band heterotopia. Eur J Hum Genet 17:911, 2009.

Sossey-Alaoui K, Hartung AJ, Guerrini R, et al.: Human *doublecortin (DCX)* and the homologous gene in mouse encode a putative Ca²⁺-dependent signaling protein which is mutated in human X-linked neuronal migration defects. Hum Mol Genet 7:1327, 1998.

Srivastava AK, Ross ME, Allen KM, et al.: X-linked lissencephaly and SBH (XLIS): Mapping of a novel neuronal migration gene. Am J Hum Genet 59(Suppl):A55, 1996.

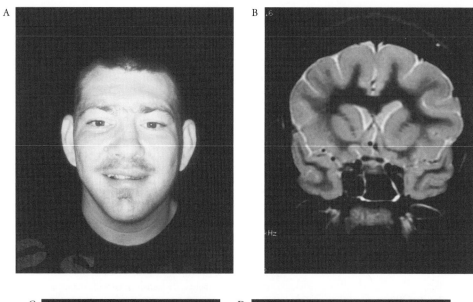

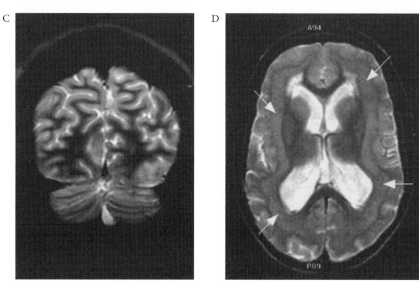

Lissencephaly, X-linked. Microcephaly, upslanted palpebral fissures, and otherwise normal facies in a 32-year-old male (A); coronal section of frontal cortex as seen with MRI showing pachygyria (B); coronal section from posterior parietal cortex showing normal gyral pattern (C); axial section from carrier female showing subcortical band heterotopia [*arrows*] (D).   Illustration D Courtesy of Dr. Joseph Gleeson, Beth Israel Deaconess Medical Center, Boston.

Syndrome	Dysgenesis of Corpus Callosum	Seizures	Neuronal Migration Disturbance	Comments
Lissencephaly, X-linked	+	+	+	Hypotonia, spasticity, genital hypoplasia, subcortical band heterotopia in carrier females
Aicardi	+	+	+	Ocular dysgenesis, lacunar retinopathy, costovertebral anomalies
Lissencephaly and Abnormal Genitalia (*ARX*-Associated XLID)	+	+	+	Abnormal genitalia, hypotonia, early childhood death
Bertini	+	+	0	Macular degeneration, hypotonia, ataxia, childhood death, hypoplasia of cerebellar vermis and corpus callosum, developmental delays and regression, postnatal growth impairment
Juberg-Marsidi-Brooks	+	+	0	Microcephaly, short stature, deep-set eyes, blepharophimosis, cupped ears, bulbous nose, small mouth, thin upper lip, pectus excavatum, flexion contractures
Kang	+	+	0	Microcephaly, frontal prominence, telecanthus, small nose, short hands, downslanted mouth, brachydactyly
Proud (*ARX*-Associated XLID)	+	+	0	Microcephaly, hearing loss, vision loss, cryptorchidism, inguinal hernias, ataxia, spasticity
Pyruvate Deyhdrogenase Deficiency	+	+	0	Microcephaly, ataxia, dysarthria, structural brain anomalies, hypotonia, lactic acidosis
CK	0	+	+	Microcephaly, long thin face, scoliosis, asthenic build, seizures, hypotonia, behavior problems

LOWE SYNDROME
(OCULO-CEREBRO-RENAL SYNDROME)

OMIM 309000

Xq25

OCRL1

Definition. XLID with short stature, cataracts, renal tubular dysfunction, and hypotonia. The gene, *OCRL1*, encodes for phosphotidylinisotol 4,5-bisphospate 5-phosphatase.

Somatic Features. Congenital cataracts provide the initial diagnostic lead in almost all cases. The eyes may appear deepset and in time may develop glaucoma and corneal keloids. These ocular features, frontal prominence with normal head circumference, marked hypotonia, and areflexia comprise the phenotype in infancy and early childhood. Progressive renal disease ultimately leads to death. During childhood, tubular dysfunction is manifest by urinary loss of protein, amino acids, carnitine, and phosphate. Glomerular function is little affected during childhood but steadily declines during the adult years. Metabolic disturbances from the renal dysfunction may result in undermineralization, fractures, and rickets. Renal failure occurs during the fourth decade.

Growth and Development. Intrauterine growth appears normal, but linear growth falls below the 3rd centile by age 1 to 3 years. Weight follows a similar pattern, although normal weight may persist for the first few years. Head circumference may remain in the mid-centiles in the preschool years, fall to or below the lower centiles in late childhood, but thereafter gain toward the mean.

Cognitive Function. Moderate-to-severe impairment generally occurs, although one-fourth of cases will score 70 or higher on IQ tests.

Behavior. Maladaptive behavior consisting of stubbornness, temper tantrums, and repetitive shaking of the limbs occurs in many cases.

Heterozygote Expression. Carrier females can be identified by fine opacities in the lens. Slit lamp examination may be required.

Laboratory. Proteinuria, aminoaciduria, and low urine osmolality are the first evidence of tubular dysfunction. There are subsequent excess renal losses of bicarbonate phosphate, potassium, and carnitine. Metabolic acidosis, hypophosphatemia, hypokalemia, and low serum carnitine

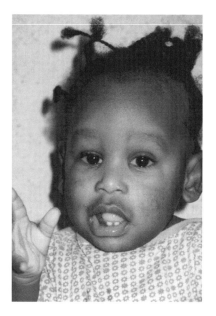

Lowe Syndrome. Fifteen-month-old male with cataracts, epicanthus, and hypotonia.

result. With glomerular involvement, there is progressive evidence of renal insufficiency.

Comment. Manifestations are present from birth and follow a predictable course. Because of the cataracts and renal tubular dysfunction, Lowe syndrome may be readily differentiated from other hypotonia syndromes. Abnormalities of the actin cytoskeleton have been documented in patients with Lowe syndrome.

REFERENCES

Attree O, Olivos IM, Okabe I, et al.: The Lowe's oculocerebrorenal syndrome gene encodes a protein highly homologous to inositol polyphosphate-5-phosphatase. Nature 358:239, 1992.

Charnas LR, Bernardini I, Rader D, et al.: Clinical and laboratory findings in the oculocerebrorenal syndrome of Lowe, with special reference to growth and renal function. New Eng J Med 324:1318, 1991.

Lowe CU, Terrey M, MacLachlan EA: Organic-aciduria, decreased renal ammonia production, hydrophthalmos, and mental retardation: A clinical entity. Am J Dis Child 83:164, 1952.

Mueller OT, Hartsfield JK Jr, Gallardo LA, et al.: Lowe oculocerebrorenal syndrome in a female with a balanced X;20 translocation: Mapping of the X chromosome breakpoint. Am J Hum Genet 49:804, 1991.

Suchy SF, Nussbaum RL: The deficiency of PIP2 5-phosphatase in Lowe syndrome affects actin polymerization. Am J Hum Genet 71:1420, 2002.

DIFFERENTIAL MATRIX

Syndrome	Ocular Anomaly	Renal Dysfunction or Anomalies	Hypotonia	Comments
Lowe	+	+	+	Short stature, cataracts, aminoaciduria, progressive renal failure
Wittwer	+	+	+	Microcephaly, short stature, microphthalmia, hearing loss, vision loss, hypertelorism, genitourinary anomalies, seizures
Cerebro-Oculo-Genital	+	+	0	Microcephaly, hydrocephaly, short stature, agenesis of corpus callosum, microphthalmia, ptosis, hypospadias, cryptorchidism, clubfoot, spasticity
Goltz	+	+	0	Cataracts, ocular dysgenesis, linear areas of dermal aplasia, cutaneous adipose herniations, dystrophic nails, abnormal teeth and hair, vertebral anomalies, limb reduction defects, genitourinary anomalies
Lenz Microphthalmia	+	+	0	Microcephaly, microphthalmia, ocular dysgenesis, malformed ears, cleft lip/palate, cardiac and genitourinary anomalies, thumb duplication or hypoplasia, narrow shoulders
Arts	+	0	+	Growth deficiency, poor muscle development, areflexia, ataxia, deafness, vision loss, seizures, childhood death
Bertini	+	0	+	Macular degeneration, ataxia, seizures, childhood death, hypoplasia of cerebellar vermis and corpus callosum, developmental delays and regression, postnatal growth impairment
Cerebro-Cerebello-Coloboma	+	0	+	Hydrocephaly, cerebellar vermis hypoplasia, retinal coloboma, seizures, abnormal respiratory pattern
Roifman	+	0	+	Microcephaly, short stature, spondyloepiphyseal dysplasia, retinal pigmentary deposits, antibody deficiency, eczema

LUJAN SYNDROME

(LUJAN-FRYNS SYNDROME, XLID-MARFANOID HABITUS)

OMIM 309520

Xq13

MED12 (HOPA)

Definition. XLID with marfanoid skeletal habitus and behavioral aberrations. The gene, *MED12*, is a member of the large Mediator Complex which is required for activation and suppression of RNA Polymerase II. The condition is allelic with Optiz FG syndrome.

Somatic Features. Patients are generally tall and thin with stature and head circumference in the upper centiles. The face is long with prominent forehead, high nasal bridge, high palate, low-set retroverted but normal-length ears, and micrognathia. Hands and feet are long and thin with long digits. Pectus excavatum and joint hyperextensibility may be present. One patient had an extra row of upper teeth at 17 years and another had an atrial septal defect. Speech is high-pitched and hypernasal, but velopharyngeal incompetence or submucous cleft palate has not been reported. Seizures, hyperactivity, and aggressiveness have been significant management issues. Testicular enlargement has been noted in several cases.

Growth and Development. From early childhood, height and head circumference measure in the upper growth centiles. Weight is usually below the 50th centile. Speech

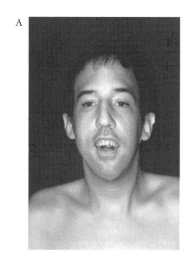
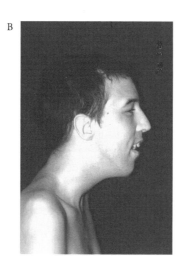
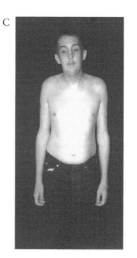
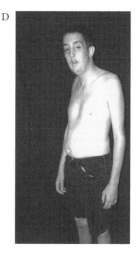

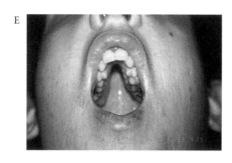

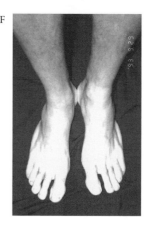

Lujan Syndrome. Twenty-eight-year-old with prominent forehead and long face, high nasal bridge, receding chin, and low-set, simply formed ears (**A, B**). Thirty-three-year-old brother showing tall face, ptosis, simple ears, large mandible, and pectus exacavatum (**C, D**); narrow arched palate (**E**); long feet and toes with spacing between toes 1 and 2 (**F**).   Courtesy of Dr. Hubert Lubs, University of Miami School of Medicine, Miami.

and motor milestones are delayed, but the severity varies considerably.

Cognitive Function. A wide range of cognitive function accompanies the prominent behavioral manifestations. In most cases, mild to moderate cognitive impairment occurs.

Behavior. Various males have exhibited hyperactive, aggressive, autistic, and psychotic behaviors, as well as shyness and joviality.

Neurological Findings. None

Heterozygote Expression. One carrier female with normal intellect has marfanoid habitus and high-pitched nasal speech.

Imaging. One case with agenesis of corpus callosum and one with suspected partial absence of corpus callosum were present in the original Lujan syndrome family.

Comment. A number of cases and a few families have been reported since the Lujan et al. report of 1984. It is clear that genetic heterogeneity is represented in those reports. A mutation in *MED12* (p.N1007S) has been found only in the original family. Lujan syndrome is allelic with Opitz FG syndrome with which it shares some clinical findings.

REFERENCES

Fryns J-P, Buttiens M: X-linked mental retardation with Marfanoid habitus. Am J Med Genet 28:267, 1987.

Lacombe D, Bonneau D, Verloes A, et al.: Lujan-Fryns syndrome (X-linked mental retardation with Marfanoid habitus): Report of three cases and review. Genet Couns 4:193, 1993.

Lalatta F, Livini E, Selicorni A, et al.: X-linked mental retardation with Marfanoid habitus: First report of four Italian patients. Am J Med Genet 38:228, 1991.

Lujan JE, Carlin ME, Lubs HA: A form of X-linked mental retardation with Marfanoid habitus. Am J Med Genet 17:311, 1984.

Schwartz CE, Tarpey PS, Lubs HA, et al.: The original Lujan syndrome family has a novel missense mutation (p.N1007S) in the MED12 gene. J Med Genet 44:472, 2007.

DIFFERENTIAL MATRIX

Syndrome	Marfanoid Habitus	Behavioral Disturbance	Seizures	Comments
Lujan	+	+	+	Asthenic build, long face, prominent forehead, high palate, micrognathia, long digits, pectus excavatum, joint hyperextensibility, hyperactivity
Ornithine Transcarbamoylase Deficiency	0	+	+	Chronic or intermittent hyperammonemia, microcephaly, protein-induced vomiting and lethargy, ataxia

MARTIN-PROBST SYNDROME

OMIM 300519

Xq22.2

RAB40AL

Definition. XLID associated with microcephaly, short stature, telecanthus, umbilical hernia, telangiectasias, excessive fingerprint arches, and sensorineural hearing loss.

Somatic Features. In addition to microcephaly, affected males have telecanthus, broad nasal root, epicanthus, low-set ears, malar hypoplasia, broad mouth, dental malocclusion, and micrognathia. The nipples are hypoplastic and widely spaced. Small kidneys, genital hypoplasia and umbilical hernias occur. Telangiectasias, abnormal distal interphalangeal creases, and an excessive number of arch fingerprints may be present. Cleft soft palate was seen in one case; frontal upsweep in one case; and pancytopenia in two adult cases.

Growth and Development. Statural growth slows during childhood and adult stature is short. Global developmental delay occurs, and cognitive function is variably affected with hearing loss possibly contributing to impairment in speech and learning. Hypothyroidism occurred in one case.

Neurological Findings. Hypotonia may be present.

Heterozygote Expression. None

Comment. The phenotype is based on one family with three affected males. Affected males have some manifestations seen in patients with Noonan, Costello, and CFC syndromes. A missence mutation has been found in *RAB40AL*, which encodes a RAS-like GTPase protein that contains a suppression of cytokine signaling (SOCS) box.

REFERENCES

Bedoyan JK, Schaibley V, Peng W, et al.: Mutations in *RAB40AL* cause Martin-Probst syndrome, an X-linked disorder characterized by sensorineural hearing loss, cognitive impairment, short stature, and craniofacial dysmorphisms. American Society of Human Genetics Annual Meeting, Montreal, Oct 11–15, 2011.

Martin DM, Probst FJ, Camper SA, Petty EM: Characterisation and genetic mapping of a new X linked deafness syndrome. J Med Genet 37:836, 2000.

Saito-Ohara F, Fukuda Y, Ito M, et al.: The Xq22 inversion breakpoint interrupted a novel Ras-like GTPase gene in a patient with Duchenne Muscular Dystrophy and profound mental retardation. Am J Hum Genet 71:637, 2002.

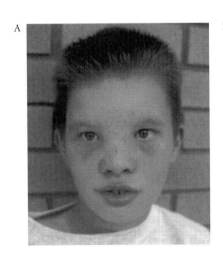
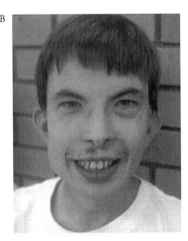

Martin-Probst Syndrome. Microcephaly, upsweep of frontal hair, hypertelorism, broad nasal root, low-set ears, and broad mouth in a 12-year-old boy (A) and his 31-year-old uncle (B). Courtesy of Dr. Donna Martin, Ann Arbor, Michigan.

Syndrome	Microcephaly	Telecanthus or Hypertelorism	Hearing Loss	Comments
Martin-Probst	+	+	+	Short stature, excessive arch fingerprints
Wittwer	+	+	+	Short stature, microphthalmia, hypertelorism, genitourinary anomalies, hypotonia
Gustavson	+	0	+	Short stature, optic atrophy with blindness, large ears, joint contractures, rockerbottom feet, brain undergrowth, hydrocephaly
Juberg-Marsidi-Brooks	+	0	+	Short stature, dysgenesis of corpus callosum, deep-set eyes, blepharophimosis, cupped ears, bulbous nose, small mouth, thin upper lip, pectus excavatum, flexion contractures
Paine	+	0	+	Short stature, optic atrophy
Schimke	+	0	+	Sunken eyes, downslanting palpebral fissures, narrow nose, wide spacing of teeth, cupped ears, hypotonia, choreoathetosis, contractures

MEHMO SYNDROME

(INTELLECTUAL DISABILITY-EPILEPTIC SEIZURES-HYPOGONADISM AND HYPOGENITALISM-MICROCEPHALY-OBESITY SYNDROME, XLID-MICROCEPHALY-OBESITY-HYPOGONADISM-SEIZURES)

OMIM 300148

Xp21

EIF2S3

Definition. XLID with short stature, microcephaly, hypogonadism, obesity, seizures, and early childhood death. A mutation in *EIF2S3*, a gene involved in initiation of translation, has been reported.

Somatic Features. Major malformations do not occur. Microcephaly and facial features suggestive of hypotonia (thick helices with upturned earlobes, thick alae nasi, tented upper lip with downturned angles of the mouth, and puffy cheeks) were present in the child described most completely. The penis was small and the testes undescended. Hands and feet were edematous, fingers were tapered, and the feet had equinovarus deformation. Generalized obesity was present. Death occurs during infancy or early childhood.

Growth and Development. At birth, growth parameters measure in the lower percentiles. Thereafter, head growth and stature are further slowed, but weight gain is excessive. No significant developmental milestones are achieved.

Cognitive Function. Severe impairment.

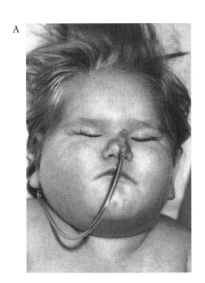

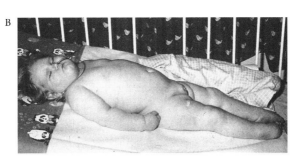

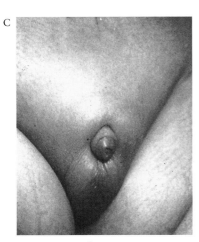

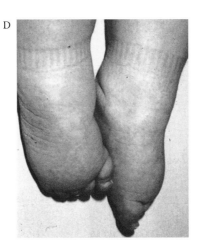

MEHMO Syndrome. Microcephaly, full rounded face, downturned corners of the mouth, obesity, hypogenitalism, and talipes in a boy age 2 years.
Courtesy of Dr. Ulrich Müller, Institut für Humangenetik, Universität Giessen, Giessen, Germany.

Neurological Findings. Details of the neurological examination are not available.

Heterozygote Expression. None

Comment. This XLID syndrome suffers profound developmental failure, seizures, and death in infancy or early childhood, and in this regard differs from other XLID syndromes with hypotonia, hypogonadism, and obesity. In 1989, DeLozier-Blanchet et al. reported a patient and suggested that Steinmüller's patient may have the same disorder. Mitochondrial abnormalities documented by markedly reduced activities of respiratory chain enzymes were reported by Leshinsky-Silver et al. (2002), who suggested that MEHMO may represent an X-linked mitochondrial disorder. A mutation in the gene, *EIF2S3*, which encodes subunit 3 of eukaryotic translation initiation factor 2, has been identified by Kalscheuer et al. (2011).

REFERENCES

DeLozier-Blanchet CD, Haenggeli CA, Bottani A: MEHMO, a novel syndrome: assignment of disease locus to Xp21.1-p22.13. Eur J Hum Genet 7:621, 1999.

DeLozier-Blanchet CD, Haenggeli CA, Engel E: [Microencephalic nanism, severe retardation, hypertonia, obesity, and hypogonadism in two brothers: a new syndrome?] J Genet Hum 37:353, 1989.

Kalscheuer VM, Hu H, Haas SA, et al.: Fragile X and Early Onset Cognitive Disorder Workshop. Berlin, Sept 4–7, 2011.

Leshinsky-Silver E, Zinger A, Bibi CN, et al.: MEHMO (mental retardation, epileptic seizures, hypogenitalism, microcephaly, obesity): a new X-linked mitochondrial disorder. Eur J Hum Genet 10:226, 2002.

Steinmüller R, Steinberger D, Müller U: MEHMO (mental retardation, epileptic seizures, hypogonadism and -genitalism, microcephaly, obesity), a novel syndrome: assignment of disease locus to Xp21.1-p22.13. Eur J Hum Genet 6:201, 1998.

DIFFERENTIAL MATRIX

Syndrome	Obesity	Hypotonia	Hypogonadism	Comments
MEHMO	+	+	+	Short stature, microcephaly, edematous hands and feet, equinovarus deformity, seizures, early childhood death
Börjeson-Forssman-Lehmann	+	+	+	Microcephaly, short stature, coarse face, large ears, gynecomastia, narrow sloped shoulders, visual impairment, tapered digits
Vasquez	+	+	+	Microcephaly, short stature, gynecomastia
Wilson-Turner	+	+	+	Normal growth, small hands and feet, tapered digits, gynecomastia, emotional lability
Urban	+	0	+	Short stature, small hands and feet, digital contractures, osteoporosis
XLID-Panhypopituitarism	+	0	+	Short stature, hypogenitalism, small sella turcica, deficiency of pituitary, thyroid, adrenal, and gonadal hormones
XLID-Hypogonadism-Tremor	+	0	+	Short stature, prominent lower lip, muscle wasting of legs, abnormal gait, seizures, tremor
Young-Hughes	+	0	+	Short stature, small palpebral fissures, cupped ears, ichthyosiform scaling
ATRX-Associated XLID	0	+	+	Microcephaly, short stature, telecanthus/hypertelorism, small triangular nose, tented upper lip, open mouth, wide spacing of teeth, abnormal genitalia, minor musculoskeletal anomalies, erythrocyte HbH inclusions in some
Pettigrew	0	+	+	Dandy-Walker malformation, spasticity, microcephaly or hydrocephaly, long face with macrostomia and prognathism, small testes, contractures, choreoathetosis, iron deposits in basal ganglia, seizures

MENKES SYNDROME

(XLID-KINKY HAIR, XLID-COPPER TRANSPORT DEFECT)

OMIM 309400

Xq21.1

ATP7A

Definition. XLID with growth deficiency, full cheeks, sparse kinky hair, metaphyseal changes, limited spontaneous movement, hypertonicity, seizures, hypothermia, lethargy, arterial tortuosity, and death in early childhood, associated with low serum copper and ceruloplasmin and deficient cellular transport of copper. The gene, *ATP7A*, encodes a Cu(2+)-transporting ATPase. The protein functions in the homeostatic maintenance of cellular copper levels and copper transport, which leads to deficient function of several cuproenzymes.

Somatic Features. Although the face may be pale, expressionless, and with full cheeks, it is the hair that is most distinctive. Cranial hair is sparse and hypopigmented, often with the shafts broken near the skin. Eyebrows are similarly sparse, horizontal, and twisted in appearance. The characteristic twisting of pili torti is the only structurally visible change in the hair shafts. The skin is also hypopigmented and tends to be lax. Seborrheic dermatitis, predominantly affecting the face and scalp, may persist throughout life. Major malformations do not occur. The arteries are tortuous, with irregularly narrowed lumens. Wormian bones may be found in the sagittal and lambdoid sutures. Metaphyses of the ribs and long bones are widened, and spurs may occur at the metaphyses of the long bones.

Growth and Development. Although premature delivery occurs commonly, intrauterine growth is normal or nearly so. Postnatal growth appears variable, with some infants maintaining normal growth velocity while others lag behind and eventually fall below –2SD in head circumference and stature. Development is profoundly delayed, with most infants never progressing beyond smiling and control of the head position, skills that are quickly lost.

Cognitive Function. In the usual case, no significant cognitive skills are attained. Milder variants with less severe impairments have been described.

Neurological Findings. From the early days or weeks of life, these infants appear lethargic, with little spontaneous movement and very little progress in development. They become mildly hypertonic, often exhibit hypothermia, and develop seizures of generalized or myoclonic types. Death occurs within the first few years.

Natural History. The classic presentation is early and lethal. The hair is fine but normal microscopically at birth. Hypothermia, hyperbilirubinemia, frequent infections, poor feeding, and hypotonia may complicate the first days and weeks of life. After several months of limited development, relentless developmental and neurological deterioration ensues, manifested in the form of myoclonic seizures, spasticity, limited movement, and minimal responsiveness. The facial, cutaneous, hair, and joint findings become apparent in the first months. Death occurs in the first

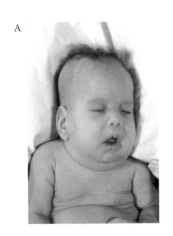
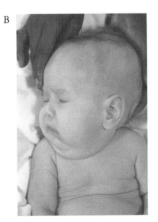
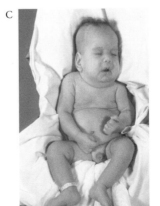
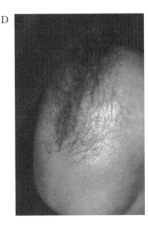

A   B   C   D

Menkes Syndrome. Four-month-old infant with generalized hypotonia, puffiness and sagging of the cheeks, and sparse hair.   Courtesy of Dr. Arthur S. Aylsworth, University of North Carolina School of Medicine, Chapel Hill.

3 years of life. The few survivors beyond early childhood have profound mental and neurological impairments.

Several milder variants with *ATP7A* mutations have been described. In some cases, milder developmental delay and intellectual disability, ataxia, dysarthria, seizures, pili torti, facial, and connective tissue features are described. In the occipital horn syndrome, connective tissue (lax skin, loose joints, diverticula of bladder, hernias) and skeletal changes (occipital exostoses, expansion of the lateral clavicles, wavy long bone cortices) predominate, but intelligence is low normal, borderline, or in the mild ID range. Mutations in *ATP7A* have also been reported in X-linked distal spinal muscular atrophy-3.

Heterozygote Expression. Carrier females may have pili torti, but this is not an obligate finding. Neurological or cognitive abnormalities do not occur.

Imaging. Cerebral and cerebellar atrophy and deficient myelination.

Neuropathology. The brain is moderately undergrown and has diffuse neuronal loss, gliosis, and areas of microcystic degeneration. There appears to be a predisposition to subdural hematomas. Cerebral arteries may be thin-walled, tortuous, and dilated.

Laboratory. Low levels of copper and ceruloplasmin may be demonstrated in the serum. Defective intracellular trafficking of copper leads to deficient movement of copper transplacentally, decreased intestinal absorption of copper, and excessive accumulation of copper in the tissues.

Comment. Various clinical manifestations appear as a result of deficient activities of enzymes requiring copper (lysyl oxidase, cytochrome C oxidase, dopamine β-hydroxylase, and superoxide mutase). The hope that parenteral administration of copper would be curative in most patients has not been fulfilled. Parenteral copper administration can normalize serum copper and ceruloplasmin. Success in modifying the clinical course appears, in part, because of the age at which therapy begins. When initiated prior to the onset of neurological signs, subcutaneous copper-histidine treatment may prevent altogether the neurological manifestations and intellectual disability in some patients. Other cases do not respond so beneficially. Long-term treatment, however, does not prevent development, progression, and complications of occipital horn syndrome. The success of treatment may depend, in part, on the type of *ATP7A* mutation.

REFERENCES

Amador E, Domene R, Fuentes C, et al.: Long-term skeletal findings in Menkes disease. Pediatr Radiol 40:1426, 2010.

Chelly J, Türner Z, Tønnesen T, et al.: Isolation of a candidate gene for Menkes disease that encodes a potential heavy metal binding protein. Nat Genet 3:14, 1993.

Christodoulou J, Danks DM, Bibidhendra S, et al.: Early treatment of Menkes disease with parenteral copper-histidine: Long-term follow-up of four treated patients. Am J Med Genet 76:154, 1998.

Danks DM, Campbell PE, Stevens BJ, et al.: Menkes's kinky hair syndrome. An inherited defect in copper absorption with widespread effects. Pediatrics 50:188, 1972.

Madsen E, Gitlin JD: Copper and iron disorders of the brain. Ann Rev Neurosci 30:317, 2007.

Menkes JH, Alter M, Steigleder GK, et al.: A sex-linked recessive disorder with retardation of growth, peculiar hair and focal cerebral and cerebellar degeneration. Pediatrics 29:764, 1962.

Mercer JFB, Livingston J, Hall B, et al.: Isolation of a partial candidate gene for Menkes disease by positional cloning. Nat Genet 3:20, 1993.

Proud VK, Mussell HG, Kaler SG, et al.: Distinctive Menkes disease variant with occipital horns: Delineation of natural history and clinical phenotype. Am J Med Genet 65:44, 1996.

Vulpe C, Levinson B, Whitney S, et al.: Isolation of a candidate gene for Menkes disease and evidence that it encodes a copper transporting ATPase. Nat Genet 3:7, 1993.

Syndrome	Hair Abnormality	Skeletal Abnormalities	Seizures	Comments
Menkes	+	+	+	Growth deficiency, hypothermia, pallor, limited movement, hypertonicity, metaphyseal widening and spurs, arterial tortuosity, childhood death
Oral-Facial-Digital I	+	+	+	Sparse scalp hair, dystopia canthorum, flat midface, hypoplastic alae nasi, hypertrophic and aberrant oral frenuli, intraoral clefts and pseudoclefts, lingual hamartomas, brachydactyly, syndactyly, clinodactyly, structural brain anomalies, polycystic kidneys
Fitzsimmons	+	+	0	Pes cavus, hyperkeratosis of palms and soles, dystrophic nails, spastic paraplegia
Goltz	+	+	0	Cataracts, ocular dysgenesis, linear areas of dermal aplasia, cutaneous adipose herniations, dystrophic nails, abnormal teeth and hair, vertebral anomalies, limb reduction defects, genitourinary anomalies
Hereditary Bullous Dystrophy, X-linked	+	+	0	Microcephaly, short stature, upslanting palpebral fissures, protruding ears, short and tapered digits, cardiac defects, bullous dystrophy, small testes, early death from pulmonary infection
Cantu	+	0	+	Microcephaly, short stature, alopecia, follicular keratosis, cortical atrophy
XLID-Nail Dystrophy-Seizures	+	0	+	Distinctive face, small penis, dry skin, nail dystrophy

MIDAS SYNDROME

(MICROPHTHALMIA-DERMAL APLASIA-SCLEROCORNEA SYNDROME,
MICROPHTHALMIA-LINEAR SKIN DEFECTS SYNDROME)

OMIM 309801

Xp22.2

HCCS

Definition. XLID in females with microphthalmia, corneal opacification, and linear areas of dermal aplasia on the face, neck, and upper torso. The gene, holocytochrome C synthase (*HCCS*), functions in mitochondrial oxidative phosphorylation and apoptosis.

Somatic Features. At birth, infants have irregular linear skin defects of the face and upper torso, generalized facial erythema, microphthalmia, and corneal opacification. Additional ocular findings may include glaucoma, iris coloboma, embryotoxin, cataracts, retinopathy, retinal detachment, and orbital cysts. Vision is limited to light perception. The skin defects heal over the initial months of life, leaving linear atrophic scars.

Aside from the ocular and cutaneous manifestations, the facial appearance is usually normal. Hypertelorism, abnormally formed ears, and micrognathia have been described. A wide variety of other structural anomalies have been described. Central nervous system and cardiac malformations are most notable. Dysgenesis of the corpus callosum, absent septum pellucidum, cystic lesions of the cerebrum, and enlarged ventricles number among the CNS anomalies. Structural cardiac defects include ASD, VSD, and overriding aorta. Arrhythmias have also been described. Bird et al. (1994) have pointed out the particular association with oncocytic cardiomyopathy. Diaphragmatic hernia and anterior placement of the anus have been seen in one or more cases.

Growth and Development. Short stature is obvious by a few months. Microcephaly has been noted in only one case.

Cognitive Function. Cognitive impairment seems to be restricted to those who have associated CNS anomalies.

Imaging. Dysgenesis of the corpus callosum, absent septum pellucidum, cystic lesions of the cerebrum, and enlarged ventricles may be seen.

Comment. Translocations, deletions, or other rearrangements involving the X chromosome have been documented in most cases. Because all cases reported have been females, MIDAS syndrome is considered lethal in males. Among cases not associated with X-chromosome rearrangements, an alternative explanation may be the emergence in females of paternal germline mutations. Wimplinger et al. (2006) have suggested that chromosomal mosaicism and/or nonrandom X-inactivation could affect the clinical phenotype.

REFERENCES

Al-Gazali LI, Mueller RF, Caine A, et al.: Two 46,XX,t(X;Y) females with linear skin defects and congenital microphthalmia: a new syndrome at Xp22.3. J Med Genet 27:59, 1990.

Bird LM, Krous HF, Eichenfield LF, et al.: Female infant with oncocytic cardiomyopathy and microphthalmia with linear skin defects (MLS): A clue to the pathogenesis of oncocytic cardiomyopathy? Am J Med Genet 53:141, 1994.

Wimplinger I, Morleo M, Rosenberger G, et al.: Mutations of the mitochondrial holochrome C-type synthase in X-linked dominant microphthalmia with linear skin defects syndrome. Am J Hum Genet 79:878, 2006.

Wimplinger I, Rauch A, Orth U, et al.: Mother and daughter with a terminal Xp deletion: implication of chromosomal mosaicism and X-inactivation in the high clinical variability of the microphthalmia with linear skin defects (MLS) syndrome. Eur J Med Genet 50:421, 2007.

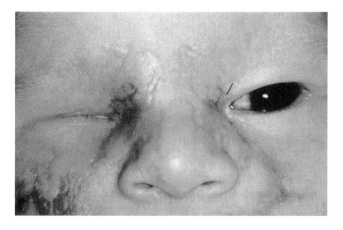

MIDAS Syndrome. Female infant with a de novo X;Y translocation with irregular areas of erythematous skin hypoplasia in the periocular area, microphthalmia, and corneal opacity.   Courtesy of Dr. Robert Mueller, Leeds General Infirmary, England.

DIFFERENTIAL MATRIX

Syndrome	Ectodermal Dysplasia	Ocular Anomaly	CNS Anomaly	Comments
MIDAS	+	+	+	Microphthalmia, ocular dysgenesis, corneal opacification, dermal aplasia, dysgenesis of corpus callosum, cardiac defects, cardiomyopathy
Goltz	+	+	0	Cataracts, ocular dysgenesis, linear areas of dermal aplasia, cutaneous adipose herniations, dystrophic nails, abnormal teeth and hair, vertebral anomalies, limb reduction defects, genitourinary anomalies
Incontinentia Pigmenti	+	+	0	Cutaneous vesicles, verrucous lesions, irregular hyperpigmentation, microcephaly, ocular anomalies, oligodontia, abnormally shaped teeth, spasticity, seizures
Aicardi	0	+	+	Ocular dysgenesis, lacunar retinopathy, costovertebral anomalies, agenesis of corpus callosum, seizures
Cerebro-Oculo-Genital	0	+	+	Microcephaly, hydrocephaly, short stature, agenesis of corpus callosum, microphthalmia, ptosis, hypospadias, cryptorchidism, clubfoot, spasticity
Wittwer	0	+	+	Microcephaly, short stature, microphthalmia, hearing loss, vision loss, hypertelorism, genitourinary anomalies, hypotonia, seizures

MILES-CARPENTER SYNDROME

(MRXS4, MILES SYNDROME, XLID WITH CONGENITAL CONTRACTURES
AND LOW FINGERTIP ARCHES)

OMIM 309605

Xq13-q22

Definition. XLID with short stature, microcephaly, exotropia, long hands, digit contractures, rockerbottom feet, arch fingerprints, and spasticity. The gene has not been identified but is localized to proximal Xq.

Somatic Features. Craniofacial, skeletal, and cutaneous features distinguish the Miles-Carpenter syndrome. Microcephaly is present but not so marked as to cause craniofacial disproportion. Facial characteristics include medial flair of the eyebrows, exotropia, ptosis, small palpebral fissures, maxillary hypoplasia, thick alae nasi, open mouth with arched palate and thick alveolar ridges, and obtuse mandibular angle. Facial asymmetry, bitemporal narrowing, and small teeth with irregular placement may be present. Ear size and architecture is not remarkable. The axial skeleton shows pectus excavatum and thoracic scoliosis. Hands are long (especially the palms), hyperextensible at the MCP joints, and have proximal thumb placement, fifth-finger camptodactyly, abnormal palmar creases, cupping of the palms, and hyperconvex nails. Mild cutaneous syndactyly may be present. Feet are equally distinctive with rockerbottom configuration resulting from vertical talus and show valgus positioning of the great toes and contractures of toes 4 and 5. The legs taper distally, the elbows and knees hyperextend, and stature may be shortened by flexed knee posture and scoliosis. The constant presence of 10 low fingerprint arches adds a distinctive and diagnostically helpful manifestation.

Growth and Development. Birth weights range from 2.4 kilograms to 3.2 kilograms. Postnatal growth shows short stature and microcephaly. Genitalia appear normal, although secondary sexual characteristics may be underdeveloped.

Cognitive Function. Affected males have severe intellectual disability; carrier females may be mildly impaired.

Neurological Findings. Mild spasticity, toe walking, and unsteady gait

Heterozygote Expression. Carrier females may have both somatic features and cognitive impairment although milder than in males. Microcephaly and craniofacial features may be present. The long cupped hands with digital contractures, hyperextensible MCP joints, and proximally placed thumbs typically occur in carrier females, but rockerbottom feet do not, although toe contractures and lateral deviation of the great toes may be present. Arches predominate the fingerprint pattern.

Imaging. Radiographs of one male demonstrated thickened calvaria, hyperostosis frontalis interna, bifid sternum, coxa valga, narrow diaphyses of the long bones, and epiphyseal delay.

Comment. The phenotype is based on observation in a single family with four affected males and six carrier females. Hoefnagel reported a brother and sister with similar findings. Four other XLID syndromes have an excess of arch fingerprints or a low total ridge count: Chudley-Lowry, XLID-Arch Fingerprints-Hypotonia, Coffin-Lowry, and Prieto syndromes, the first two resulting from *ATRX* mutations.

REFERENCES

Hoefnagel D: Malformation syndromes with mental deficiency. Birth Defects: Orig Art Ser V(2):11, 1969.

Miles JH, Carpenter NJ: Unique X-linked mental retardation syndrome with fingertip arches and contractures linked to Xq21.31. Am J Med Genet 38:215, 1991.

Tackels D, Schwartz CE, Carpenter NJ, et al.: Refined gene localization for the Miles-Carpenter syndrome (MCS). Am J Med Genet 85:221, 1999.

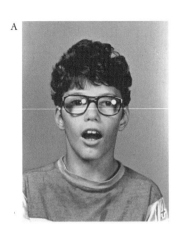

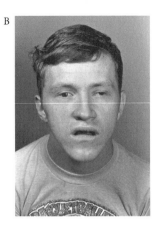

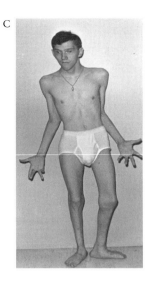

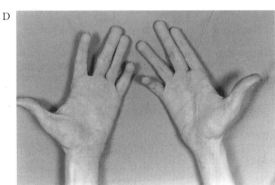

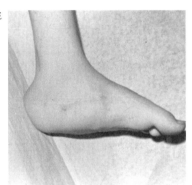

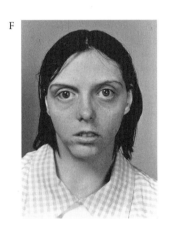

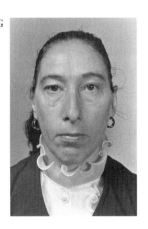

Miles-Carpenter Syndrome. Twenty-two-year-old male with exotropia, smooth philtrum, and tented upper lip (A); 31-year-old male cousin with facial asymmetry, left exotropia, and ptosis (B); 32-year-old male with slender build, pectus excavatum, scoliosis, high nasal bridge, long palms, accessory hypothenar crease, camptodactyly of fifth fingers, proximally placed thumbs, and pes planus with prominent heel (C–E); 25-year-old carrier female with microcephaly, facial asymmetry, proptosis, and small mandible (F); 36-year-old carrier female with long face and high nasal bridge (G).   Courtesy of Dr. Judith Miles, University of Missouri Health Sciences Center, Columbia.

Syndrome	Microcephaly	Skeletal Manifestations	Spasticity	Comments
Miles-Carpenter	+	+	+	Short stature, ptosis, small palpebral fissures, open mouth, pectus excavatum, scoliosis, long hands, camptodactyly, rockerbottom feet, arch fingerprints, unsteady gait
Cerebro-Oculo-Genital	+	+	+	Hydrocephaly, short stature, agenesis of corpus callosum, microphthalmia, ptosis, hypospadias, cryptorchidism, clubfoot
Gustavson	+	+	+	Short stature, optic atrophy with blindness, large ears, deafness, joint contractures, rockerbottom feet, brain undergrowth, hydrocephaly, cerebellar hypoplasia, seizures
Kang	+	+	+	Frontal prominence, telecanthus, small nose, short hands, dysgenesis of corpus callosum, seizures, downslanted mouth, brachydactyly
Pettigrew	+	+	+	Dandy-Walker malformation, microcephaly or hydrocephaly, long face with macrostomia and prognathism, small testes, contractures, choreoathetosis, iron deposits in basal ganglia, seizures
Proud (*ARX*-Associated XLID)	+	+	+	Hearing loss, vision loss, agenesis of corpus callosum, cryptorchidism, inguinal hernias, ataxia, seizures
Schimke	+	+	+	Sunken eyes, downslanting palpebral fissures, narrow nose, wide spacing of teeth, cupped ears, hypotonia, abducens palsy, hearing loss, vision loss, choreoathetosis, contractures
Roifman	+	+	O	Short stature, spondyloepiphyseal dysplasia, retinal pigmentary deposits, antibody deficiency, eczema, hypotonia

MOHR-TRANEBJAERG SYNDROME

(DYSTONIA-DEAFNESS SYNDROME (DDS), DEAFNESS-DYSTONIA-OPTIC ATROPHY SYNDROME, MOHR SYNDROME, MOHR-MAGEROY SYNDROME, OPTIC ACOUSTIC NERVE ATROPHY WITH DEMENTIA, JENSEN SYNDROME)

OMIM 304700

Xq22.1

TIMM8A (DDP)

Definition. XLID with progressive deafness, blindness, and neurological deterioration with onset in early childhood. The gene encodes an inner membrane protein, which mediates importation of mitochondrial proteins.

Somatic Features. Normal growth and craniofacial appearance. Fractures are common and are perhaps related to the predisposition to injury because of unsteady gait.

Growth and Development. Intrauterine and postnatal growth is normal. Early developmental milestones are normal, but verbal abilities may be impaired because of hearing loss.

Cognitive Function. Progressive loss of cognitive skills eventually leads to severe impairment. The onset coincides with other neurological findings, usually by late childhood or early adult life.

Behavior. Restlessness, irritability, and aggressiveness may occur in childhood. Following the onset of dementia, there may be confusion, unsociable behavior, paranoid ideation, and aggressiveness.

Neurological Findings. Hearing loss develops after birth and rapidly worsens. Speech develops among those with hearing loss delayed beyond the first few years. Vision becomes impaired and is lost at a later age, generally becoming symptomatic in the 30s and progressively worsening. Photophobia and scotomas may precede vision loss by a number of years. Retinal changes are compatible with central choroidal areolar dystrophy with central scotomas. Retinal dysfunction is usually not seen on ERG. Motor skills become impaired early in life, in some cases before age 10 years. Ataxia, dystonia, and spasticity interfere with speech, feeding, and ambulation. Some cases become opisthotonic. Mental deterioration coincides with the other neurological impairments. Irritability, aggressiveness, and paranoia occur in some cases. Mild neurogenic muscle atrophy has been verified by EMG and muscle biopsy.

An allelic disorder, Optic Acoustic Nerve Atrophy with Dementia (Jensen syndrome), presents with infantile profound sensorineural hearing loss, adolescent optic nerve atrophy, and blindness as well as progressive dementia in adulthood.

Heterozygote Expression. Mild hearing loss, pallor, or the optic discs and possible signs of motorsensory neuropathy have been noted in several obligate carriers.

Imaging. Cerebral atrophy occurs as early as age 7 years.

A

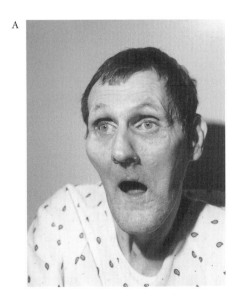

B

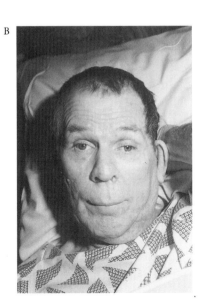

Mohr-Tranebjaerg Syndrome. Fifty-five-year-old male with wasting of facial muscles and sunken eyes (A); 62-year-old with facial asymmetry, upslanting palpebral fissures, and blindness (B).

Neuropathology. Generalized brain atrophy is the typical post mortem finding.

Laboratory. Long-chain fatty acids, phytanic acid, plasmalogens, and muscle staining for amyloid are normal.

Comment. The initial family was reported as isolated X-linked deafness (DFN-1). The neurodegenerative manifestations were recognized on later follow-up. Progressive sensorineural hearing loss has onset between 1 and 5 years, usually after acquisition of some speech. Loss of vision and onset of neurological abnormalities and dementia are often delayed until adult life but may begin in late childhood. Neurodegeneration appears relentless, with eventual loss of motor skills, lack of contact with the environment, dysphagia, spasticity, and psychosis. Although rapid progression to death occurred in one teenage patient, life expectancy does not appear shortened in most cases.

REFERENCES

Jensen PKA: Nerve deafness, optic nerve atrophy and dementia: A new X-linked recessive syndrome? Am J Med Genet 9:55, 1981.

Jin H, May M, Tranebjaerg L, et al.: A novel X-linked gene, DDP, shows mutations in families with deafness (DFN-1), dystonia, mental deficiency and blindness. Nat Genet 14:177, 1996.

Mohr J, Magerøy K: Sex-linked deafness of a possibly new type. Acta Genet Stat Med 10:54, 1960.

Ponjavic V, Andreasson S, Tranebjaerg L, et al.: Full-field electroretinograms in a family with Mohr-Tranebjaerg syndrome. Acta Ophthalmol Scand 74:632, 1996.

Tranebjaerg L, Hamel BCJ, Gabreels FJM, et al.: A de novo missense mutation in a critical domain of the X-linked DDP gene causes the typical deafness-dystonia-optic atrophy syndrome. Eur J Hum Genet 8:464, 2000.

Tranebjaerg L, Schwartz C, Eriksen H, et al.: A new X linked recessive deafness syndrome with blindness, dystonia, fractures, and mental deficiency is linked to Xq22. J Med Genet 32:257, 1995.

Tranebjaerg L, van Ghelue M, Nilssen O, et al.: Jensen syndrome is allelic to Mohr-Tranebjaerg syndrome and both are caused by stop mutations in the DDP gene. Am J Hum Genet 61(suppl):A349, 1997.

DIFFERENTIAL MATRIX

Syndrome	Vision Loss	Hearing Loss	Spasticity, Dystonia, or Ataxia	Comments
Mohr-Tranebjaerg	+	+	+	Neurological deterioration with childhood onset
Gustavson	+	+	+	Microcephaly, short stature, optic atrophy, large ears, joint contractures, rockerbottom feet, brain undergrowth, hydrocephaly, cerebellar hypoplasia, seizures
Paine	+	+	+	Microcephaly, short stature, optic atrophy, seizures
Proud (*ARX*-Associated XLID)	+	+	+	Microcephaly, agenesis of corpus callosum, cryptorchidism, inguinal hernias, seizures
Schimke	+	+	+	Microcephaly, sunken eyes, downslanting palpebral fissures, narrow nose, wide spacing of teeth, cupped ears, hypotonia, abducens palsy, choreoathetosis, contractures
Ataxia-Deafness-Dementia, X-linked	+	+	+	Optic atrophy, spastic paraplegia, hypotonia, seizures, childhood death
Norrie	+	+	0	Ocular dysplasia and degeneration
Wittwer	+	+	0	Microcephaly, short stature, microphthalmia, hypertelorism, genitourinary anomalies, hypotonia, seizures
Arts	+	0	+	Growth deficiency, poor muscle development, hypotonia, areflexia, seizures, childhood death
Bertini	+	0	+	Macular degeneration, hypotonia, seizures, childhood death, hypoplasia of cerebellar vermis and corpus callosum, developmental delays and regression, postnatal growth impairment
XLID-Spastic Paraplegia, type 7	+	0	+	Nystagmus, reduced vision, absent speech and ambulation, bowel and bladder dysfunction, spastic quadriplegia
Juberg-Marsidi-Brooks	0	+	+	Microcephaly and hydrocephaly, short stature, dysgenesis of corpus callosum, deep-set eyes, blepharophimosis, cupped ears, bulbous nose, small mouth, thin upper lip, pectus excavatum, flexion contractures, seizures

MONOAMINE OXIDASE-A DEFICIENCY

(BRUNNER SYNDROME)

OMIM 309850

Xp11.23

MAO-A

Definition. X-linked behavioral disorder and borderline intelligence secondary to monoamine oxidase-A deficiency. A truncating mutation in the *MAO-A* gene was found in the large family described by Brunner et al. (1993).

Somatic Features. No distinctive facial features have been reported.

Growth and Development. Normal growth. Early development progress is not notably abnormal.

Cognitive Function. Normal to borderline-low cognitive function.

Behavior. A withdrawn and shy demeanor punctuated by disordered behavior, particularly aggressive and violent behavior out of proportion to provocation, is typical. Recurrent clusters of aggressive behavior, insomnia and night terrors last several days. Additional behaviors include setting fires, exhibitionism, voyeurism, rape, and unwelcome embracing.

Neurological Findings. Stereotypical hand movements occur commonly, but neurological examination is grossly normal.

Heterozygote Expression. None described

Laboratory. Urine analysis shows elevated monamine substrates (normetanephrine, 3 methoxytyramine, and tyramine) and reduced monamine products (vanilacetic acid, vanilglycolic acid, 5 hydroxy-indole-3-acetic acid, and 3 methyoxy-4-hydroxy-phenyl-glycol). MAO-B activity is normal in platelets.

Comment. MAO-A and MAO-B are isoenzymes of monoamine oxidase, and MAO-A is much more important in biogenic amine metabolism. Whereas deletion of both genes has been associated with severe mental retardation, deletion of the *MAO-B* gene alone does not appear to cause any disability. Several subsequent studies have failed to document mutations in the *MAO-A* gene even in populations enriched for aggressive behavior. Thus, this is likely a rare etiology for this phenotype.

REFERENCES

Brunner HG, Nelen M, Breakefield XO, et al.: Abnormal behavior associated with a point mutation in the structural gene for monoamine oxidase A. Science 262:578, 1993.

Brunner HG, Nelen MR, van Zandvoort P, et al.: X-linked borderline mental retardation with prominent behavioral disturbance: phenotype, genetic localization, and evidence for disturbed monoamine metabolism. Am J Hum Genet 52:1032, 1993.

Lenders JWM, Eisenhofer G, Abeling NGGM, et al.: Specific genetic deficiencies of the A and B isoenzymes of monoamine oxidase are characterized by distinct neurochemical and clinical phenotypes. J Clin Invest 97:1010, 1996.

Mejia JM, Ervin FR, Palmour RM, et al.: (Letter to the Editor) Aggressive behavior and Brunner syndrome: No evidence for the C936T mutation in a population sample. Am J Med Genet 105:396, 2001.

DIFFERENTIAL MATRIX

Syndrome	Aggressive or Violent Behavior	Stereotypic Movements	Metabolic Disturbance	Comments
Monoamine Oxidase-A Deficiency	+	+	+	—
Mucopolysaccharidosis IIA	+	0	+	Macrocephaly, short stature, coarse facies, hepatosplenomegaly, hernias, joint stiffness, thick skin, hirsutism
Lowe	0	+	+	Short stature, cataracts, hypotonia, aminoaciduria, progressive renal failure

MUCOPOLYSACCHARIDOSIS IIA

(HUNTER SYNDROME, MPS IIA, IDURONATE 2-SULFATASE DEFICIENCY)

OMIM 309900

Xq28

IDS

Definition. XLID with generalized mucopolysaccharide storage caused by sulfoiduronate sulfatase deficiency. Gene deletions and nonsense mutations are associated with severe disease (IIA).

Somatic Features. Two somewhat less distinctive types of mucopolysaccharidosis II are recognized clinically. In the "severe form" (MPS IIA), profound intellectual disability becomes obvious by late childhood. In the "mild form" (MPS IIB), mentation may be normal and deterioration of mental function only slowly progressive. At birth, infants usually appear normal. Some patients appear to have an intermediate phenotype. There is a paucity of clinical signs with the exception of respiratory symptoms (noisy breathing from upper airway obstruction, recurrent rhinorrhea), large scaphoid head, and herniae (inguinal and umbilical) during infancy. Coarsening of facial features with thickening of the nostrils, lips, and tongue; joint stiffness; growth failure; excessive growth of fine body hair; and hepatosplenomegaly become obvious at about age 2 years and progress in severity. Thick skin, short neck, widely spaced teeth, hearing loss of some degree, and papilledema are commonly present. Nodular skin lesions on the arms or posterior chest wall, retinal pigmentation, mild pectus excavatum, pes cavus, mucoid diarrhea, and seizures occur less commonly.

Valvular and coronary heart diseases develop during childhood, and mental function, hearing, and joint mobility deteriorate steadily. The spine is straight, and corneas are not cloudy.

Growth and Development. Patients experience normal or excessive growth during the first 1 to 2 years. Adult height is decreased. Motor and intellectual development are delayed, more severely in MPS IIA.

Cognitive Function. Function is severely impaired prior to the end of the first decade.

Behavior. Affected individuals typically develop aggressive and destructive behavior in late childhood.

Neurological Findings. Progressive hearing loss, neurodegeneration in type IIA

Heterozygote Expression. Rare, but severe in affected females

Imaging. Roentgenological findings include scaphoid skull, enlarged sella with anterior excavation, skeletal findings of dysostosis multiplex, minimal vertebral changes, and precocious osteoarthritis of femoral head. Cranial MRI demonstrates white matter changes, atrophy, and hydrocephalus.

Neuropathology. Gliosis in white matter

Laboratory. Excessive urinary excretion of dermatan sulfate and heparan sulfate; leukocytes fibroblasts and serum

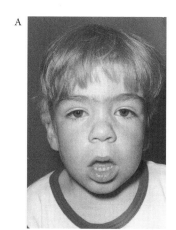
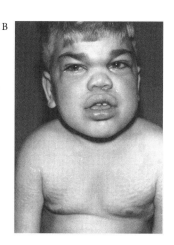
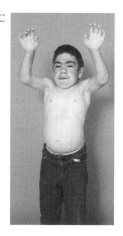

Mucopolysaccharidosis IIA. Coarse facies, depressed nasal bridge, full lower face, thickened lips, facial acne, and joint contractures at ages 4 and 16 years (**A, C**); 14-year-old with prominent lower face, depressed nasal bridge, full lips, and nodular skin lesions over the chest and arms (**B**).

are deficient in the enzyme iduronate sulfatase; metachromatic staining of leukocyte granules and fibroblasts

Comment. Hunter syndrome is the only X-linked mucopolysaccharidosis. The two types (MPS IIA and MPS IIB) are examples of allelic variation, which result in remarkably different neurobehavioral phenotypes but the same somatic phenotype. Enzyme replacement therapy has been commercially available since 2006. The incidence is 1:110,000–132,500. Iduronate sulfatase (IDS) gene contains nine exons and more than 300 different mutations have been described.

REFERENCES

Hunter C: A rare disease in two brothers. Proc Roy Soc Med 10:104, 1917.

Muenzer J, Beck M, Eng CM, et al.: Multidisciplinary management of Hunter syndrome. Pediatrics 124:e1228, 2009.

Wilson PJ, Morris CP, Anson DS, et al.: Hunter syndrome: Isolation of an iduronate-2-sulfatase cDNA clone and analysis of patient DNA. Proc Natl Acad Sci 87:8531, 1990.

Wraith JE: Enzyme replacement therapy for the management of the mucopolysaccharidoses. Int J Clin Pharmacol Ther 47 Suppl 1:563, 2009.

DIFFERENTIAL MATRIX

Syndrome	Short Stature	Coarse Facies	Macrocephaly	Comments
Mucopolysaccharidosis IIA	+	+	+	Hepatosplenomegaly, hernias, joint stiffness, thick skin, hirsutism, behavioral disturbance
Atkin-Flaitz	+	+	+	Hypertelorism, downslanting palpebral fissures, broad nasal tip, thick lower lip, brachydactyly, seizures
Börjeson-Forssman-Lehmann	+	+	0	Obesity, hypotonia, hypogonadism, microcephaly, large ears, gynecomastia, narrow shoulders, visual impairment, tapered digits
Coffin-Lowry	+	+	0	Hypertelorism, anteverted nares, tented upper lip, prominent lips and large mouth, large ears, soft hands with tapered digits, pectus carinatum, hypotonia
XLID-Hypogonadism-Tremor	+	+	0	Prominent lower lip, muscle wasting of legs, abnormal gait, hypogonadism, obesity, seizures, tremor

MYOTUBULAR MYOPATHY

(CENTRONUCLEAR MYOPATHY, MTMX)

OMIM 310400

Xq28

MTM1

Definition. XLID associated with hypotonia, weakness, and absent deep tendon reflexes secondary to myotubular myopathy. Truncating mutations in Myotubularin cause a severe phenotype, and missense mutations may be associated with milder forms.

Somatic Features. A craniofacial phenotype, resulting in large measure from hypotonia, may be recognized. Ptosis, arched upper lip, high palate, open mouth, thick alae nasi, and auricular helices accent an elongated and immobile face. The head tends to be large and elongated in its anteroposterior diameter. Hydrocephalus has been demonstrated in patients with intracranial hemorrhage in the perinatal period and in patients without this complication. Long slender digits are typical, contractures may be present, and cryptorchidism is commonly noted. The limbs are thin with decreased muscle mass.

Growth and Development. Birth length and head circumference, but not birth weight, tend to be large. Hydrocephaly contributes to the increased head circumference in some cases. The hydrocephaly is communicating and may arrest spontaneously or remain progressive. The tendency toward increased body length persists among those who survive the early months of life. Pervasive delay of motor milestones is typical in these usually ventilator-dependent children.

Cognitive Function. Severe motor impairment, ventilator dependency, and early death prevent adequate assessment of cognitive function.

Neurological Findings. Profound hypotonia, weakness, and areflexia exist from birth and presumably from early in fetal life. Respiratory efforts are insufficient, generally requiring ventilator support.

Heterozygote Expression. Although rarely clinically weak, some females have presented with weakness in the third to fourth decades. Carriers may show myopathic changes on muscle histology, however this finding is inconsistent.

Imaging. Hydrocephaly is present in some cases. Intracranial hemorrhage and evidence of ischemia may also be present.

Neuropathology. None

Laboratory. Small muscle fibers with centralization of nuclei and absence of central myofibrils can be demonstrated by light and electron microscopy suggesting a failure of myofiber maturation.

Comment. Myotubular myopathy has been suspected in at-risk pregnancies by the paucity of fetal movement and the appearance, often only in the third trimester, of polyhydramnios. Most patients die in the first few months of life. Survival is possible, but many require early and continued ventilator support. Autosomal dominant centronuclear myopathy is caused by mutations in the dynamin-2

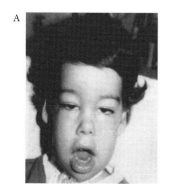
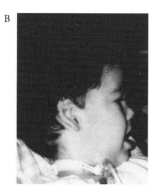
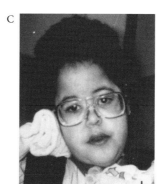
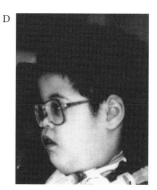

Myotubular Myopathy. Four-year-old with macrocephaly and myopathic facies, including ptosis, thickening of the alae nasi, and tenting of the upper lip (**A, B**); 6-year-old with macrocephaly, narrow bifrontal area, long facies, and tented upper lip (**C, D**).   Courtesy of Dr. Shashidhar Pai, Medical University of South Carolina, Charleston.

(*DMM2*) and a recessive form results from mutations in amphiphysin 2 (*BIN1*).

REFERENCES

DeAngelis MS, Palmucci L, Leone M, et al.: Centronuclear myopathy: clinical morphologic and genetic characters. A review of 288 cases. J Neurol Sci 103:2, 1991.

Joseph M, Pai GS, Holden KR, et al.: X-linked myotubular myopathy: clinical observations in ten additional cases. Am J Med Genet 59:168, 1995.

Jungbluth H, Wallgren-Petterson C, Laporte J: Centronuclear (myotubular) myopathy. Orphanet 3:26, 2008.

Romero NB: Centronuclear myopathies: a widening concept. Neuromuscul Disord 20:223, 2010.

Van Wijngaarden GK, Fleury P, Bethlem J, et al.: Familial myotubular myopathy. Neurology 19:901, 1969.

DIFFERENTIAL MATRIX

Syndrome	Muscle Wasting	Hypotonia	Areflexia, Hyporeflexia	Comments
Myotubular Myopathy	+	+	+	Open mouth, tented upper lip, hydrocephaly, long digits, cryptorchidism, weakness
Arts	+	+	+	Growth deficiency, poor muscle development, ataxia, deafness, vision loss, seizures, childhood death
Charcot-Marie-Tooth Neuropathy, Cowchock variant	+	0	+	Peripheral motor and sensory neuropathy, deafness, pes cavus, weakness
Charcot-Marie-Tooth Neuropathy, Ionasescu variant	+	0	+	Peripheral motor and sensory neuropathy, wasting of intrinsic hand muscles, enlarged ulnar nerves, pes cavus, weakness
Duchenne Muscular Dystrophy	+	0	+	Hypertrophy of calf muscles, elevated muscle enzymes, progressive weakness, contractures
Phosphoglycerate Kinase Deficiency	+	0	+	Expressionless face, weakness, seizures, myoglobinuria, hemolytic anemia

N-ALPHA-ACETYLTRANSFERASE DEFICIENCY

OMIM 300013

Xq28

NAA10

Definition. XLID with growth failure, hypotonia, aged facial appearance, cardiac arrhythmias, and early childhood death. Mutations have been found in *NAA10*, which encodes the subunit of an enzyme that modifies proteins by N-terminal acetylation.

Somatic Features. The face appears distinctive with aged appearance, arched brow, large palpebral fissures, and ptosis. There is increased body hair, lax skin and irregular fat deposition. Cardiac structure appears normal but arrhythmias develop ultimately leading to death in infancy or early childhood.

Growth and Development. Prenatal growth is normal. Postnatally, growth slows dramatically and global developmental delay is typical. Early lethality precludes long term observation.

Cognitive Function. Presumed to be severely impaired.

Heterozygote Expression. None

Comment. This lethal XLID syndrome is distinctive in having an aged facial appearance, lax skin, and cardiac arrhythmias. Impaired acetylation of the N-terminus of multiple proteins is the plausible cause of the syndrome findings.

REFERENCES

Bird LM, Jones MC, Johnston JJ, et al.: An X-linked malformation syndrome with infantile lethality due to mutation in NAA10. David W. Smith Workshop on Malformations and Morphogenesis, Lake Arrowhead, CA, September 9–14, 2011.

Rope AF, Tandell M, Arnesen T, et al.: A new syndrome caused by N-acetylation deficiency. David W. Smith Workshop on Malformations and Morphogenesis, Lake Arrowhead, CA, September 9–14, 2011.

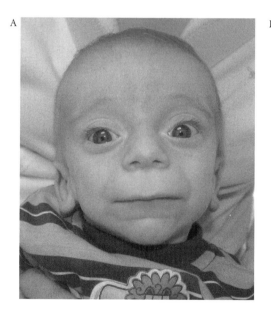 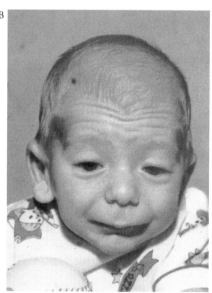

N-Alpha-Acetyltransferase Deficiency. Seven-month-old infant showing raised eyebrows, low-set ears, long philtrum with poorly formed ridges, thin upper lip and horizontal crease on chin (A). Uncle at 8 months showing horizontal furrows on forehead, raised eyebrows, excessively folded helices with large uplifted lobes, thin upper lip, and worried expression (B). Courtesy of Lynne M. Bird, MD, Rady Children's Specialists of San Diego, California.

DIFFERENTIAL MATRIX

Syndrome	Cutaneous Findings	Cardiac Malformation/ Arrhythmias	Hypotonia	Comments
N-Alpha-Acetyltransferase Deficiency	+	+	+	Aged facial appearance, growth failure, lax skin
Fitzsimmons	+	+	0	Alopecia/sparse hair, spastic paraplegia, pes cavus, dystrophic nails
Hereditary Bullous Dystrophy, X-linked	+	+	0	Microcephaly, short stature, upslanting palpebral fissures, protruding ears, digits short and tapered, small testes, early death from pulmonary infection
MIDAS	+	+	0	Ocular anomaly, CNS anomaly, microphthalmia, ocular dysgenesis, corneal opacification, dermal aplasia
XLID-Psoriasis	+	0	+	Hypogenitalism, ectodermal changes, hypertelorism, open mouth, large ears, seizures
TARP	0	+	+	Micrognathia, cleft palate, talipes equinovarus, persistence of left superior vena cava, hearing loss, visual impairment, arrhythmia, early childhood death

NANCE-HORAN SYNDROME
(XLID-CATARACT-DENTAL SYNDROME)

OMIM 302350

Xp22.13

NHS

Definition. XLID with congenital cataracts, microcorneas, dental anomalies, and brachydactyly. The gene encodes the NHS protein, a regulator of actin remodelling.

Somatic Features. Congenital cataracts almost invariably bring this condition to attention at birth or in early infancy. The dense bilateral nuclear cataracts may be detected on routine examination or in the course of evaluating the accompanying nystagmus. Microcornea and, less frequently, microphthalmia and glaucoma may be present. Vision is severely impaired. Dental anomalies include supernumerary maxillary medical incisors (mesiodens), peg-shaped teeth, notching of the incisors, and increased spacing of the central incisors (diastema). The ears are frequently cupped, prominent, and simply formed. Other facial features include long facies, prominent nasal bridge and nose, prominent mandible, retracted midface, and high-arched palate. Short fourth metacarpals and short broad fingers complete the phenotype.

Growth and Development. Growth appears to be normal. Development is delayed and cognition is impaired in about 20% of males. The visual impairment is contributory but does not appear to be the sole cause.

Cognitive Function. Mild-to-moderate cognitive impairment has been suspected in a minority of cases.

Heterozygote Expression. Young females may have posterior sutural cataracts that are only detected by slit lamp and do not limit vision. Increasing lens opacity with age has been reported. Tapering, notching, and increased spacing of the incisors have been observed.

Comment. X-linked cataracts are allelic to Nance-Horan syndrome.

REFERENCES

Brooks SP, Coccia M, Tang HR, et al.: The Nance-Horan syndrome protein encodes a functional WAVE homology domain (WHD) and is important in actin remodelling and maintaining cell morphology. Hum Mol Genet 19:2421, 2010.

Burden KP, McKay JD, Sale MM, et al.: Mutations in a novel gene, NHS, cause the pleiotropic effects of Nance-Horan syndrome, including severe congenital cataract, dental anomalies, and mental retardation. Am J Hum Genet 73:1120, 2003.

Horan MB, Billson FA: X-linked cataract and Hutchinsonian teeth. Aust Paediatr J 10:98, 1974.

Nance WE, Warburg M, Bixler D, et al.: Congenital X-linked cataract, dental anomalies and brachymetacarpalia. Birth Defects: Orig Art Ser X(4):285, 1974.

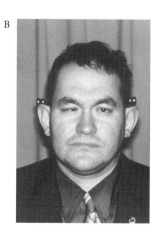

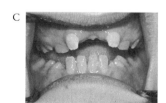
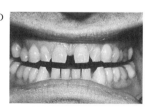

Nance-Horan Syndrome. Nine-year-old male with cupped ears, microcornea, and congenital cataracts (**A**); 38-year-old with cupped ears, microcornea, and congenital cataracts (**B**). Teeth of patient in **A** showing spacing of incisors and narrow incisal edges (**C**); teeth of patient in **B** showing spacing of incisors and tapering of incisal edges (**D**). Courtesy of Dr. Walter Nance, Medical College of Virginia, Richmond.

DIFFERENTIAL MATRIX

Syndrome	Cataracts	Dental Anomalies	Digital Anomalies	Comments
Nance-Horan	+	+	+	Microcornea, nystagmus, cupped ears, short fourth metacarpals
Armfield	+	+	+	Short stature, cataracts or glaucoma, small hands and feet, hydrocephaly, joint stiffness, seizures
Goltz	+	+	+	Ocular dysgenesis, linear areas of dermal aplasia, cutaneous adipose herniations, dystrophic nails, vertebral anomalies, limb reduction defects, genitourinary anomalies
Lenz Microphthalmia	+	+	+	Microcephaly, microphthalmia, ocular dysgenesis, malformed ears, cleft lip/palate, cardiac and genitourinary anomalies, thumb duplication or hypoplasia, narrow shoulders
Incontinentia Pigmenti	+	+	0	Cutaneous vesicles, verrucous lesions, irregular hyperpigmentation, microcephaly, ocular anomalies, oligodontia, spasticity, seizures

NORRIE DISEASE

(NORRIE RETINAL DYSPLASIA)

OMIM 310600

Xp11.3

NDP

Definition. XLID with a progressive ophthalmopathy (iris atrophy, uveal ectropion, anterior and posterior synechiae, cataract, hyperplastic vitreous, and retrolental mass) and adult-onset hearing loss. The gene codes for a cysteine knot-containing growth factor. Missense mutations – especially in the C-terminal portion – result in a less severe phenotype.

Somatic Features. Ocular dysplasia and degeneration dominate the physical phenotype. Apart from the ocular findings, major malformations and facial manifestations do not occur. Binocular blindness is present from birth. The corneas vary in size and in clarity. The anterior chamber is likewise variable in depth. Iris atrophy occurs in most and is associated with anterior and posterior synechiae. Cataracts will develop in many but not all cases. Retinal dysplasia manifests as impaired vascularization, aplasia of sensory cells, and hyperplasia of pigment cells, combined with hyperplasia of the vitreous to form a yellowish-gray retrolental mass constituting an obligatory finding. The degeneration may ultimately progress to collapse of the ocular globe. Moderate to severe sensorineural hearing loss appears in the second or third decade in about one-third of patients.

Growth and Development. Intrauterine and postnatal growth is normal. Developmental delay in childhood identifies those who will be intellectually disabled.

Cognitive Function. Cognitive impairment of varying severity affects the majority but not all cases.

Neurological Findings. Aside from blindness and deafness, neurological abnormalities do not occur.

Heterozygote Expression. None

Imaging. Abnormalities of brain structure have not been described.

Comment. The X-chromosome hosts a disproportionate share of genes that disturb formation and function of the eye. Mutations in these genes also produce CNS malformations or functional impairments but do so quite inconsistently. As yet, reasons for the variable expression have not been found. Missense mutations in the Norrie disease gene have also been found in X-linked familial exudative vitreoretinopathy and in X-linked recessive primary retinal dysplasia, entities in which intellectual disability and hearing loss do not occur. Vision loss appears later and may be unilateral and less severe.

REFERENCES

Chen Z-Y, Battinelli EM, Fielder A, et al.: A mutation in the Norrie disease gene (NDP) associated with X-linked familial exudative vitreoretinopathy. Nat Genet 5:180, 1993.

Chen Z-Y, Battinelli EM, Kendriks RW, et al.: Norrie disease gene: characterization of deletions and possible function. Genomics 16:533, 1993.

Norrie G: Causes of blindness in children. Acta Ophth 5:7, 1927.

Shastry BS, Hejtmancik JF, Trese MT: Identification of novel missense mutations in the Norrie disease gene associated with one X-linked and four sporadic cases of familial exudative vitreoretinopathy. Hum Mutat 9:396, 1997.

Strasberg P, Liede HA, Stein T, et al.: A novel mutation in the Norrie disease gene predicted to disrupt the cystine knot growth factor motif. Hum Mol Genet 4:2179, 1995.

Warburg M: Norrie's disease. A new hereditary bilateral pseudotumour of the retina. Acta Ophth 39:757, 1961.

Wu WC, Drenser K, Trese M, et al.: Retinal phenotype-genotype correlation of pediatric patients expressing mutations in the Norrie disease gene. Arch Ophthalmol 125:225, 2007.

Syndrome	Ocular Dysgenesis	Vision Loss	Hearing Loss	Comments
Norrie	+	+	+	Adult-onset hearing loss
Wittwer	+	+	+	Microcephaly, short stature, microphthalmia, hypertelorism, genitourinary anomalies, hypotonia, seizures
Cerebro-Oculo-Genital	+	+	0	Microcephaly, hydrocephaly, short stature, agenesis of corpus callosum, microphthalmia, ptosis, hypospadias, cryptorchidism, clubfoot, spasticity
Goltz	+	+	0	Cataracts, linear areas of dermal aplasia, cutaneous adipose herniations, dystrophic nails, abnormal teeth and hair, vertebral anomalies, limb reduction defects, genitourinary anomalies
Lenz Microphthalmia	+	+	0	Microcephaly, microphthalmia, malformed ears, cleft lip/palate, cardiac and genitourinary anomalies, thumb duplication or hypoplasia, narrow shoulders
MIDAS	+	+	0	Microphthalmia, corneal opacification, dermal aplasia, dysgenesis of corpus callosum, cardiac defects, cardiomyopathy
Nance-Horan	+	+	0	Microcornea, nystagmus, cupped ears, short fourth metacarpals, cataracts, dental anomalies, digital anomalies

ATLAS OF X-LINKED INTELLECTUAL DISABILITY SYNDROMES

OPITZ FG SYNDROME

(FG SYNDROME, OPITZ-KAVEGGIA SYNDROME)

OMIM 305450

Xq13.1

MED12

Definition. XLID with macrocephaly, tall forehead, broad flat thumbs, imperforate anus or constipation, and hypotonia.

Somatic Features. The facial characteristics include macrocephaly or large head in comparison to height, broad forehead, frontal hair upsweep, hypertelorism, epicanthus, downslanted palpebral fissures, open mouth with thick alae nasi, small cupped simply formed ears, high arched palate, and everted lower lip. Hypotonia is notable and may be responsible for some of the facial features. A wide variety of structural anomalies of the CNS, heart, and urinary tract have been described. Complete or partial agenesis of the corpus callosum is the most common CNS anomaly, but dilated ventricles, pachygyria, and cerebral heterotopias have been noted. Cardiac defects, present in one-third of cases, include ventricular septal defect and hypoplastic left heart. Dilation of the urinary system, cryptorchidism, and hypospadias are the most common urinary tract abnormalities. Pyloric stenosis and hernias have been reported. Imperforate anus or severe childhood constipation without imperforate anus appears to be a distinguishing feature found in most cases. Musculoskeletal manifestations include broad flat thumbs and great toes, cutaneous syndactyly of fingers 2 and 3, horizontal palmar creases, camptodactyly, pectus excavatum, kyphoscoliosis, and large joint contractures. Joint hyperextensibility is typical. Split hand and polydactyly have been noted in exceptional cases.

Growth and Development. Intrauterine growth is usually normal or only mildly impaired. Stature usually remains in lower centiles but in some cases falls below the third centile. The head grows disproportionately, becoming macrocephalic or at least large in comparison to stature. The anterior fontanel may be large and delayed in closure. Motor and language development lags from the outset.

Cognitive Function. Severe impairment is the rule, although milder impairment has been seen occasionally.

Behavior. An affable personality with excessive talkativeness and hyperactivity has been described in some.

Neurological Findings. Hypotonia dominates the neurological examination but in some cases gives way to spasticity, contractures, and unsteadiness during adult life. Seizures and sensorineural hearing loss occur in a minority.

Heterozygote Expression. No consistent manifestations are present in carrier females, although broad forehead, hypertelorism, and anterior upsweep of the scalp hair have been noted.

Imaging. Partial or complete agenesis of the corpus callosum occurs most commonly. In some cases, the ventricles may be dilated. Pachygyria and cerebral heterotopias have been described in a few cases.

Comment. Genetic heterogeneity exists among the many cases that have been given this diagnosis and perhaps explains, in part, the clinical difficulty in diagnosis. The diagnosis is most compelling in the presence of macrocephaly, hypotonia, and imperforate anus. Diagnosis on the basis of the rather subtle and variable craniofacial manifestations requires an experienced eye. The vast majority of patients clinically diagnosed with Opitz FG syndrome do not, in fact, have this X-linked syndrome but other phenotypically similar conditions caused by gene mutations or genomic changes on the autosomes or the X-chromosome.

Most cases, including the original family described by Opitz and Kaveggia (1974), have a single mutation, R961W. Several other mutations in *MED12* have been described, resulting in Opitz FG syndrome or at least some of the key findings. Notably, a N1007S mutation has been described in the original family with Lujan syndrome.

The assignment of multiple loci on the X-chromosome to Opitz FG syndrome seems ill-conceived. These conditions are in themselves distinctive, although they may share one or more features with Opitz FG syndrome. Such cases in point are the XLID macrocephaly syndromes reported by Unger et al. (2007) and Tarpey et al. (2007).

REFERENCES

Briault S, Hill R, Shrimpton A, et al.: A gene for FG syndrome maps in the Xq12–21.31 region. Am J Med Genet 73:87, 1997.
Clark RD, Graham JM, Friez MJ, et al.: FG syndrome, an X-linked multiple congenital anomaly syndrome: the clinical phenotype and an algorithm for diagnostic testing. Genet Med 11:769, 2009.

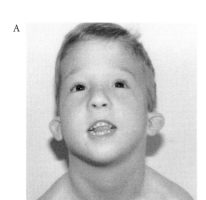
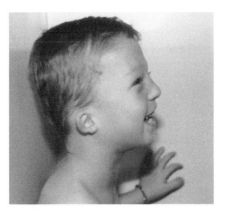

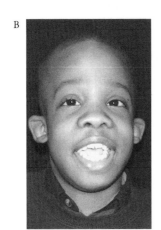
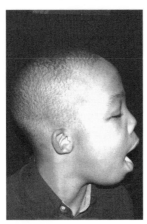

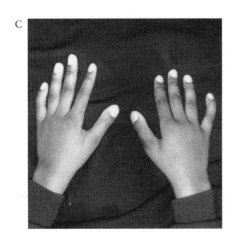
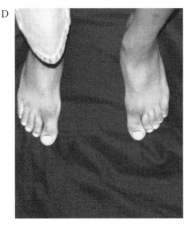

Optiz FG Syndrome. Turricephaly, hypertelorism, downslanting palpebral fissures, small and low-set simply formed ears, and tented and thin upper lip in a 5-year-old male (A); macrocephaly, dolichocephaly, hypertelorism, downslanting palpebral fissures, tented upper lip, maxillary overbite, notching of the upper central incisors, and broad thumbs and great toes in an 8-year-old boy (B–D). Illustration **A** courtesy of Dr. John Graham, Cedars-Sinai Medical Center, Los Angeles.

Graham JM, Tackels D, Dibbern K, et al.: FG syndrome: report of three new families with linkage to Xq12-q21.31. Am J Med Genet 80:145, 1998.

Lyons MJ, Graham JM Jr., Neri G, et al.: Clinical experience in the evaluation of 30 patients with a prior diagnosis of FG syndrome. J Med Genet 46:9, 2009.

Opitz JM, Kaveggia EG: Studies of malformation syndromes of man XXXIII: The FG syndrome. An X-linked recessive syndrome of multiple congenital anomalies and mental retardation. Z Kinderheilk 117:1, 1974.

Opitz JM, Richieri-da Costa A, Aase JM, et al.: FG syndrome update 1988: note of 5 new patients and bibliography. Am J Med Genet 30:309, 1988.

Risheg H, Graham JM Jr., Clark RD, et al.: A recurrent mutation in MED12 leading to R961W causes Opitz-Kaveggia syndrome. Nat Genet 39:451, 2007.

Schwartz CE, Tarpey PS, Lubs HA, et al.: The original Lujan syndrome family has a novel missense mutation (p.N1007S) in the MED12 gene. J Med Genet 44:472, 2007.

Sorge G, Polizzi A, Ruggieri M, et al.: Early fatal course in three brothers with FG syndrome. Clin Pediatr 35:365, 1996.

Tarpey PS, Raymond FL, Nguyen LS, et al.: Mutations in UPF3B, a member of the nonsense-mediated mRNA decay complex, cause syndromic and nonsyndromic mental retardation. Nat Genet 39:1127, 2007.

Unger S, Mainberger A, Spitz C, et al.: Filamin A mutation is one cause of FG syndrome. Am J Med Genet 143A:1876, 2008.

Syndrome	Macrocephaly	Digital Anomalies	Hypotonia	Comments
Opitz FG	+	+	+	Broad forehead, downslanted palpebral fissures, everted lower lip, dysgenesis of corpus callosum, cardiac defects, imperforate anus, constipation, broad flat thumbs and great toes
Simpson-Golabi-Behmel	+	+	+	Somatic overgrowth, supernumerary nipples, polydactyly
Atkin-Flaitz	+	+	0	Short stature, hypertelorism, downslanting palpebral fissures, broad nasal tip, thick lower lip, brachydactyly, seizures
Mucopolysaccharidosis IIA	+	+	0	Short stature, coarse facies, hepatosplenomegaly, hernias, joint stiffness, thick skin, hirsutism, behavioral disturbance
ATRX-Associated XLID	0	+	+	Microcephaly, short stature, small testes, telecanthus, small triangular nose, tented upper lip, open mouth, wide spacing of teeth, genital anomalies, musculoskeletal anomalies, hemoglobin H inclusions in erythrocytes
Coffin-Lowry	0	+	+	Microcephaly, short stature, hypertelorism, anteverted nares, tented upper lip, prominent lips and large mouth, large ears, soft hands with tapered digits, pectus carinatum
Miles-Carpenter	0	+	+	Microcephaly, short stature, ptosis, small palpebral fissures, open mouth, pectus excavatum, scoliosis, long hands, camptodactyly, rockerbottom feet, arch fingerprints, spasticity, unsteady gait

OPTIC ATROPHY, X-LINKED

(WENT SYNDROME, OPTIC ATROPHY-2)

OMIM 311050

Xp11.4-p11.21

Definition. XLID with optic atrophy, ataxia, tremors, absent ankle deep tendon reflexes, and emotional liability. The gene has not been identified.

Somatic Features. Major malformations or craniofacial manifestations do not occur. Ocular and neurological findings predominate. Bilateral optic atrophy begins early, perhaps being present at birth, and is slowly progressive. The optic discs appear pale and commonly are cupped. Retinal vessels may have abnormal origin and course. Peripheral visual fields are normal, but central scotomas or enlarged physiological blind spots have been demonstrated. Color vision may be defective as a secondary phenomenon. Neurological dysfunction presents in the form of gait disturbance, ataxia, tremors, dysdiadochokinesis, hyperactive deep tendon reflexes at the knees, but absent ankle reflexes and Babinski signs. The Achilles tendon may be short. Clubfoot or kyphosis may occur.

Growth and Development. Details of growth have not been reported.

Cognitive Features. Early schooling difficulties, in part related to visual impairment. Adults show mild cognitive impairment.

Behavior. Emotional lability has been described in some cases.

Neurological Findings. Neurological abnormalities, primarily involuntary movements, pathological reflexes, gait disturbances, dysdiadochokinesis, and dysarthria, vary in severity and time of onset. Typically, the deep tendon reflexes at the knees are hyperactive and depressed or absent at the ankles.

Heterozygote Expression. Carrier females have normal ocular and neurological findings.

Comment. The phenotype is based on a single family with eight affected males in three generations. It is possible that this entity stems from a contiguous gene deletion syndrome rather than a single gene mutation.

REFERENCES

Assink JJ, Tijmes NT, ten Brink JB, et al.: A gene for X-linked optic atrophy is closely linked to the Xp11.4-Xp11.2 region of the X chromosome. Am J Hum Genet 61:934, 1997.

Katz BJ, Zhao Y, Warner JE, et al.: A family with X-linked optic atrophy linked to the OPA2 locus Xp11.4-Xp11.2. Am J Med Genet A 140A:2207, 2006.

Völker-Dieben HJ, Van Lith GHM, Went LN, et al.: A family with sex-linked optic atrophy (ophthalmological and neurological aspects). Doc Ophthalmologica 37:307, 1974.

Went LN, De Vries-De Mol EC, Völker-Dieben HJ: A family with apparently sex-linked optic atrophy. J Med Genet 12:94, 1975.

DIFFERENTIAL MATRIX

Syndrome	Vision Loss	Tremors	Abnormal Deep Tendon Reflexes	Comments
Optic Atrophy, X-linked	+	+	+	Optic atrophy, ataxia, dysarthria, gait disturbance, emotional lability
Ataxia-Deafness-Dementia, X-linked	+	+	+	Optic atrophy, hearing loss, spastic paraplegia, ataxia, hypotonia, seizures, childhood death
Arts	+	0	+	Growth deficiency, poor muscle development, hypotonia, areflexia, ataxia, deafness, seizures, childhood death
Gustavson	+	0	+	Microcephaly, short stature, large ears, deafness, joint contractures, rockerbottom feet, brain undergrowth, hydrocephaly, cerebellar hypoplasia, spasticity, seizures
Mohr-Tranebjaerg	+	0	+	Hearing loss, neurological deterioration with childhood onset, dystonia, spasticity
Paine	+	0	+	Microcephaly, short stature, optic atrophy, hearing loss, spasticity, seizures
Proud (*ARX*-Associated, X-linked)	+	0	+	Microcephaly, hearing loss, agenesis of corpus callosum, cryptorchidism, inguinal hernias, ataxia, spasticity, seizures
Schimke	+	0	+	Microcephaly, sunken eyes, downslanting palpebral fissures, narrow nose, wide spacing of teeth, cupped ears, hypotonia, abducens palsy, hearing loss, spasticity, choreoathetosis, contractures

ORAL-FACIAL-DIGITAL SYNDROME I
(OROFACIODIGITAL SYNDROME I, OFD-1)

OMIM 311200

Xp22.2

OFD1 (CXORF5)

Definition. XLID associated with dystopia canthorum, midface anomalies, intraoral clefts and pseudoclefts, lingual hamartomas, hypertrophied oral frenuli, structural anomalies of the brain, polycystic kidneys, brachydactyly, and syndactyly manifest predominantly in females.

Somatic Features. Craniofacial manifestations – especially those involving the oral structures – predominate. Externally obvious facial features are transient facial milia, dystopia canthorum, flattening of the midface, hypoplasia of alar cartilages, and midline pseudocleft of the lip. Intra-oral anomalies include high arch or cleft (often irregular) of the palate, pseudocleft or lobation of the tongue, hamartomas on the tongue, hypertrophied and aberrant frenuli, malocclusion, and hypodontia. The fingers are asymmetrically short with proximal cutaneous syndactyly and clinodactyly, especially of fingers 2 and 5. Polydactyly rarely occurs. Other anomalies include dry, sparse scalp hair, alopecia, agenesis of corpus callosum, hydrocephaly, porencephaly, and adult-type polycystic kidneys.

Growth and Development. Growth is usually normal, but developmental milestones may be delayed.

Cognitive Function. About half of cases have cognitive impairment.

Neurological Findings. The presence and type of neurological symptoms and signs presumably depend on cerebral involvement, which is variable. Findings include seizures, ataxia, dysarthria, dysmetria, and trembling of the hands.

Imaging. Structural anomalies of the brain include agenesis of corpus callosum, neuronal heterotopias, hydrocephaly, porencephaly, cerebral infarcts, cerebral cysts, brain

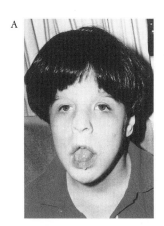

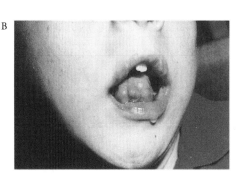

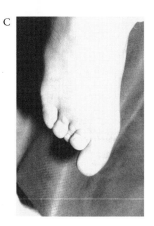

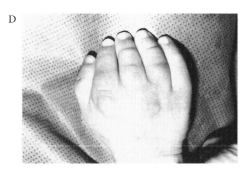

Oral-Facial-Digital I Syndrome. Seventeen-year-old girl with epicanthus, downslanting palpebral fissures, nasal deformation, gaping mouth, tongue nodule, and brachydactyly.   Courtesy of Dr. Arthur S. Aylsworth, University of North Carolina School of Medicine, Chapel Hill.

atrophy, cerebellar hypoplasia/dysplasia, and hypothalamic hamartomas.

Comment. OFD I represents one of the X-linked conditions that have been found almost exclusively in females. Most cases (up to 75%) are sporadic, perhaps arising from mutations in the paternal germline. Available pedigrees are also consistent with X-linked dominant inheritance with lethality in hemizygous males. Affected males have been reported. Some have had the karyotype 47,XXY. Others may have an orofaciodigital syndrome other than OFD I. Edwards et al. (1988) reported a family with an OFD II-like syndrome having an X-linked recessive pattern of transmission. Vallaud et al. (1968) described a family in which females with OFD I were related through unaffected transmitting males.

REFERENCES

Budny B, Chen W, Omran H, et al.: A novel X-linked recessive mental retardation syndrome comprising macrocephaly and ciliary dysfunction is allelic to oral-facial-digital type I syndrome. Hum Genet 120:171, 2006.

Edwards M, Mulcahy D, Turner G: X-linked recessive inheritance of an orofaciodigital syndrome with partial expression in females and survival of affected males. Clin Genet 34:325, 1988.

Feather SA, Woolf AS, Donnai D, et al.: The oral-facial-digital syndrome type I (OFDI), a cause of polycystic kidney disease and associated malformations, maps to Xp22.2-Xp22.3. Hum Mol Genet 6:1163, 1997.

Ferrante MI, Giorgio G, Feather SA, et al.: Identification of the gene for oral-facial-digital type I syndrome. Am J Hum Genet 68:569, 2001.

Gorlin RJ, Anderson VE, Scott CR: Hypertrophied frenuli, oligophrenia, familial trembling and anomalies of the hand. New Eng J Med 264:486, 1961.

Leão MJ, Ribeiro-Silva ML: Orofaciodigital syndrome type I in a patient with severe CNS defects. Pediatr Neurol 13:247, 1995.

Papillon-Léage, Mme., Psaume J: Une malformation héréditaire de la muqueuse buccale brides et freins anormaux. Rev Stomatol (Paris) 55:209, 1954.

Thauvin-Robinet C, Cossée M, Cormier-Daire V, et al.: Clinical, molecular, and genotype-phenotype correlation studies from 25 cases of oral-facial-digital syndrome type 1: a French and Belgian collaborative study. J Med Genet 43:54, 2006.

Vaillaud JC, Martin J, Szepetowski G, et al.: Le syndrome oro-facial-digital. Etude clinique et génétique à propos de 10 cas observés dans une même famille. Rev Pédiat 5:383, 1968.

Wettke-Schäfer R, Kantner G: X-linked dominant inherited diseases with lethality in hemizygous males. Hum Genet 64:1, 1983.

DIFFERENTIAL MATRIX

Syndrome	Orofacial Clefting	Oral Frenula/ Tongue Hamartomas	Brachydactyly	Comments
Oral-Facial-Digital I	+	+	+	Sparse scalp hair, dystopia canthorum, flat midface, hypoplastic alae nasi, syndactyly, clinodactyly, structural brain anomalies, polycystic kidneys
Armfield	+	O	+	Short stature, cataracts or glaucoma, dental anomalies, small hands and feet, hydrocephaly, joint stiffness, seizures
Otopalatodigital I (*FLNA*-Associated XLID)	+	O	+	Short stature, conductive hearing impairment, prominent brow, broad nasal root, apparent ocular hypertelorism, downslanting palpebral fissures, cleft palate, blunted distal phalanges, irregular curvature and spacing of digits, limitation of elbow movement
Otopalatodigital II (*FLNA*-Associated XLID)	+	O	+	Short stature, hearing impairment, prominent forehead, flat/broad nasal bridge, ocular hypertelorism, downslanting palpebral fissures, flat midface, blunted flexed overlapping fingers, rockerbottom feet, hypoplastic fibulas, subluxed or dislocated joints

ORNITHINE TRANSCARBAMOYLASE DEFICIENCY
(ORNITHINE CARBAMOYLTRANSFERASE DEFICIENCY, OTC DEFICIENCY)

OMIM 311250

Xp11.4

OTC

Definition. XLID condition caused by chronic or intermittent hyperammonemia resulting from deficiency of ornithine transcarbamoylase.

Somatic Features. Malformations and other distinctive somatic manifestations do not occur.

Growth and Development. Intrauterine growth is normal. Those who experience hyperammonemic encephalopathy early in infancy have subsequent growth failure including microcephaly. Delay of developmental milestones may likewise be related to early hyperammonemia.

Cognitive Function. Neonatal hyperammonemia causes intellectual disability. Later onset hyperammonemic encephalopathy results in some cognitive impairment. Even those with intermittent, self-limited episodes and asymptomatic females may have lower IQs than expected.

Behavioral Manifestations. Agitation or irritability followed by disorientation and lethargy may be associated with hyperammonemia.

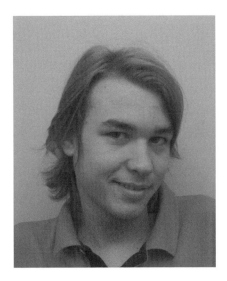

Ornithine Transcarbamoylase Deficiency. Eighteen-year-old with normal craniofacial appearance.

Neurological Findings. Cerebral edema and subsequent compromise of cerebral perfusion lead to a variety of neurological findings including changes in sensorium, ataxia, hemiparesis, slurred speech, seizures, amblyopia, and coma.

Natural History. Presentation is variable depending on the residual enzyme activity and, in heterozygotes, on Lyonization in hepatocytes. With negligible enzyme activity, presentation occurs early, in the second or third day of life, with poor feeding, vomiting, lethargy, and hyperventilation progressing to coma, respiratory arrest, and death. Survivors have intellectual disability and often cerebral palsy.

Presentation is more variable in the later onset group. Symptoms may present in infancy with advancement to a higher protein diet in children and adults with a high-protein meal, and at any age with an infection or with no apparent precipitating event. Symptoms include vomiting, headache, hyperventilation, and changes in sensorium or behavior in the form of irritability, agitation, lethargy, or disorientation. Slurred speech, hemiparesis, seizures, ataxia, and amblyopia may appear. If left untreated, coma, respiratory arrest, and death may ensue. All survivors of hyperammonemic encephalopathy have some cognitive impairment.

Heterozygote Expression. Expression in females depends on residual enzyme activity and on Lyonization of enzyme activity in hepatocytes. Females have been reported with early presentation, but this is unusual. Usually expressing females have later onset and episodic symptoms. Two-thirds of asymptomatic women have elevated plasma ammonia and glutamine compared to controls.

Imaging. Cerebral imaging reveals edema acutely and atrophy with prolonged or repeated episodes.

Neuropathology. Neurological symptoms and signs stem from cerebral edema and compromise of cerebral blood flow. This appears to primarily result from high glutamine concentrations in glial cells with subsequent osmotic swelling of the cells.

Laboratory. Chronically in the early onset and intermittently in the late onset, there is respiratory alkalosis, hyperammonemia, and oroticaciduria. Plasma glutamine and alanine may be elevated. In neonatal presentation, plasma citrulline is absent or very low. Allopurinol challenge test may detect mildly affected patients between episodes and asymptomatic heterozygotes. Direct mutational analysis of the *OTC* gene is possible.

Treatment. Prevention of encephalopathic episodes offers the best prognosis. Hyperammonemic encephalopathy causes brain damage. Even asymptomatic or mildly symptomatic episodes may cause mild but permanent cerebral dysfunction. Elevated plasma glutamine may predict an impending encephalopathy. Those infants diagnosed prenatally should be started on treatment at birth. Treatment for all ages consists of a low-protein diet, citrulline or arginine as a source of arginine, and sodium phenylbutyrate for alternative nitrogen excretion. Hemodialysis is the best form of ammonia/glutamine removal in encephalopathic coma.

REFERENCES

Bachmann C: Ornithine carbamoyl transferase deficiency: findings, models and problems. J Inher Met Dis 15:578, 1992.

Brusilow SW: Urea cycle disorders: diagnosis, pathophysiology, and therapy. Adv Pediatr 43:127, 1996.

Lindgren V, De Martinville B, Horwich AL, et al.: Human ornithine transcarbamylase locus mapped to band Xp21.1 near the Duchenne muscular dystrophy locus. Science 226:698, 1984.

Tuchman M: The clinical, biochemical, and molecular spectrum of ornithine transcarbamylase deficiency. J Lab Clin Med 120:836, 1992.

DIFFERENTIAL MATRIX

Syndrome	Metabolic Disturbance	Sensorium Change	Ataxia	Comments
Ornithine Transcarbamoylase Deficiency	+	+	+	Chronic or intermittent hyperammonemia, microcephaly, protein-induced vomiting and lethargy, seizures
Pyruvate Dehydrogenase Deficiency	+	+	+	Microcephaly, ataxia, dysarthria, structural brain anomalies, hypotonia, lactic acidosis

OTOPALATODIGITAL SYNDROME I (*SEE ALSO FLNA*-ASSOCIATED XLID)

(OTOPALATODIGITAL SYNDROME, OPD SYNDROME, OPD 1, *FLNA* SPECTRUM)

OMIM 311300

Xq28

FLNA

Definition. XLID with distinctive facial appearance, cleft palate, conductive hearing impairment, short stature, skeletal dysplasia, and, in some cases, mild cognitive impairment.

Somatic Features. A "pugilistic" facial appearance and digital anomalies suggest OPD I. Craniofacial features include occipital prominence, frontal bossing, overhanging brow, broad depressed nasal bridge, apparent ocular hypertelorism, downslanting palpebral fissures, small mouth, micrognathia, and cleft palate. The trunk is short with pectus excavatum. The thumbs and halluces are short and broad. The terminal fingers and toes are blunted and bulbous with short nails.

The digits are also irregular in curvature and the toes widely spaced. The long bones of the limbs may be involved, with limitation of elbow movement, bowing, and abnormal modeling. Some of the facial and skeletal findings are mirrored in the radiographs – thick skull base, prominent supraorbital ridges, hypoplastic facial bones, small mandible with obtuse angle, hypoplastic/aplastic paranasal sinuses, short broad distal phalanges of digits, accessory ossification centers at bases of metacarpals and metatarsals, and abnormal configurations and coalitions of carpals and tarsals.

Growth and Development. Stature is generally less than the 10th centile. Development may be delayed. Delay in speech development may be a manifestation of the general cognitive impairment or secondary to conductive hearing impairment resulting from malformed middle ear ossicles and chronic middle ear effusions.

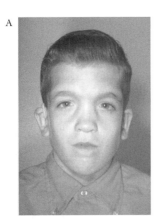
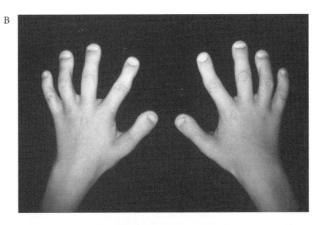
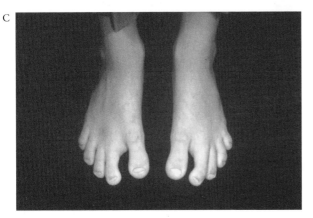
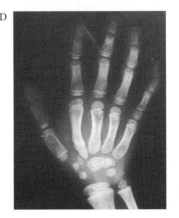
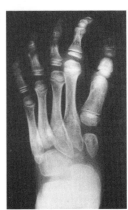

Otopalatodigital Syndrome I. Teenage boy with downslanting palpebral fissures, broad nasal base, underdeveloped malar area, and small mouth (**A**); hands with brachydactyly and expansion of distal phalanges (**B**); feet with expansion of distal phalanges and increased space between toes 1 and 2 (**C**); radiograph of hand showing short thumb, accessory ossification center of proximal metacarpal 2, abnormal size and orientation of carpal bones and abnormal middle phalanx of finger 5 (**D**); radiograph of foot showing short first metatarsal and great toe and accessory ossification centers fused with proximal metatarsals 2, 3, and 4 (**E**).   Courtesy of Dr. Robert J. Gorlin, University of Minnesota School of Dentistry, Minneapolis.

Cognitive Function. IQs are usually 75 to 90.

Heterozygote Expression. Females may have prominent supra-orbital ridges, apparent hypertelorism, flat maxillary and malar areas, depressed broad nasal bridge, fifth finger clinodactyly, short nails, toe spacing, and radiographic findings.

Comment. Diagnosis is based on clinical and radiographic features and confirmed with *FLNA* testing. OPD I has craniofacial and digital manifestations similar to those in Craniorodigital syndrome (OPD II). OPD I is the milder of the two conditions, but both result from mutations in *FLNA*, as are Periventricular Nodular Heterotopia, Frontometaphyseal Dysplasia, and Melnick-Needles syndrome. OPD I and OPD II are caused by gain-of-function mutations in contrast to the loss-of-function mutations found in the allelic disorders with disturbed neuronal migration.

REFERENCES

Biancalana V, LeMarec B, Odent S, et al.: Oto-palato-digital syndrome type I: Further evidence for assignment of the locus to Xq28. Hum Genet 88:228, 1991.

Clark AR, Sawyer GM, Robertson SP, et al.: Skeletal dysplasias due to filamin A mutations result from a gain-of-function mechanism distinct from allelic neurological disorders. Hum Mol Genet 18:4791, 2009.

Dudding BA, Gorlin RJ, Langer LO: The oto-palato-digital syndrome, a new symptom-complex consisting of deafness, dwarfism, cleft palate, characteristic facies, and generalized bone dysplasia. Am J Dis Child 113:214, 1967.

Fox JW, Lamperti ED, Ekşioğlu YZ, et al.: Mutations in filamin 1 prevent migration of cerebral cortical neurons in human periventricular heterotopia. Neuron 21:1315, 1998.

Gall JC, Stern AM, Poznanski AK, et al.: Oto-palato-digital syndrome: Comparison of clinical and radiographic manifestations in males and females. Am J Hum Genet 24:24, 1972.

Langer LO: The roentgenographic features of the oto-palato-digital (OPD) syndrome. Am J Roentgen 100:63, 1967.

Poznanski AK, MacPherson RI, Dijkman DJ, et al.: Otopalatodigital syndrome: Radiologic findings in the hand and foot. Birth Defects: Orig Art Ser X(5):125, 1974.

Robertson SP: Otopalatodigital syndrome spectrum disorders: otopalatodigital syndrome types 1 and 2, frontometaphyseal dysplasia and Melnick-Needles syndrome. Eur J Hum Genet 15:3, 2007.

Robertson SP, Twigg SR, Sutherland-Smith AJ, et al.: Localized mutations in the gene encoding the cytoskeletal protein filamin A cause diverse malformations in humans. Nat Genet 33:487, 2003.

Sheen VL, Dixon PH, Fox JW, et al.: Mutations in the X-linked filamin 1 gene cause periventricular nodular heterotopia in males as well as in females. Hum Mol Genet 10:1775, 2001.

Taybi H: Generalized skeletal dysplasia with multiple anomalies. Am J Roentgen 88:450, 1962.

DIFFERENTIAL MATRIX

Syndrome	Cleft Palate	Hearing Impairment	Digital Anomalies	Comments
Otopalatodigital I (*FLNA*-Associated XLID)	+	+	+	Short stature, prominent brow, broad nasal root, apparent ocular hypertelorism, downslanting palpebral fissures, blunted distal phalanges, irregular curvature and spacing of digits, limitation of elbow movement
Otopalatodigital II (*FLNA*-Associated XLID)	+	+	+	Short stature, prominent forehead, flat/broad nasal bridge, ocular hypertelorism, downslanting palpebral fissures, flat midface, blunted flexed overlapping fingers, rockerbottom feet, hypoplastic fibulae, subluxed or dislocated joints
Oral-Facial-Digital I	+	0	+	Sparse scalp hair, dystopia canthorum, flat midface, hypoplastic alae nasi, hypertrophic and aberrant oral frenuli, intraoral clefts and pseudoclefts, lingual hamartomas, brachydactyly, syndactyly, clinodactyly, structural brain anomalies, polycystic kidneys
Pallister W	+	0	+	Short stature, prominent forehead, wide nasal tip, incomplete cleft lip/palate, spasticity, contractures

OTOPALATODIGITAL SYNDROME II (*SEE ALSO FLNA*-ASSOCIATED XLID)

(CRANIOORODIGITAL SYNDROME, OPD II SYNDROME, OPD2, FACIOPALATOOSSEOUS SYNDROME)

OMIM 304120

Xq28

FLNA

Definition. XLID with facial features similar to OPD I but more severe skeletal anomalies and with variable intellectual disability. This condition is allelic to Otopalatodigital syndrome I, Frontometaphyseal Dysplasia, Melnick-Needles syndrome, and Periventricular Nodular Heterotopia.

Somatic Features. Craniofacial features include prominent forehead, flat midface, flat/broad nasal bridge, hypertelorism, downslanting palpebral fissures, small mouth, marked micrognathia, cleft palate, low-set rotated ears, wide sutures, and large anterior fontanel with delayed closure. The thumbs and halluces are short and blunted. The halluces may be absent. The fingers are blunted, flexed, and overlapping. There is variable syndactyly, clinodactyly, and postaxial polydactyly of fingers and toes. The feet may be rockerbottom. The fibulae are small or absent. The other long bones are bowed and the elbows, wrists, knees, and hips may be subluxed/dislocated. The thorax is narrow with pectus excavatum.

The membranous calvarium is underossified, and the base of the skull, the supraorbital ridges, and the long bones are osteosclerotic. These findings may resolve with age. Sinuses are absent or underaerated. The mandible and malar areas are hypoplastic. Phalanges (particularly distal), metacarpals, and metatarsals are short. Toe phalanges may not be visualized radiographically. The first metatarsals and halluces may be absent. Phalangeal bone maturation is advanced and carpal maturation delayed. The clavicles are thin and wavy. The ribs are narrow centrally and widened at the ends. Vertebral bodies may be flat.

Growth and Development. Survivors are undergrown.

Cognitive Function. Most of the few survivors have some degree of intellectual disability, but normal intellect has been reported. Mixed hearing impairment may affect speech development.

Natural History. The majority are stillborn or die in the first year of life, usually from pulmonary infections and aspiration. Survivors are undergrown and may have orthopedic problems. Facial appearance, bone mineralization, and bowing improve with age.

Heterozygote Expression. Heterozygotes may have mild facial, digital, and radiographic features. Features reported in females include frontal bossing, skull sclerosis, poorly aerated sinuses, hypertelorism, downslanting palpebral fissures, low-set ears, high arch palate, bifid uvula, micrognathia, syndactyly, and clinodactyly.

Comment. OPD II may be considered a severe variant of OPD I. Mutations in *FLNA* have been found in both entities as well as in Melnick-Needles syndrome, Periventricular Nodular Heterotopia, and Frontometaphyseal Dysplasia.

REFERENCES

Fitch N, Jequier S, Gorlin R: The oto-palato-digital syndrome, proposed type II. Am J Med Genet 15:655, 1983.

Fitch N, Jequier S, Papageorgiou A: A familial syndrome of cranial, facial, oral and limb anomalies. Clin Genet 10:226, 1976.

Fox JW, Lamperti ED, Ekşioğlu YZ, et al.: Mutations in filamin 1 prevent migration of cerebral cortex neurons in human periventricular heterotopia. Neuron 21:315, 1998.

Holder SE, Winter RM: Otopalatodigital syndrome type II. J Med Genet 30:310, 1993.

Preis S, Kemperdick H, Majewski F: Oto-palato-digital syndrome type II in two unrelated boys. Clin Genet 45:154, 1994.

Robertson SP, Twigg SR, Sutherland-Smith AJ, et al.: Localized mutations in the gene encoding the cytoskeletal protein filamin A cause diverse malformations in humans. Nat Genet 33:487, 2003.

Sheen VL, Dixon PH, Fox JW, et al.: Mutations in the X-linked filamin 1 gene cause periventricular nodular heterotopia in males as well as in females. Hum Mol Genet 10:1775, 2001.

Stratton RF, Bluestone DL: Oto-palato-digital syndrome type II with X-linked cerebellar hypoplasia/hydrocephalus. Am J Med Genet 41:169, 1991.

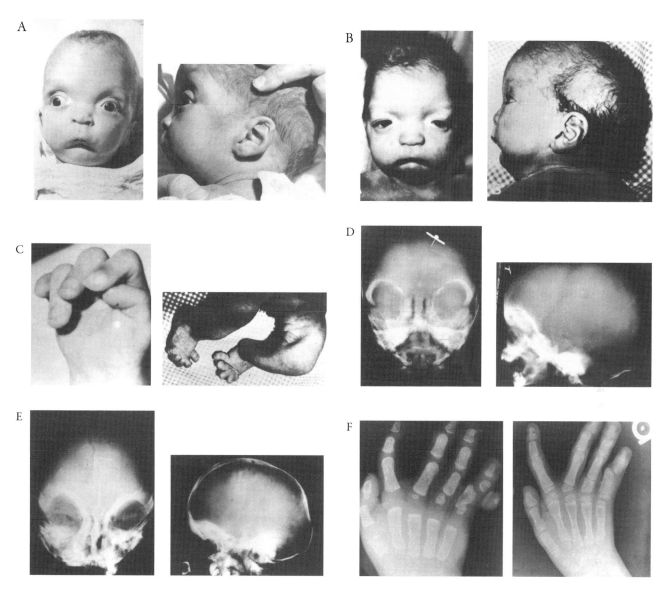

Otopalatodigital Syndrome II. Hypertelorism, downslanting palpebral fissures, flattened nose, prominence of the philtrum, small mouth, micrognathia, and excessively folded helices in infants reported by Fitch et al. (1983) **(A)** and Andrea et al. (1981) **(B)**. Spreading, malposition, and syndactyly of toes, and flexion and overlapping of fingers in patient reported by Andre et al. (1981) **(C)**; skull X-rays at 1 month showing wide intra-orbital distance, unusual ossification of the lateral orbital ridges, large calvarium with prominent occiput, and dense base of the skull **(D)**.
Courtesy of the *American Journal of Medical Genetics*, Copyright 1983, Alan R. Liss, Inc.

DIFFERENTIAL MATRIX

Syndrome	Cleft Palate	Hearing Impairment	Hypoplastic Fibulae	Comments
Otopalatodigital II (*FLNA*-Associated XLID)	+	+	+	Short stature, prominent forehead, flat/broad nasal bridge, ocular hypertelorism, downslanting palpebral fissures, flat midface, blunted, flexed, overlapping fingers, rockerbottom feet, subluxed or dislocated joints
Otopalatodigital I (*FLNA*-Associated XLID)	+	+	+	Short stature, prominent brow, broad nasal root, apparent ocular hypertelorism, downslanting palpebral fissures, blunted distal phalanges, irregular curvature and spacing of digits, limitation of elbow movement

PAINE SYNDROME
(PAINE-SEEMANOVÁ SYNDROME)

OMIM 311400

Definition. XLID with microcephaly, optic atrophy, spastic diplegia, and seizures. Genetic heterogeneity is likely. No gene has been identified.

Somatic Features. Microcephaly and short stature, possibly of postnatal onset, in the company of optic atrophy and spastic diplegia, dominate the clinical phenotype. Impaired vision and hearing are probable. Major malformations do not occur. Dermatoglyphics in one family showed an excess of arches or low loops and distal displacement of the palmar triradius. Death in infancy or early childhood is the rule.

Growth and Development. Intrauterine growth may be normal, but all parameters of postnatal growth are impaired. Microcephaly and short stature become obvious early in infancy if not at birth. No significant developmental milestones are achieved.

Cognitive Function. Severe impairment is obvious from early infancy.

Neurological Findings. Generalized spasticity with increased muscle tone, hyperreflexia, grimacing, opisthotonic body positioning, and myoclonic/opisthotonic seizures.

Imaging. The brain shows global undergrowth or atrophy. The ventricles and extra cerebral spaces may be enlarged. Radiographs show no calcifications.

Neuropathology. Autopsy on a 15-month-old child showed generalized undergrowth of the brain with decreased cerebral neurons but without gliosis.

Laboratory. A mild aminoaciduria and elevated alpha-amino nitrogen level in the cerebrospinal fluid originally reported by Paine (1960) could not be confirmed in later studies or in the patients reported by Seemanová et al. (1973).

Comment. Genetic heterogeneity is almost certain. Although similar in many respects to the cases reviewed by Reardon et al. (1994), CNS calcifications and neonatal thrombocytopenia have not been reported in Paine syndrome. Other XLID syndromes with death during childhood include Arts, Bertini, Gustavson, Holmes-Gang,

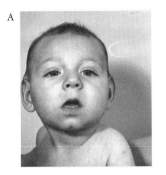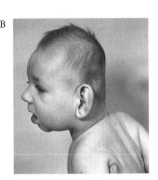
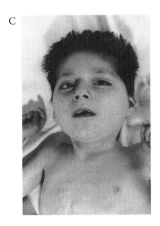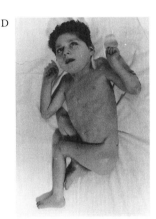

Paine Syndrome. Ten-month-old with microcephaly **(A, B)**; 7½-year-old with microcephaly and spasticity **(C, D)**. Courtesy of Dr. E Seemanová, University Children's Hospital of Charles University, Prague, Czech Republic.

Hydrocephaly-Cerebellar Agenesis, Hereditary Bullous Dystrophy, VACTERL-Hydrocephalus, X-Linked Ataxia-Deafness-Dementia, and X-Linked Lissencephaly. Specific gene or genomic changes are now known for several of these XLID syndromes.

REFERENCES

Paine RS: Evaluation of familial biochemically determined mental retardation in children, with special reference to aminoaciduria. New Eng J Med 262:658, 1960.

Reardon W, Hockey A, Silberstein, et al.: Autosomal recessive congenital intrauterine infection-like syndrome of microcephaly, intracranial calcifications, and CNS disease. Am J Med Genet 52:58, 1994.

Seemanová E, Lesný I, Hyánek J, et al.: X-chromosomal recessive microcephaly with epilepsy, spastic tetraplegia and absent abdominal reflexes. New variety of "Paine Syndrome"? Humangenetik 20:113, 1973.

DIFFERENTIAL MATRIX

Syndrome	Blindness and/ or Deafness	Spasticity	Seizures	Comments
Paine	+	+	+	Microcephaly, short stature, optic atrophy
Juberg-Marsidi-Brooks	+	+	+	Microcephaly and hydrocephaly, short stature, dysgenesis of corpus callosum, deep-set eyes, blepharophimosis, cupped ears, bulbous nose, small mouth, thin upper lip, pectus excavatum, flexion contractures
Proud (ARX-Associated XLID)	+	+	+	Microcephaly, agenesis of corpus callosum, cryptorchidism, inguinal hernias, ataxia
Schimke	+	+	+	Microcephaly, sunken eyes, downslanting palpebral fissures, narrow nose, wide spacing of teeth, cupped ears, abducens palsy, choreoathetosis, contractures
Mohr-Tranebjaerg	+	+	0	Neurological deterioration with childhood onset, dystonia
Bertini	+	0	+	Macular degeneration, hypotonia, childhood death, hypoplasia of cerebellar vermis and corpus callosum, developmental delays and regression, postnatal growth impairment
Wittwer	+	0	+	Microcephaly, short stature, microphthalmia, hypertelorism, genitourinary anomalies, hypotonia

PALLISTER W SYNDROME

(W SYNDROME)

OMIM 311450

Definition. XLID with short stature, characteristic facies (high forehead, frontal upsweep, prominent brow, hypertelorism, downslanting palpebral fissures, depressed and broad nasal bridge, wide nasal tip, incomplete cleft lip and palate, short high mandible), absent central maxillary incisors, elbow limitation, and spasticity. A gene locus has not been determined.

Somatic Features. All components of the face share in the distinctive characteristics. Head circumference is normal, but the forehead is tall and the brow prominent. Midfacial manifestations include hypertelorism, small and downslanting palpebral fissures, depression or broadness of the nasal bridge, and wide nasal tip with thick alae nasi and columella. The lower face is defined by simple short philtrum with thin upper lip, partial cleft or notching of the upper lip with extension to the alveolar ridge or anterior palate, absent central maxillary incisors and vertically tall mandible but not prognathism. Facial asymmetry is typical. Skeletal manifestations include general asthenia with cubitus valgus, limited movement or dislocation of the elbow, pectus excavatum, camptodactyly of fingers 4 and 5, limited movement of MCP joint of finger 1, and pes cavus or pes planus with midfoot varus. Muscle tone may be decreased, but there is general spasticity with hyperactive deep tendon reflexes. A coarse tremor of the upper limbs was noted in two brothers.

A 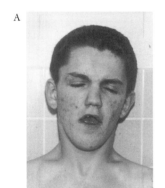 B 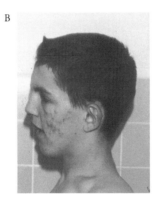 C 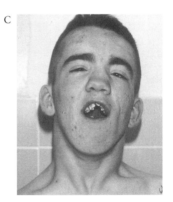 D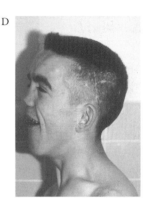

E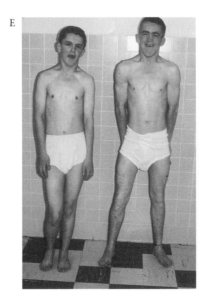

Pallister W Syndrome. Brothers at ages 20 and 22 years showing high forehead, frontal upsweep, prominent brow, hypertelorism, downslanting palpebral fissures, wide nasal tip, and short tall mandible (A-E).   Courtesy of Dr. Philip Pallister, Boulder, Montana.

Growth and Development. Intrauterine growth is variable. The head circumference remains normal, but stature falls below -2SD during childhood. Delay of developmental milestones is obvious from early infancy.

Cognitive Function. Severe impairment

Neurological Findings. Hypotonia was present in the one case in which the early childhood history was known. Spasticity with increased deep tendon reflexes and seizures of various types become the dominant neurological manifestation.

Heterozygote Expression. In the original family, carrier females had high forehead, hypertelorism, downslanting palpebral fissures, strabismus, short philtrum and vertically tall mandible, and possibly showed cognitive or neurobehavioral abnormality.

Imaging. Pneumoencephalography has shown ventricular enlargement and agenesis of the corpus callosum in one case.

Comment. A total of seven patients have been reported. Confirmation that the responsible gene is located on the X-chromosome has not been possible. Pallister et al. (1974) noted resemblance of the facial manifestations to those of Otopalatodigital syndrome, another X-linked disorder.

REFERENCES

Bottani A, Schinzel A: A third patient with median cleft upper lip, mental retardation and pugilistic facies (W syndrome): corroboration of a hitherto private syndrome. Clin Dysmorphol 2:225, 1993.

Goizet C, Bonneau D, Lacombe D: W syndrome: report of three cases and review. Am J Med Genet, 87:446, 1999.

Pallister PD, Herrmann J: Pallister-W syndrome. In Birth Defects Encyclopedia. Buyse ML, ed. Center for Birth Defects Information Services, Inc., Dover, 1990, p. 1354.

Pallister PD, Herrmann J, Spranger JW, et al.: The W syndrome. Studies of malformation syndromes of man XXVIII. Birth Defects: Orig Art Ser X(7):51, 1974.

DIFFERENTIAL MATRIX

Syndrome	Short Stature	Orofacial Clefting	Seizures	Comments
Pallister W	+	+	+	Prominent forehead, wide nasal tip, incomplete cleft lip/palate, spasticity
Armfield	+	+	+	Cataracts or glaucoma, dental anomalies, small hands and feet, hydrocephaly, joint stiffness
FLNA-Associated XLID	+	+	0	Prominent brow or forehead, hypertelorism, downslanting palpebral fissures, blunting of distal phalanges, irregular spacing of digits, limited/subluxed/dislocated joints, hypoplastic fibulas, periventricular nodular heterotopias

PARTINGTON SYNDROME (*SEE ALSO ARX*-ASSOCIATED XLID)

(MRXS1, XLID-DYSTONIA SYNDROME, *ARX* SPECTRUM)

OMIM 309510

Xp21.3

ARX

Definition. XLID with dysarthria, dystonia, hyperreflexia, and seizures. On the basis of molecular studies, Partington syndrome has been found to be allelic to West syndrome, Proud syndrome, and X-Linked Lissencephaly with Abnormal Genitalia. Several families with nonsyndromal XLID have mutations in *ARX* as well.

Somatic Features. Major malformations do not occur and craniofacial findings are not consistent. The face tends to be elongated, especially after childhood. Flexed posture and scoliosis may be present.

Growth and Development. Cranial and statural growth follows a normal course. Early childhood milestones lag behind but are quite variable. Difficulty in articulation is the major speech disability. The most severely affected individuals do not speak or seldom do so.

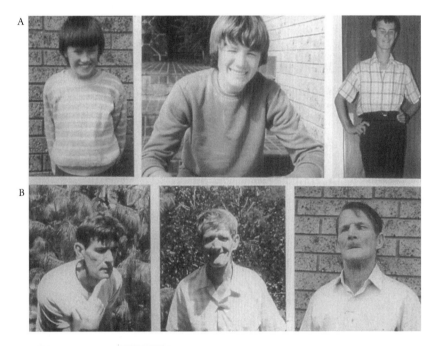

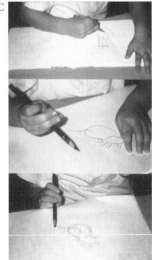

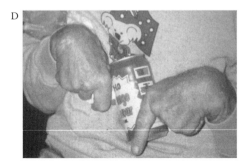

Partington Syndrome. Affected males at ages 12, 16, and 15 years showing normal facies **(A)**; adult males at ages 37, 47, and 57 years **(B)**; dystonic hand positions at ages 12 years **(C)** and 67 years **(D)**. Courtesy of Dr. Michael Partington, Human Genetics, New South Wales, Australia.

Cognitive Function. Variable from borderline to moderate impairment

Neurological Findings. Recurrent dystonic spasms involving the hands and dysarthria become obvious prior to school age and progress slowly, if at all. The gait appears awkward, and the deep tendon reflexes are brisk. Seizures occur in a minority of cases.

Heterozygote Expression. None

Laboratory. Normal nerve conduction velocity and electromyography

Comment. Dystonia limited to the hands and nonprogressive, or only slowly progressive, appears unique to the Partington syndrome. Other XLID-dystonia syndromes have been mapped to Xq, which is helpful in distinguishing them from Partington syndrome. This distinction can be confirmed by mutational analysis of *ARX*. The range of clinical presentation of individuals with *ARX* mutations is great with nonsyndromal XLID being the mildest and X-linked Lissencephaly with Abnormal Genitalia being most severe. Some individuals initially considered to have nonsyndromal XLID have been found to have dystonia on subsequent examination.

REFERENCES

Bienvenu T, Poirier K, Friocourt G, et al.: ARX, a novel Prd-class-homeobox gene highly expressed in the telencephalon, is mutated in X-linked mental retardation. Hum Mol Genet 11:981, 2002.

Frints SGM, Froyen G, Marynen P, et al.: Re-evaluation of MRX36 family after discovery of an ARX gene mutation reveals mild neurological features of Partington syndrome. Am J Med Genet 112:427, 2002.

Kitamura K, Yanazawa M, Sugiyama N, et al.: Mutation of ARX causes abnormal development of forebrain and testes in mice and X-linked lissencephaly with abnormal genitalia in humans. Nat Genet 32:359, 2002.

Nawara M, Szczaluba K, Poirier K, et al.: The ARX mutations: a frequent cause of X-linked mental retardation. Am J Med Genet A 140:727, 2006.

Partington MW, Mulley JC, Sutherland GR, et al.: X-linked mental retardation with dystonic movements of the hands. Am J Med Genet 30:251, 1988.

Strømme P, Mangelsdorf ME, Shaw MA, et al.: Mutations in the human ortholog of Aristaless cause X-linked mental retardation and epilepsy. Nat Genet 30:441, 2002.

Turner G, Partington M, Kerr B, et al.: Variable expression of mental retardation, autism, seizures, and dystonic hand movements in two families with an identical ARX gene mutation. Am J Med Genet 112:405, 2002.

DIFFERENTIAL MATRIX

Syndrome	Dystonia or Choreoathetosis	Hyperreflexia	Seizures	Comments
Partington (*ARX*-Associated XLID)	+	+	+	Scoliosis, flexed posture, dysarthria
Lesch-Nyhan	+	+	+	Spasticity, self-mutilation, hyperuricemia
Pettigrew	+	+	+	Dandy-Walker malformation, spasticity, microcephaly or hydrocephaly, long face with macrostomia and prognathism, small testes, contractures, iron deposits in basal ganglia
XLID-Spastic Paraplegia-Athetosis	+	+	+	Nystagmus, weakness, dysarthria, spastic paraplegia, muscle wasting
Allan-Herndon-Dudley	+	+	0	Large ears with cupping or abnormal architecture, muscle hypoplasia, childhood hypotonia, contractures, dysarthria, athetosis, ataxia, spastic paraplegia
Mohr-Tranebjaerg	+	+	0	Hearing loss, vision loss, neurological deterioration with childhood onset, spasticity
Goldblatt Spastic Paraplegia	0	+	+	Optic atrophy, exotropia, nystagmus, ataxia, spastic paraplegia, dysarthria, muscle hypoplasia, contractures
Gustavson	0	+	+	Microcephaly, short stature, optic atrophy with blindness, large ears, deafness, joint contractures, rockerbottom feet, brain undergrowth, hydrocephaly, cerebellar hypoplasia, spasticity
Paine	0	+	+	Microcephaly, short stature, optic atrophy, vision loss, hearing loss, spasticity
Ataxia-Deafness-Dementia, X-linked	0	+	+	Optic atrophy, vision loss, hearing loss, spastic paraplegia, ataxia, hypotonia, childhood death

PELIZAEUS-MERZBACHER SYNDROME

(X-LINKED SPASTIC PARAPLEGIA, PELIZAEUS-MERZBACHER TYPE; COMPLICATED X-LINKED SPASTIC PARAPLEGIA 2; SPG2; ARENA SYNDROME)

OMIM 312080

Xq22.1

PLP1

Definition. XLID with nystagmus, truncal hypotonia, progressive spastic paraplegia, ataxia, and dystonia associated with CNS dysmyelination.

Somatic Features. Neurological manifestations dominate the phenotype. Malformations and distinctive craniofacial features do not occur. Optic atrophy is found in most cases by school age. Contractures may result from the neurological impairment.

Arena et al. (1992) reported a family with severe cognitive impairment, hypotonia of the lower limbs, club foot, spasticity, ataxia, dystonia, rigidity, and MRI findings of small brain with macrogyria, diffuse white matter deficiency, and evidence of iron deficiency in the thalamus and basal ganglia. They considered this to represent a new XLID syndrome, but a missense mutation in *PLP1* was subsequently identified.

Growth and Development. Intrauterine and postnatal growth appears normal in most cases. Short stature of mild degree has been reported in a minority of cases. Developmental milestones may be globally delayed with motor skills lagging further behind than language development.

Cognitive Function. Considerable variability in cognitive function ranging from normal to moderate impairment

has been noted, even among affected males of the same family.

Neurological Findings. Nystagmus generally precedes other neurological findings, appearing in the early months of life, is multidirectional in nature, and often becomes less pronounced in childhood. Respiratory stridor has also been noted during infancy in many cases. Truncal hypotonia and pyramidal signs appear during early childhood, manifested variably by increased tone in the lower limbs, hyper-reflexia, awkward gait, and Babinski sign. The spastic paraplegia is progressive and may be accompanied by ataxia, upper limb tremors, dystonic movements, dysarthria, and dysmetria. Seizures occur in a minority. Ambulation may be sufficiently impaired in the teen or early adult years to require wheelchair or other support. In the most severe cases, speech is absent or limited to indistinct phrases, and continence of bladder and bowel is not achieved.

Heterozygote Expression. Although two of the cases reported by Pelizaeus were females, there is no convincing evidence of carrier manifestation.

Imaging. Global or spotty decrease in density of the white matter appears during childhood. Overall brain atrophy and ventricular dilation are mild. There may be dense deposits in the basal ganglia.

Laboratory. Visual-evoked responses and brainstem auditory-evoked responses are often abnormal. Histological examination of the brain has documented a deficiency of

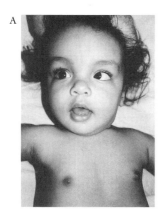
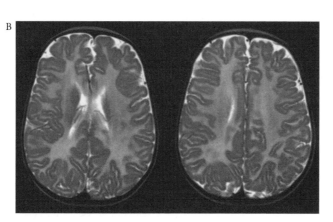

Pelizaeus-Merzbacher Syndrome. Seven-month-old male with nystagmus, developmental delay, and normal facies (**A**); axial MRI at age 44 months showing increased signal of white matter indicating deficient myelination (**B**). Courtesy of Dr. Arthur S. Aylsworth, University of North Carolina School of Medicine, Chapel Hill.

oligodendrocytes, the myelin producing cells of the CNS. Consequently, axons lack myelin sheaths.

Comment. Pelizaeus-Merzbacher syndrome was the first of the X-linked spastic paraplegias to be described (1885 and 1910), the first to be regionally mapped (1985), and the first to be attributed to mutations in the proteolipid protein gene, *PLP1* (1987). Complicated spastic paraplegia (SPG2) was shown to be allelic in 1994 and Arena syndrome in 2009.

REFERENCES

Arena JF, Schwartz C, Stevenson R, et al.: Spastic paraplegia with iron deposits in the basal ganglia: a new X-linked mental retardation syndrome. Am J Med Genet 43:479, 1992.

Boulloche J, Aicardi J: Pelizaeus-Merzbacher Disease: Clinical and Nosological Study. J Child Neurol 1:233, 1986.

Gencic S, Abuelo D, Ambler M, et al.: Pelizaeus-Merzbacher disease: an X-linked neurologic disorder of myelin metabolism with a novel mutation in the gene encoding proteolipid protein. Am J Hum Genet 45:435, 1989.

Merzbacher L: Eine eigenartige familiäre Erkrankungsform (aplasia axialis extracorticalis congenita) - Z Gesamte. Neurol Psychiatr 3:1, 1910.

Pelizaeus F: Über eine eigenthümliche Form spastischer Lähmung mit Cerebralerscheinungen auf hereditärer Grundlage (multiple Sklerose). Arch Psychiatr Nervenkr 16:698, 1885.

Saugier-Veber P, Munnich A, Bonneau D, et al.: X-linked spastic paraplegia and Pelizaeus-Merzbacher disease are allelic disorders at the proteolipid protein locus. Nat Genet 6:257, 1994.

Stevenson RE, Tarpey P, May MM, et al.: Arena syndrome is caused by a missense mutation in PLP1. Am J Med Genet A 149A:1081, 2009.

Trofatter JA, Dlouhy SR, De Meyer W, et al.: Pelizaeus-Merzbacher diseases: tight linkage to proteolipid protein gene exon variant. Proc Nat Acad Sci 86:9427, 1989.

DIFFERENTIAL MATRIX

Syndrome	Ataxia	Spastic Paraplegia	Nystagmus	Comments
Pelizaeus-Merzbacher	+	+	+	Optic atrophy, hypotonia, dystonia, CNS dysmyelination
Apak Ataxia-Spastic Diplegia	+	+	+	Short stature, muscle hypoplasia, contractures
Goldblatt Spastic Paraplegia	+	+	+	Optic atrophy, exotropia, dysarthria, contractures, muscle hypoplasia
XLID-Spastic Paraplegia-Athetosis	+	+	+	Weakness, dysarthria, muscle wasting, contractures
Adrenoleukodystrophy	+	+	0	Adrenal insufficiency, diffuse skin pigmentation, progressive neurological deterioration and dementia, elevated very-long-chain fatty acids in plasma
Allan-Herndon-Dudley	+	+	0	Childhood hypotonia, dysarthria, athetosis, large ears with cupping or abnormal architecture, contractures
Hydrocephaly-MASA Spectrum	+	+	0	Hydrocephaly, adducted thumbs, dysgenesis of corpus callosum
Pettigrew	+	+	0	Microcephaly or hydrocephaly, long face with macrostomia and prognathism, Dandy-Walker malformation, small testes, contractures, choreoathetosis, iron deposits in basal ganglia, seizures
Ataxia-Deafness-Dementia, X-linked	+	+	0	Optic atrophy, vision loss, hearing loss, hypotonia, seizures, childhood death
XLID-Ataxia-Dementia	+	+	0	Adult-onset dementia
XLID-Nystagmus-Seizures	+	0	+	Variable head circumference, vision loss, dysgenesis of corpus callosum, neuronal migration disturbance, cerebellar and midbrain hypoplasia, seizures
Cerebro-Oculo-Genital	0	+	+	Microcephaly, hydrocephaly, short stature, agenesis of corpus callosum, microphthalmia, ptosis, hypospadias, cryptorchidism, clubfoot
XLID-Spastic Paraplegia, type 7	0	+	+	Reduced vision, absent speech and ambulation, bowel and bladder dysfunction

PERIVENTRICULAR NODULAR HETEROTOPIA (*SEE ALSO FLNA*-ASSOCIATED XLID)

(HEREDITARY NODULAR HETEROTOPIA)

OMIM 300049

Xq28

FLNA

Definition. XLID with seizures and bilateral periventricular nodular heterotopias in female gene carriers. Although considered to be lethal in males, there have been exceptions to this generalization. Allelic conditions include OPDI, OPDII, Frontometaphyseal Dysplasia, and Melnick-Needles syndrome.

Somatic Features. Multiple subependymal nodules of heterotopic gray matter, usually bilateral, are the major somatic abnormality. Enlargement of the cisterna magna has been described in several cases. The findings are usually found in females with at least one pedigree suggesting gestational lethality of males.

Growth and Development. Normal

Cognitive Function. If cognitive impairment occurs, it is mild. Normal intelligence is usual.

Neurological Findings. Seizures of multiple clinical types occur with the usual onset during the teen years but, in some cases, beginning in early childhood or in adult life. Complex partial and tonic-clonic seizures are particularly common.

Imaging. Periventricular nodular heterotopias are best demonstrated by magnetic resonance imaging. They appear isointense with gray matter.

Comment. The finding of periventricular nodules in a child with seizures usually leads to the diagnosis of tuberous sclerosis. Bilateral periventricular nodular heterotopias can be differentiated from tuberous sclerosis by the absence of skin lesions, cortical lesions, and hamartomas in other organs. Further, the lesions do not calcify and retain the density of gray matter. Intellectual disability, if it occurs at all, is mild. Demonstration of *FLNA* mutations in males indicates that all mutations are not male-lethal. Periventricular nodular heterotopia has also been reported in a male with *PQBP1* mutation.

REFERENCES

Eksioglu YZ, Scheffer IE, Cardenas P, et al.: Periventricular heterotopia: An X-linked dominant epilepsy locus causing aberrant cerebral cortical development. Neuron 16:77, 1996.

Fox JW, Lamperti ED, Ekşioğlu YZ, et al.: Mutations in filamin 1 prevent migration of cerebral cortical neurons in human periventricular heterotopia. Neuron 21:1315, 1998.

Huttenlocher PR, Taravath S, Mojtahedi S: Periventricular heterotopia and epilepsy. Neurology 44:51, 1994.

Jardine PE, Clarke MA, Super M: Familial bilateral periventricular nodular heterotopia mimics tuberous sclerosis. Arch Dis Child 74:244, 1996.

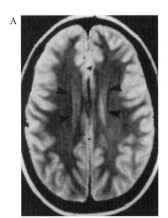 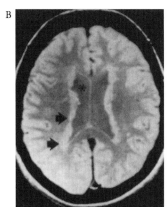 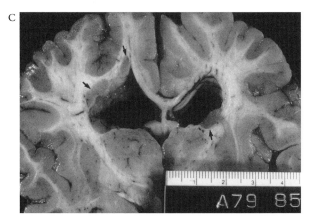

Periventricular Nodular Heterotopia. T$_1$-weighted MRI from normal individual showing good definition of white matter and the periventricular zone [*arrowheads*] is extremely thin and indistinct (A); T$_1$-weighted MRI from a female showing heterotopias with signal characteristics identical to that of gray matter in the periventricular zone [*arrows*] and distortion of the lateral ventricles [*asterisk*] (B). Coronal section of brain showing bilateral periventricular heterotopias [*arrows*] (C). Illustrations A and B courtesy of Dr. Peter Huttenlocher, Department of Pediatrics and Neurology, University of Chicago, and *Neuron*, Copyright 1996, Cell Press; illustration C courtesy of Dr. Alasdair G.W. Hunter and the Department of Pathology, Children's Hospital of Eastern Ontario, Ottawa.

Oda T, Nagai Y, Fujimoto S, et al.: Hereditary nodular heterotopia accompanied by mega cisterna magna. Am J Med Genet 47:268, 1993.

Parrini E, Mei D, Wright M, et al.: Mosaic mutations of the FLN1 gene cause a mild phenotype in patients with periventricular heterotopia. Neurogenetics 5:191, 2004.

Robertson SP, Twigg SR, Sutherland-Smith AJ, et al.: Localized mutations in the gene encoding the cytoskeletal protein filamin A cause diverse malformations in humans. Nat Genet 33:487, 2003.

Sheen VL, Dixon PH, Fox JW, et al.: Mutations in the X-linked filamin 1 gene cause periventricular nodular heterotopia in males as well as in females. Hum Mol Genet 10:1775, 2001.

Sheen VL, Torres AR, Du X, et al.: Mutation in PQBP1 is associated with periventricular heterotopia. Am J Med Genet 152A:2888, 2010.

Walsh CA, Cardenas P, Ji B, et al.: Linkage of cerebral cortical periventricular heterotopia and epilepsy to markers in Xq28. Neurology 45(Suppl 4):A440, 1995.

DIFFERENTIAL MATRIX

Syndrome	Neuronal Migration Disturbance	Seizures	Female-Limited Expression	Comments
Periventricular Nodular Heterotopia	+	+	+	Bilateral subependymal nodular heterotopias
Aicardi	+	+	+	Ocular dysgenesis, lacunar retinopathy, costovertebral anomalies, agenesis of corpus callosum
CK	+	+	0	Microcephaly, asthenic build, hypotonia, long thin face, scoliosis, behavior problems
Lissencephaly, X-linked	+	+	0	Dysgenesis of corpus callosum, hypotonia, spasticity, genital hypoplasia
Rett	0	+	+	Acquired microcephaly, developmental regression, truncal ataxia, repetitive hand movements, autistic features
XLID-Epilepsy	0	+	+	Developmental regression, repetitive stereotypic hand movements, hyporeflexia

PETTIGREW SYNDROME

(XLID-DANDY-WALKER MALFORMATION-BASAL GANGLIA DISEASE-SEIZURES)

OMIM 304340

Definition. XLID with long narrow face, microcephaly or hydrocephaly, Dandy-Walker malformation, seizures, spasticity, choreoathetosis, and iron deposition in the basal ganglia. The location of the gene is not known, the originally reported localization based on linkage analysis having been withdrawn.

Somatic Features. Although variable, the face tends to be long and narrow with high forehead, large bulbous nose, variable coarsening of facial features, macrostomia, and large lips. Strabismus may be present. Lacking hydrocephaly, patients are microcephalic. Tower skull was present in several cases. Contractures and kyphoscoliosis appear with progressive spasticity. Other skeletal findings include long, thin digits; pectus deformation; pes planus; and pes equinovarus. Cystic dilation of the fourth ventricle or Dandy-Walker malformation is present in half of patients. Hypotonia, present from infancy, becomes overlaid with choreoathetosis, ataxia, spasticity, and seizures in early childhood. Testicular volume appears small.

Growth and Development. Head growth is slow unless complicated by hydrocephaly. Growth parameters are otherwise normal.

Cognitive Function. Severe impairment

Neurological Findings. Hypotonia is present in early infancy. Within the first few years, choreoathetosis and spasticity of progressive nature become superimposed. Increased deep tendon reflexes are demonstrable in all limbs, and contractures occur by young adult life. Seizures may begin at any age.

Heterozygote Expression. Some carrier females have dull mentation. One carrier experienced early dementia and at autopsy had a small brain with iron deposition in basal ganglia and cerebellum.

Imaging. Hydrocephaly, posterior fossa cyst or Dandy-Walker malformation, hypoplasia of the cerebellum, underdeveloped frontal cortex, and iron deposits in the basal ganglia have been demonstrated.

Neuropathology. Postmortem examination has documented hydrocephaly with Dandy-Walker malformations or cystic dilation of the fourth ventricle and cerebellar hypoplasia (vermis and hemispheres). Iron deposition has been found in scattered areas of the midbrain but most prominently in the basal ganglia. In absence of hydrocephaly, the brain has been small with iron deposition.

Laboratory. Hemosiderin deposits can be found in liver and spleen.

Comment. Various forms of underdevelopment of the cerebellum include total absence of the cerebellum with the exception of a small remnant, aplasia or hypoplasia of the vermis, aplasia or hypoplasia of one or both cerebellar hemispheres, and generalized hypoplasia of the entire

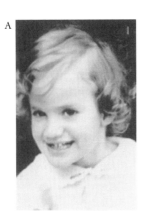 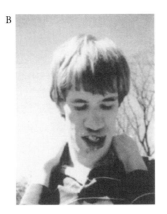 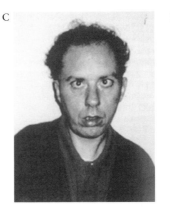 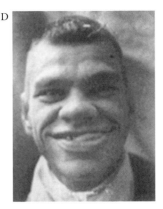

Pettigrew Syndrome. Prominent forehead and bulbous nose in childhood (**A**); long face with broad nose and thick lips at age 25 years (**B**); tall forehead, narrow face, broadening of the nasal tip, and small jaw at age 39 years (**C**); coarse facies with broad nose, large mouth, and thick lower lip at age 25 years (**D**).   Courtesy of Dr. David Ledbetter, University of Chicago and the *American Journal of Medical Genetics*, Copyright 1991, Wiley-Liss, Inc.

cerebellum. Dandy-Walker malformation may occur, particularly among those cases with aplasia or hypoplasia of the vermis. Mutations in one or more X-linked genes may lead to underdevelopment of the cerebellum and – especially among those cases with other central nervous system anomalies – may have associated intellectual disability.

REFERENCES

Huang TH-M, Hejtmancik JF, Edwards A, et al.: Linkage of the gene for an X-linked mental retardation disorder to a hypervariable $(AGAT)_n$ repeat motif within the human hypoxanthine phosphoribosyltransferase (HPRT) locus (Xq26). Am J Hum Genet 49:1312, 1991.

Pettigrew AL, Jackson LG, Ledbetter DH: New X-linked mental retardation disorder with Dandy-Walker malformation, basal ganglia disease, and seizures. Am J Med Genet 38:200, 1991.

DIFFERENTIAL MATRIX

Syndrome	Cerebellar Hypoplasia	Spastic Paraplegia	Iron Deposits or Calcification of Basal Ganglia	Comments
Pettigrew	+	+	+	Dandy-Walker malformation, microcephaly or hydrocephaly, long face with macrostomia, small testes, contractures, choreoathetosis, seizures
Christianson	+	+	+	Short stature, microcephaly, general asthenia, contractures, seizures, ophthalmoplegia
Gustavson	+	+	+	Microcephaly, short stature, optic atrophy with blindness, large ears, deafness, joint contractures, rockerbottom feet, brain undergrowth, hydrocephaly, seizures
Pelizaeus-Merzbacher	+	+	+	Optic atrophy, nystagmus, hypotonia, ataxia, dystonia, CNS dysmyelination
Schimke	+	+	+	Microcephaly, sunken eyes, downslanting palpebral fissures, narrow nose, wide spacing of teeth, cupped ears, hypotonia, abducens palsy, hearing loss, vision loss, choreoathetosis, contractures
Paine	+	+	0	Microcephaly, short stature, optic atrophy, vision and hearing loss, seizures
AP1S2-Associated XLID	0	+	+	Hydrocephaly, muscle hypoplasia, sensory impairment

PHOSPHOGLYCERATE KINASE DEFICIENCY

(PGK DEFICIENCY)

OMIM 311800

Xq21.1

PGK1

Definition. XLID with muscle weakness, diminished deep tendon reflexes, seizures, and recurrent myoglobinuria caused by phosphoglycerate kinase deficiency.

Somatic Features. Major malformations do not occur. The face may be relatively expressionless. Muscle bulk and distribution are not unusual.

Growth and Development. Intrauterine and postnatal growth progress normally, but mild to moderate delay of motor and speech development occurs.

Cognitive Function. Moderate impairment

Neurological Findings. Seizures may precipitate episodes of generalized muscle pain, weakness, hemolytic anemia, and myoglobinuria. Deep tendon reflexes are depressed.

Imaging. Normal

Laboratory. Phosphoglycerate kinase activity in muscle measures below 10% of normal levels. Nonetheless, glycogen accumulation is not demonstrably increased. During episodes of myoglobinuria, creatine kinase and LDH are elevated.

Comment. Phosphoglycerate kinase, phosphoglycerate mutase, and lactic dehydrogenase M-subunit deficiency constitute a group of muscle glycogenoses that may be associated with recurrent episodes of myoglobinuria. PGK alone is X-linked.

REFERENCES

Flanagan JM, Rhodes M, Wilson M, et al.: The identification of a recurrent phosphoglycerate kinase mutation associated with chronic haemolytic anaemia and neurological dysfunction in a family from USA. Br J Haematol 134:233. 2006.

Spiegel R, Gomez EA, Akman HO, et al.: Myopathic form of phosphoglycerate kinase (PGK) deficiency: a new case and pathogenic considerations. Neuromuscul Disord 19:207 2009.

Sugie H, Sugie Y, Nishida M, et al.: Recurrent myoglobinuria in a child with mental retardation: phosphoglycerate kinase deficiency. J Child Neurol 4:95, 1989.

DIFFERENTIAL MATRIX

Syndrome	Muscle Weakness	Areflexia, Hypo-reflexia	Seizures	Comments
Phosphoglycerate Kinase Deficiency	+	+	+	Expressionless face, decreased deep tendon reflexes, myoglobinuria, hemolytic anemia
Arts	+	+	+	Growth deficiency, poor muscle development, hypotonia, ataxia, deafness, vision loss, childhood death
Charcot-Marie-Tooth Neuropathy, Cowchock variant	+	+	0	Peripheral motor and sensory neuropathy, deafness, pes cavus
Charcot-Marie-Tooth Neuropathy, Ionasescu variant	+	+	0	Peripheral motor and sensory neuropathy, wasting of intrinsic hand muscles, enlarged ulnar nerves, pes cavus
Duchenne Muscular Dystrophy	+	+	0	Hypertrophy of calf muscles, elevated muscle enzymes, progressive weakness, muscle wasting, contractures
Myotubular Myopathy	+	+	0	Hypotonic facies, open mouth, tented upper lip, hydrocephaly, long digits, cryptorchidism, hypotonia

PLOTT SYNDROME

(XLID WITH LARYNGEAL ABDUCTOR PALSY)

OMIM 308850

Definition. XLID with laryngeal abductor palsy. The gene has not been localized.

Somatic Features. Expressionless facies result from a paucity of spontaneous movement of the facial muscles. Volitional movement, however, appears normal, and electromyography of facial muscles is normal. No malformations occur. Respiratory stridor is present from the first breath and does not resolve. It may become less symptomatic or may worsen, leading to tracheotomy or death. Stridor results from paralysis of the posterior cricoarytenoid muscle, which leaves the vocal cords in the adducted position. During crying, the vocal cords close completely; during quiet respiration, the vocal cords are relaxed with a slit-like opening. Abductor palsy has been attributed to dysgenesis of the nucleus ambiguus. One case had unilateral abducens palsy and unilateral deafness.

Growth and Development. Although birth weights in some cases register in the lower centiles, in other cases intrauterine growth is normal. Postnatal growth proceeds at a normal rate. Early motor development is characterized by clumsiness, awkward gait, and poor hand-eye coordination. Muscle strength and tone are normal.

Cognitive Function. Mild cognitive impairment occurred in three cases in the original report (IQ 56–73).

Comment. Three males in a second family reported by Watters and Fitch (1973) had more severe laryngeal stridor associated with sucking and swallowing difficulties, poor weight gain, apneic episodes, floppiness and stiffening, nystagmus, blindness, optic atrophy and early death, or survival with profound psychomotor and neurological impairments.

Perinatal hypoxia may be a significant factor in the mental impairment. Alternatively, the dysgenetic process, presumed to cause faulty development of the medulla, may also affect other areas of the brain.

REFERENCES

Plott D: Congenital laryngeal-abductor paralysis due to nucleus ambiguus dysgenesis in three brothers. New Eng J Med 271:593, 1964.

Watters GV, Fitch N: Familial laryngeal abductor paralysis and psychomotor retardation. Clin Genet 4:429, 1973.

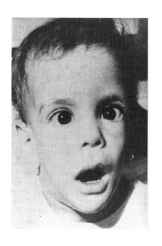 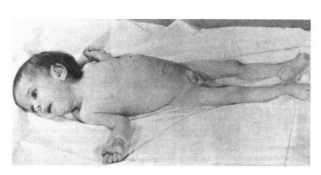

Plott Syndrome. Seventeen-month-old male with expressionless and staring facies with open mouth, opisthotonus, and tonic posturing of hands and feet.
Courtesy of Dr. Gordon Watters, Montreal Children's Hospital, Montreal.

DIFFERENTIAL MATRIX

Syndrome	Respiratory Difficulty from Birth	Expressionless Face	Normal Muscle Strength	Comments
Plott	+	+	+	Laryngeal abductor paralysis
Myotubular Myopathy	+	+	0	Hypotonic facies, open mouth, tented upper lip, hydrocephaly, long digits, crypt-orchidism, hypotonia, weakness, areflexia

PORTEOUS SYNDROME (*SEE ALSO* RENPENNING SYNDROME)

Xp11.23

PQBP1

The phenotype is based on a single family in which six affected males have short stature, normal head circumference, high forehead, receding hairline, high-pitched voice, and mild-to-moderate cognitive impairment. Testicular volume was normal. Carrier females had no somatic or cognitive manifestations. A mutation in *PQBP1* was identified. Thus, Porteous syndrome is allelic to Renpenning, Hamel Cerebro-Palato-Cardiac, Sutherland-Haan, and Golabi-Ito-Hall syndromes.

REFERENCES

Porteous MEM, Johnson H, Burn J, et al.: A new mental retardation syndrome mapping to the pericentromeric region of the X-chromosome. Am J Hum Genet 51: A106, 1992.
Stevenson RE, Bennett CW, Abidi F, et al.: Renpenning syndrome comes into focus. Am J Med Genet A 134:415, 2005.

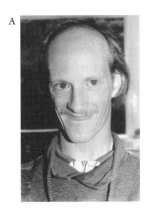
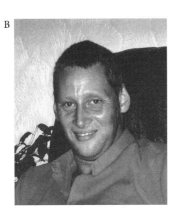

Porteous Syndrome. Cousins showing long facies, prominent forehead, receding hairline, and prominent mandible.   Courtesy of Dr. Mary Porteous, South East Scotland Clinical Genetic Service, Edinburgh.

PPM-X

(PSYCHOSIS-PYRAMIDAL SIGNS-MACROORCHIDISM SYNDROME)

OMIM 300055

Xq28

MECP2

Definition. XLID with macroorchidism, pyramidal signs, and manic-depressive psychosis.

Somatic Features. The craniofacies appear normal and head size is normal. Several males have had short stature. Macroorchidism is consistently present. Neuropsychiatric features predominate with onset in childhood. Manic and depressive episodes were periodically imposed on a background of hyperreflexia or spastic paraplegia, tremors, and Parkinsonian features.

Growth and Development. Prenatal growth is normal, but adult stature is short in some individuals. Cephalic growth is normal.

Cognitive Function. Moderate impairment

Neurological Findings. Increased muscle tone, hyperreflexia, Babinski signs, stiffness, stooped posture, shuffling gait, and resting tremors may be noted as early as age 10 years. Episodes of depression (despondency, weepiness, fearfulness, poor appetite, sleep disturbances) and episodes of irritability, overactivity, aggressiveness, insomnia, and talkativeness punctuated late childhood and adult life. A contribution of neuroleptic medications to the neurological findings was possible in some cases.

Heterozygote Expression. Female carriers have below average intelligence.

Imaging. Not known

Comment. Macroorchidism occurs in a limited number of XLID syndromes, specifically XLID-Macrocephaly-Macroorchidism, Fragile X, Clark-Baraitser, and PPM-X syndromes. In the family reported by Atkin-Flaitz, macroorchidism occurred in affected and nonaffected males. Spasticity, Parkinsonian signs, and psychosis do not

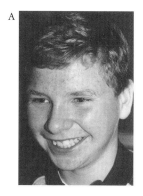
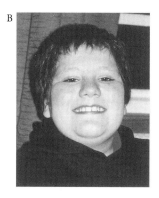
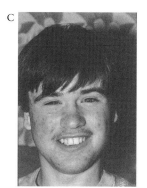
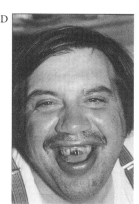
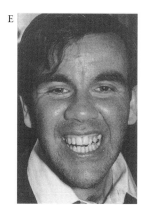
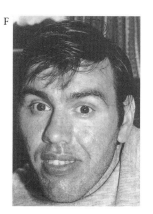

PPM-X Syndrome. Normal facial appearance in affected males at ages 11, 12, 25, 38, 39, and 41 years (A–F).   Courtesy of Dr. Susan Lindsay, University of Newcastle upon Tyne, Newcastle upon Tyne, UK.

typically occur in any of these XLID-macroorchidism syndromes, with the exception of PPM-X.

REFERENCES

Klauck SM, Lindsay S, Beyer KS, et al.: A mutation hot spot for non-specific X-linked mental retardation in the MECP2 gene causes the PPM-X syndrome. Am J Hum Genet 70:1034, 2002.

Lindsay S, Splitt M, Edney S, et al.: PPM-X: A new X-linked mental retardation syndrome with psychosis, pyramidal signs, and macroorchidism maps to Xq28. Am J Hum Genet 58:1120, 1996.

DIFFERENTIAL MATRIX

Syndrome	Macroorchidism	Spasticity	Tremors or Rigidity	Comments
PPM-X	+	+	+	Psychosis, Parkinsonian features
Gustavson	0	+	+	Microcephaly, short stature, optic atrophy with blindness, large ears, deafness, joint contractures, rockerbottom feet, brain undergrowth, hydrocephaly, cerebellar hypoplasia, seizures
Lesch-Nyhan	0	+	+	Choreoathetosis, self-mutilation, hyperuricemia
Pelizaeus-Merzbacher	0	+	+	Optic atrophy, nystagmus, hypotonia, ataxia, dystonia, CNS dysmyelination
Pettigrew	0	+	+	Dandy-Walker malformation, microcephaly or hydrocephaly, long face with macrostomia and prognathism, small testes, contractures, choreoathetosis, iron deposits in basal ganglia, seizures
Waisman-Laxova	0	+	+	Macrocephaly, strabismus
XLID-Spastic Paraplegia-Athetosis	0	+	+	Nystagmus, weakness, dysarthria, muscle wasting, contractures

PRIETO SYNDROME

OMIM 309610

Xp11

Definition. XLID with distinctive facies, optic atrophy, ventriculomegaly, hypotonia, and skeletal anomalies. The gene has not been identified, but localizes between the genes for Ornithine Transcarbamylase (OTC) and Monoamine Oxidase A Deficiency (MAO-A) in Xp11.

Somatic Features. The cranium measures within the normal range (2nd-70th centiles) but may be asymmetric. The face may be asymmetric as well, with triangular configuration, hypertelorism, prominent eyes, epicanthus, strabismus, ptosis, long narrow nose with the tip overhanging the columella, dysplastic low-set ears with small lobes, and micrognathia or retrognathia. A double row of lower incisors was present in one case. The optic discs are pale. There is generalized decrease in tone with persistent drooling, depressed reflexes, coxa valgu, dislocated patellas, pes planus, and clubfoot. Inguinal hernia and cryptorchidism may occur. Clinodactyly is present. A skin dimple is found over the lower spine. The ventricles are enlarged, secondary to cerebral atrophy. Seizures have occurred with fever during childhood.

Growth and Development. Intrauterine growth appears normal with birth weight 2.9 to 3.8 kilograms. Postnatal stature and head growth are likewise normal. Global developmental delay is obvious from early infancy.

Cognitive Function. Formal testing has not been reported, but delay of developmental milestones suggests severe intellectual disability.

Neurological Findings. Decreased muscle tone and deep tendon reflexes are typical. Independent ambulation may be achieved but lost in adult life. Generalized seizures, usually with fever, occur during childhood.

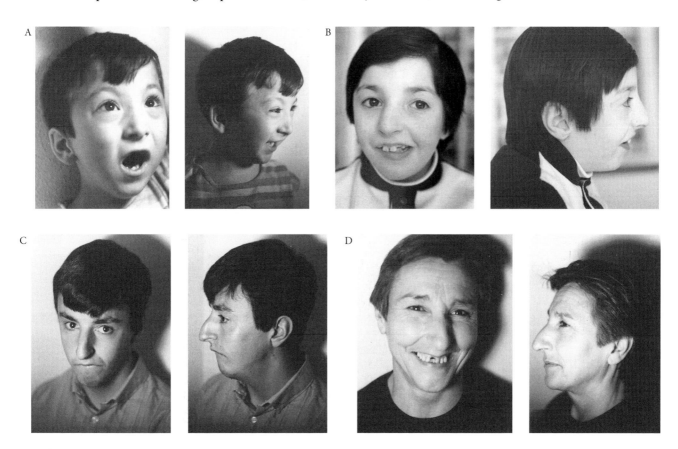

Prieto Syndrome. Triangular facies with prominent nose, absent earlobe, and retrognathia in affected males at ages 5 years **(A)** and 10 years **(B)**. Triangular faces, prominent nose, and retrognathia in an affected male at age 17 years **(C)** and in a carrier mother **(D)**.   Courtesy of Dr. Félix Prieto, La Fe University Hospital, Valencia, Spain.

Heterozygote Expression. Carrier females show no cognitive impairment.

Imaging. Pneumoencephalography and CT demonstrated enlarged ventricles with subcortical central atrophy.

Comment. Phenotype based on a single family with eight males affected in two generations.

REFERENCES

Martínez F, Prieto F, Gal A: Refined localization of the Prieto-Syndrome locus. Am J Med Genet 64:82, 1996.

Prieto F, Badia L, Mulas F, et al.: X-linked dysmorphic syndrome with mental retardation. Clin Genet 32:326, 1987.

Watty A, Prieto F, Beneyto M, et al.: Gene localization in a family with X-linked syndromal mental retardation (Prieto Syndrome). Am J Med Genet 38:234, 1991.

DIFFERENTIAL MATRIX

Syndrome	Optic Atrophy	Hydrocephaly	Hypotonia	Comments
Prieto	+	+	+	Ventricular enlargement, facial asymmetry, hypertelorism, prominent eyes, ptosis, long narrow nose, micrognathia, inguinal hernia, cryptorchidism
Juberg-Marsidi-Brooks	+	+	+	Microcephaly, short stature, dysgenesis of corpus callosum, deep-set eyes, blepharophimosis, cupped ears, bulbous nose, small mouth, thin upper lip, pectus excavatum, flexion contractures
VACTERL-Hydrocephaly	+	+	+	Vertebral anomalies, radial limb defects, tracheal and esophageal anomalies, renal malformations, anal anomalies
Gustavson	+	+	0	Microcephaly, short stature, blindness, large ears, deafness, joint contractures, rockerbottom feet, brain undergrowth, cerebellar hypoplasia, spasticity, seizures
Arts	+	0	+	Growth deficiency, poor muscle development, areflexia, ataxia, deafness, vision loss, seizures, childhood death
Pelizaeus-Merzbacher	+	0	+	Nystagmus, spasticity, ataxia, dystonia, CNS dysmyelination
Ataxia-Deafness-Dementia, X-linked	+	0	+	Vision loss, hearing loss, spastic paraplegia, ataxia, seizures, childhood death
AP1S2-Associated XLID	0	+	+	Microcephaly, calcifications in basal ganglia, long face, high forehead, long nose, spasticity, aggressive adult behavior
Cerebro-Cerebello-Coloboma	0	+	+	Cerebellar vermis hypoplasia, retinal coloboma, hypotonia, seizures, abnormal respiratory pattern
Pettigrew	0	+	+	Dandy-Walker malformation, spasticity, microcephaly or hydrocephaly, long face with macrostomia and prognathism, small testes, contractures, choreoathetosis, iron deposits in basal ganglia, seizures

PROUD SYNDROME (*SEE ALSO ARX*-ASSOCIATED XLID)

Xp22.11

ARX

Definition. XLID with short stature, microcephaly, agenesis of corpus callosum, skeletal anomalies, tapered digits, spasticity, seizures, and impairments of vision and hearing.

Somatic Features. Although normal at birth, growth of the head falls below the 3rd centile in early childhood. The facies are mildly coarse, perhaps related in part to anticonvulsant therapy. Other facial features include prominent supraorbital ridges, apparent hypertelorism, prominent ears with thick lobes, and high palate. Nystagmus, wandering eye movements, and strabismus occur. Kyphoscoliosis, lip discoloration, limb contractures, and spasticity develop. Vision and hearing are impaired. Malformations include agenesis of the corpus callosum, cryptorchidism, hypospadias, and inguinal hernia.

Cognitive Function. Males are severely and globally impaired from birth. None learn to walk or talk. Females have had variable cognitive impairment and somatic manifestation.

Neurological Findings. Intractable myoclonic and generalized seizures, nystagmus, impaired vision and hearing, spasticity, clonus, and athetosis appear in infancy or early childhood.

Natural History. Males are severely impaired from birth. Several males who were probably affected died in infancy or early childhood; others have survived to early adult life. One female carrier appeared affected to the same degree as the males; other carrier females have had less severe cognitive and physical manifestations.

Heterozygote Expression. Carrier females are cognitively impaired and may have agenesis of corpus callosum, strabismus, contractures, visual defects, and seizures.

Imaging. CT and MRI have documented agenesis of corpus callosum and ventricular dilation. One case had porencephaly. Carriers were variably affected with cerebral atrophy, ventricular dilation and partial absence of corpus callosum.

Comment. A single family with three affected males and three affected females has been described. Three other males died early, one at age 6 months as a "blue baby" and two others in early childhood with growth failures, seizures, and other features of the condition. Proud syndrome falls near the severe end of the spectrum of *ARX*-associated disorders, which include Nonsyndromal XLID, Partington

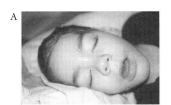
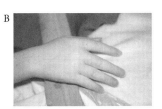
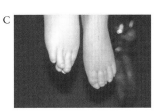
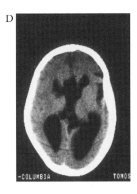
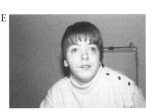

Proud Syndrome. Eight-year-old male with long face, thickened alae nasi, prominent lips, tapered fingers, and crowded and overlapping toes (A–C); cranial tomography in a 23-year-old male showing dilated ventricles and porencephaly (D); carrier female with strabismus and spasticity (E).   Courtesy of Dr. Virginia Proud, Norfolk, Virginia.

syndrome, West syndrome, and X-Linked Lissencepahly with Abnormal Genitalia (XLAG).

REFERENCES

Kitamura K, Yanazawa M, Sugiyama N, et al.: Mutation of ARX causes abnormal development of forebrain and testes in mice and X-linked lissencephaly with abnormal genitalia in humans. Nat Genet 32:359, 2002.

Proud VK, Levine C, Carpenter NJ: New X-linked syndrome with seizures, acquired micrencephaly, and agenesis of the corpus callosum. Am J Med Genet 43:458, 1992.

Strømme P, Mangelsdorf ME, Shaw MA, et al.: Mutations in the human ortholog of Aristaless cause X-linked mental retardation and epilepsy. Nat Genet 30:441, 2002.

DIFFERENTIAL MATRIX

Syndrome	Dysgenesis of Corpus Callosum	Impaired Vision and/or Hearing	Spasticity	Comments
Proud (*ARX*-Associated XLID)	+	+	+	Microcephaly, cryptorchidism, inguinal hernias, ataxia, seizures
Cerebro-Oculo-Genital	+	+	+	Microcephaly, hydrocephaly, short stature, agenesis of corpus callosum, microphthalmia, ptosis, hypospadias, cryptorchidism, clubfoot
Aicardi	+	+	0	Ocular dysgenesis, lacunar retinopathy, costovertebral anomalies, seizures
Hydrocephaly-MASA Spectrum	+	0	+	Hydrocephaly, adducted thumbs
Kang	+	0	+	Microcephaly, frontal prominence, telecanthus, small nose, short hands, seizures, downturned mouth, brachydactyly
Gustavson	0	+	+	Microcephaly, short stature, large ears, joint contractures, rockerbottom feet, brain undergrowth, hydrocephaly, cerebellar hypoplasia, seizures
Mohr-Tranebjaerg	0	+	+	Neurological deterioration with childhood onset, dystonia
Pettigrew	0	+	+	Dandy-Walker malformation, microcephaly or hydrocephaly, long face with macrostomia and prognathism, small testes, contractures, choreoathetosis, iron deposits in basal ganglia, seizures
Schimke	0	+	+	Microcephaly, sunken eyes, downslanting palpebral fissures, narrow nose, wide spacing of teeth, cupped ears, hypotonia, abducens palsy, choreoathetosis, contractures
Ataxia-Deafness-Dementia, X-linked	0	+	+	Optic atrophy, ataxia, hypotonia, seizures, childhood death
XLID-Spastic Paraplegia, type 7	0	+	+	Nystagmus, absent speech and ambulation, bowel and bladder dysfunction

PYRUVATE DEHYDROGENASE DEFICIENCY

(PYRUVATE DEHYDROGENASE E1-ALPHA DEFICIENCY, LEIGH SYNDROME
WITH PYRUVATE DEHYDROGENASE DEFICIENCY, INTERMITTENT ATAXIA
WITH PYRUVATE DEHYDROGENASE DEFICIENCY)

OMIM 312170

Xp22.13

PDHA1

Definition. XLID with variable clinical manifestations ranging from profound neuromuscular failure, developmental arrest, and early death associated with overwhelming lactic acidosis to chronic or intermittent ataxia, dysarthria, and developmental impairment with or without demonstrable lactic acidosis. Deficiency of the pyruvate dehydrogenase complex is responsible as a result of a mutation in the E1α subunit of pyruvate decarboxylase.

Somatic Features. A minority of patients will have craniofacial abnormalities, including microcephaly, bossed forehead, wide nasal bridge, upturned nose, and long philtrum – manifestations not unlike those of fetal alcohol syndrome. Dysgenesis of the corpus callosum, cerebral atrophy, and cysts of the brainstem, basal ganglia, cerebrum, and cerebral cortex have been described.

Growth and Development. Survivors usually have variable developmental delay. Growth impairment and microcephaly may result from the lactic acidosis, cerebral damage, and neurological impairment.

Cognitive Function. Survivors usually have variable degrees of intellectual disability.

Neurological Findings. Presentation may be the neurological features of Leigh Disease. Males may present with intermittent ataxia and dysarthria. Hypotonia is common and may progress to hypertonia. Seizures occur.

Natural History. In males, the severity may correlate with enzyme activity. Absent or negligible enzyme activity presumably is not compatible with prenatal survival. Low activity results in persistent severe lactic acidosis and death in the first 6 months. Survivors may have more residual enzyme activity. Their mild-to-moderate lactic acidosis may only be symptomatic with infections or may be detected in evaluation of psychomotor delay/intellectual disability. There may be a neurodegenerative course with seizures, spasticity, cortical blindness, and risk of death from apnea. An even milder form presents with intermittent or chronic ataxia/dysarthria with or without intellectual disability. The neurological symptoms and mild lactic acidosis may be precipitated by carbohydrate intake.

Heterozygote Expression. The male-to-female ratio of documented cases is about 1:1. Females predominate in the survivors and may have any presentation with the possible exception of carbohydrate-induced episodic ataxia.

Imaging. Agenesis or hypogenesis of corpus callosum, cerebral atrophy, and cysts of the cerebral cortex, basal ganglia, and brainstem. In those with ataxic episodes, neuroimaging is normal but may later reveal cystic lesions in the brainstem. Proton magnetic resonance spectroscopy of the brain demonstrates an increased signal for lactate and those for N-acetylaspartate are decreased.

Neuropathology. The brain depends on glucose as an energy (ATP) source. Pyruvate dehydrogenase is the rate-limiting step in the entry of glucose through pyruvate into the Krebs cycle and subsequently into the respiratory chain for production of ATP. Neuronal cell death results from lactic acidosis or ATP deficit and may be generalized or localized to regions of high energy utilization. The fetal brain depends on glucose oxidation, and cerebral disruption may occur *in utero*.

Laboratory. Blood lactate and pyruvate are chronically or intermittently increased, but the lactate-to-pyruvate ratio is normal. Elevations in lactate are greater in and may be limited to the cerebrospinal fluid. Decreased PDH activity is found in skin fibroblasts and other tissues. In heterozygotes, the decreased PDH activity varies in different tissues. Most mutations are unique.

Treatment. Those with episodic ataxia may benefit from a low carbohydrate ketogenic diet. A trial of thiamine and a low-carbohydrate ketogenic diet rarely are beneficial to others.

Comment. The clinical variability in males is presumably related to the level of enzyme activity, but the correlation is not always apparent in studies in vitro. Additionally in females, the capacity of normal cells to eliminate lactate, but not to supply ATP for abnormal cells, as well as lyonization contribute to the variability.

REFERENCES

Børglum AD, Flint T, Hansen LL, et al.: Refined localization of the pyruvate dehydrogenase E1α gene (PDHA1) by linkage analysis. Hum Genet 99:80, 1997.

Brown GK, Otero LJ, LeGris M, et al.: Pyruvate dehydrogenase deficiency. Med Genet 31:875, 1994.

Lissens W, De Meirleir L, Seneca S, et al.: Mutations in the X-linked pyruvate dehydrogenase (E1) alpha subunit gene (PDHA1) in patients with a pyruvate dehydrogenase complex deficiency. Hum Mutat, 15:209, 2000.

Robinson BH, MacMillan H, Petrova-Benedict R, et al.: Variable clinical presentation in patients with defective E1 component of pyruvate dehydrogenase complex. J Pediatr 111:525, 1987.

Shevell MI, Matthews PM, Scriver CR, et al.: Cerebral dysgenesis and lactic acidemia: An MRI/MRS phenotype associated with pyruvate dehydrogenase deficiency. Pediatr Neurol 11:224, 1994.

DIFFERENTIAL MATRIX

Syndrome	Microcephaly	Structural Brain Anomalies	Lactic Acidosis	Comments
Pyruvate Dehydrogenase Deficiency	+	+	+	Ataxia, dysarthria, hypotonia
CK	+	+	0	Asthenic build, neuronal migration disturbance, seizures, hypotonia, long thin face, scoliosis, behavior problems
Ornithine Transcarbamoylase Deficiency	+	0	+	Chronic or intermittent hyperammonemia, protein-induced vomiting and lethargy, ataxia, seizures

RENPENNING SYNDROME

(CEREBRO-PALATO-CARDIAC SYNDROME, SUTHERLAND-HAAN SYNDROME, GOLABI-ITO-HALL SYNDROME, PORTEOUS SYNDROME)

OMIM 309500

Xp11.23

PQBP1

Definition. XLID with short stature, microcephaly, and small testes. A number of allelic conditions (Golabi-Ito-Hall, Sutherland-Haan, Hamel Cerebro-Palato-Cardiac, and Porteous syndromes) are subsumed under this rubric.

Somatic Features. Alterations in growth contribute the major components of the phenotype. The craniofacial appearance may be distinctive only in having microcephaly or head circumference in the lower centiles. The facies may have some combination of long triangular face, sparse lateral eyebrows, upslanted palpebral fissures, large nose with overhanging columella, and prominent ears. Statural growth likewise is near or below the 3rd centile. Testicular volumes are similarly small. Major malformations do not typically occur, but cardiac malformations have occurred in several families. Ocular coloboma, choanal atresia, hypospadias, horseshoe kidney, and imperforate anus have occurred in individual cases.

Growth and Development. Intrauterine growth is mildly impaired. There is a tendency for continued slow growth with head circumference and height in the lower centiles.

Cognitive Function. Early childhood development is severely and globally delayed. Ultimate cognitive impairment is generally severe, although intra- and interfamilial variability has been documented.

Behavior. No consistent behavioral aberrations have been described.

Neurological Findings. None

Heterozygote Expression. Carrier females do not show growth or cognitive impairments.

Imaging: The brain is small overall, with the cerebellum being more diminished in size than other portions of the brain. Thin corpus callosum has also been noted.

Neuropathology. Examination of the brain in two cases has confirmed small size (780 grams and 984 grams), and in one case the neurons of the left cortex were arranged in columns, suggesting a defect in neuronal migration or maturation. A neuronal migration disturbance has not been noted on MRI.

Comment. In the 1970s, the term *Renpenning syndrome* came to be used as a generic reference to X-linked intellectual disability (Steele & Chorazy, 1974; Howard-Peebles et al., 1979; Jennings et al., 1980; Proops & Webb, 1981). This broad usage was applied to syndromal XLID, including the Fragile X syndrome, and nonsyndromal XLID. Turner et al. (1970, 1971, 1972) argued that this designation be used only for nonsyndromal XLID, specifically cases lacking macrocephaly or microcephaly, epilepsy, major malformations or more than one minor malformation, and neurological signs. We propose that these practices be abandoned and that Renpenning syndrome be reserved for that XLID condition caused by mutations in *PQBP1* and clinically characterized by cognitive impairment, microcephaly, and a tendency toward short stature and small testes. Renpenning syndrome now encompasses several allelic conditions: Hamel cerebropalatocardiac, Sutherland-Haan, Porteous, and Golabi-Ito-Hall syndromes.

Golabi, Ito, and Hall (1984) reported a family in which three males had short stature, microcephaly, narrow or triangular face, prominent glabella, telecanthus, epicanthus, upslanting palpebral fissures, long nose with high nasal root, cupped ears thin upper lip, prominent maxillary central incisors, narrow palate with wide palatine ridges, and ectodermal manifestations (dry brittle scalp hair, nail hypoplasia, and cutis marmorata). Chest asymmetry was noted in two cases and atrial septal defect in two cases. Birth weight and head circumference were normal but in the lower percentiles. Postnatally, all growth percentiles lagged, leading to microcephaly and short stature. Global developmental delay became obvious during infancy and early childhood. Abnormal neurological findings (lower limb hyperreflexia, Babinski signs, petit mal seizures, and mild sensorineural hearing loss) were described in only one case, who required resuscitation at birth.

Sutherland and associates (1988) reported a family in which males in three generations had short stature, microcephaly, small testes, and spastic diplegia. Facial manifestations included upslanted palpebral fissures, strabismus, maxillary hypoplasia, and in some cases large ears and mild prognathism. There was a tendency to lean body mass, pectus excavatum, scoliosis, stiffness of small joints, and pes cavus. One male had imperforate anus and another had anal stenosis. Intrauterine growth appeared mildly impaired, with birth weights in the lower centiles. Postnatal growth was similarly slow, with adult height and head circumference usually below –2SD. The testicular volume measured in the lower centiles and was possibly related to delay in puberty. Decreased body hair and early baldness were present. There was mild to moderate delay of speech and motor milestones. Cognitive function ranged from low-normal to moderate impairment. Several males experienced poor feeding during infancy. Increased muscle tone and hyper-reflexia of lower limbs noted by early childhood in several males was of mild to moderate severity and did not appear progressive. Prominent ventricles secondary to mild cerebral atrophy was found on CT scan in one affected male.

Porteous et al. (1992) reported a single family in which six affected males had short stature, normal head circumference, high forehead, receding hairline, high-pitched voice, and mild to moderate cognitive impairment. Testicular volume was normal. Carrier females had no somatic or cognitive manifestations.

Hamel et al. (1994) reported a family in which four affected males had microcephaly, broad nasal bridge, bulbous nose, malar hypoplasia, dysplastic cupped ears, highly arched or cleft palate, short philtrum, tented upper lip, and small mouth. The initially oval facial configuration elongated with age. Complex cardiac defects, tetralogy of Fallot in one case, atrial and ventricular septal defects and overriding aorta in another, and undiagnosed defects in two others were symptomatic in all cases. Only minor skeletal anomalies occurred, including long slender hands and feet, fifth finger clinodactyly, and contractures at the elbows and knees. Hypertonicity was present in one case and hypospadias in one case. All parameters of growth were retarded pre- and postnatally. Delay of developmental milestones became obvious in infancy. The carrier mother of two affected males had an atrial septal defect but no other manifestation. In three of the four cases, death occurred during infancy or childhood, their cardiac defect being the principal contributor. This does not appear to be the case with Renpenning syndrome nor other allelic conditions. Small brain without structural malformation was found in the single case so studied.

Germanaud et al. (2010) have reported general asthenic build and short stature with progressive atrophy of the upper back muscles, ankylosis of the first metacarpophalangeal joint, limited forearm rotation, and velopharyngeal dysfunction in their series of 7 families with 13 affected males.

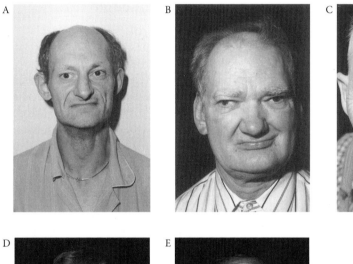
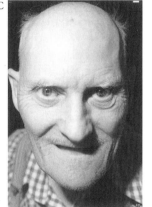
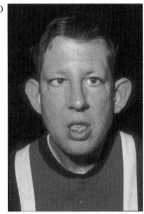
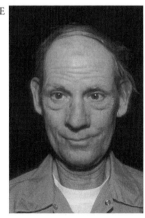

Renpenning Syndrome. Adults in original Renpenning syndrome family at ages 40, 55, and 65 years showing balding, upslanted palpebral fissures, and short philtrum. The head circumference in each measures near or below the 3rd centile (A–C). Thirty-four-year-old male from another family showing microcephaly, outfolded ears, prominent nasal root, and myopathic appearance to the face (D). Fifty-nine-year-old uncle with microcephaly, balding, prominent nasal root, mild overhanging columella, and otherwise normal appearance (E).

REFERENCES

Archidiacono N, Rocchi M, Rinaldi A, et al.: X-linked mental retardation. II. Renpenning syndrome and other types (Report of 14 families) J Génét Hum 35:381, 1987.

Filippi G, Rinaldi A, Archidiacono N, et al.: Brief Report: Linkage between G6PD and fragile-X syndrome. Am J Med Genet 15:113, 1983.

Fox P, Fox D, Gerrard JW: X-linked mental retardation: Renpenning revisited. Am J Med Genet 7:491, 1980.

Germanaud D, Rossi M, Bussy G, et al.: The Renpenning syndrome spectrum: new clinical insights supported by 13 new PQBP1-mutated males. Clin Genet 2010 [Epub ahead of print].

Gerrard JW, Renpenning HJ: Sex-linked mental retardation. Lancet 1:1346, 1974

Golabi M, Ito M, Hall BD: A new X-linked multiple congenital anomalies/mental retardation syndrome. Am J Med Genet 17:367, 1984.

Hamel BCJ, Mariman ECM, van Beersum SEC, et al.: Mental retardation, congenital heart defect, cleft palate, short stature, and facial anomalies: A new X-linked multiple congenital anomalies/mental retardation syndrome: Clinical description and molecular studies. Am J Med Genet 51:591, 1994.

Howard-Peebles PN, Stoddard GR, Mims MG: Familial X-linked mental retardation, verbal disability, and marker X chromosomes. Am J Hum Genet 31:214, 1979.

Jennings M, Hall JG, Hoehn H: Significance of phenotypic and chromosomal abnormalities in X-linked mental retardation (Martin-Bell or Renpenning Syndrome). Am J Med Genet 7:417, 1980.

Kalscheuer VM, Freude K, Musante L, et al.: Mutations in the polyglutamine binding protein 1 gene cause X-linked mental retardation. Nat Genet 35:313, 2003.

Kleefstra T, Franken CE, Arens YH, et al.: Genotype-phenotype studies in three families with mutations in the polyglutamine-binding protein 1 gene (PQBP1). Clin Genet 66:318, 2004.

Lenski C, Abidi F, Meindl A, et al.: Novel truncating mutations in the polyglutamine tract binding protein 1 gene (PQBP1) cause Renpenning syndrome and X-linked mental retardation in another family with microcephaly. Am J Hum Genet 74:777, 2004.

Lubs H, Abidi FE, Echeverri R, et al.: Golabi-Ito-Hall syndrome results from a missense mutation in the WW domain of the PQBP1 gene. J Med Genet 43:e30, 2006.

McLaughlin JF, Kriegsmann E: Developmental dyspraxias in a family with X-linked mental retardation (Renpenning syndrome). Dev Med Child Neurol 22:84, 1980.

Porteous MEM, Johnson H, Burn J, et al.: A new mental retardation syndrome mapping to the pericentromeric region of the X-chromosome. Am J Hum Genet 51:A106, 1992.

Proops R, Webb T: The 'fragile' X chromosome in the Martin-Bell-Renpenning syndrome and in males with other forms of familial mental retardation. J Med Genet 18:366, 1981.

Renpenning H, Gerrard JW, Zaleski WA, et al.: Familial sex-linked mental retardation. Canad Med Assoc J 87:954, 1962.

Richards BW: "Renpenning" syndrome. Lancet 2:520, 1970

Steele MW, Chorazy AL: Renpenning's syndrome. Lancet 2:752, 1974.

Stevenson RE, Arena JF, Ouzts E, et al.: Renpenning syndrome maps to Xp11. Am J Hum Genet 62:1092, 1998.

Stevenson RE, Bennett CW, Abidi F, et al.: Renpenning syndrome comes into focus. Am J Med Genet A 134:415, 2005.

Sutherland GR, Gedeon AK, Haan EA, et al.: Linkage studies with the gene for an X-linked syndrome of mental retardation, microcephaly and spastic diplegia. Am J Med Genet 30:493, 1988.

Turner G, Engisch B, Lindsay DG, et al.: X-linked mental retardation without physical abnormality (Renpenning's syndrome) in sibs in an institution. J Med Genet 9:324, 1972.

Turner G, Turner B, Collins E: Renpenning's syndrome - X-linked mental retardation. Lancet 2:365, 1970.

Turner G, Turner B, Collins E: X-linked mental retardation without physical abnormality: Renpenning's syndrome. Dev Med Child Neurol 13:71, 1971.

DIFFERENTIAL MATRIX

Syndrome	Microcephaly	Short Stature	Small Testes	Comments
Renpenning	+	+	+	Upslanting palpebral fissures
Abidi	+	+	+	Sloping forehead, cupped ears
ATRX-Associated XLID	+	+	+	Telecanthus/hypertelorism, small triangular nose, tented upper lip, open mouth, wide spacing of teeth, abnormal genitalia, minor musculoskeletal anomalies, hypotonia, erythrocyte HbH inclusions in some
Börjeson-Forssman-Lehmann	+	+	+	Obesity, hypotonia, hypogonadism, coarse facies, large ears, gynecomastia, narrow sloped shoulders, visual impairment, tapered digits
Hereditary Bullous Dystrophy, X-linked	+	+	+	Upslanting palpebral fissures, protruding ears, digits short and tapered, cardiac defects, bullous dystrophy, early death from pulmonary infection
XLID-Microcephaly-Testicular Failure	+	+	+	Prominent supraorbital ridges, high nasal bridge, prominent nose, macrostomia, hypogonadism
Craniofacioskeletal	+	+	0	Mild cognitive impairment, craniofacial distinctiveness, small hands and feet, excessive fingerprint arches in females. Males die in early infancy with craniofacial, cardiac, skeletal, and genital abnormalities
Miles-Carpenter	+	+	0	Ptosis, small palpebral fissures, open mouth, pectus excavatum, scoliosis, long hands, camptodactyly, rockerbottom feet, arch fingerprints, spasticity, unsteady gait
Pettigrew	+	0	+	Microcephaly or hydrocephaly, long face with macrostomia and prognathism, Dandy-Walker malformation, spasticity, seizures, contractures, choreoathetosis, iron deposits in basal ganglia, seizures

RETT SYNDROME

(ATAXIA-DEMENTIA-AUTISM SYNDROME, AUTISM-DEMENTIA-ATAXIA-LOSS OF PURPOSEFUL HAND USE SYNDROME)

OMIM 312750

Xq28

MECP2

Definition. XLID in females associated with cessation and regression of development in early childhood, truncal ataxia, autistic features, and acquired microcephaly.

Somatic Features. Major malformations do not occur. Microcephaly is evident by age 3 years but the birth head circumference is normal. The facial appearance in childhood, although not distinctive, tends to be delicate and is thereby distinguished from the facial coarseness that accompanies other developmental regression syndromes – notably the lysosomal storage disorders. A pattern of neurological deterioration dominates and defines the phenotype.

Growth and Development. Intrauterine growth appears normal; postnatal growth slows during the first year, leading to microcephaly and short stature in early childhood. A variable period of normal development follows birth but gives way first to a slowing of development and then to a loss of skills.

Cognitive Function. Progression to severe impairment occurs during the preschool years, usually with accompanying characteristics of autism.

Neurological Findings. A series of neurological stages defines the natural history of Rett syndrome. Following a period of normal developmental progress, acquisition of new skills slows and stops, hypotonia appears, interaction with the environment wanes, and the growth rates of the head and body decrease. By age 1 to 3 years, this stage merges into one of relatively rapid deterioration in which hand use, cognitive, speech, and social skills are lost, and stereotypical hand movements, jerky/apraxic limb and truncal movements, autistic mannerisms, disorganized breathing with hyperventilation and apneic episodes, and seizures appear. Thereafter, unsteadiness and seizures become more prominent, whereas cognitive impairment, autistic features, and loss of motor skills plateau. In the early school years, motor function begins to deteriorate further, eventually leading to muscle wasting, loss of mobility, hypertonicity, hyperreflexia, clonus, extensor plantar reflexes, vasomotor disturbances, and cachexia.

Imaging. Mild and nonspecific atrophy is noted on brain imaging.

Electroencephalography. In all cases, the EEG is abnormal. Although a specific pattern should not be anticipated, single or multiple epileptic foci, generalized background slowing and disorganization, and loss of normal sleep patterns occur and progressively worsen.

Comment. Rett syndrome, caused by *MECP2* mutations, occurs only in females and in this regard is similar to XLID-Infantile Spasms caused by *CDKL5* mutations, the only other X-linked condition to be considered in the differential. Because most affected females do not reproduce, the majority of cases likely represent new mutations, possibly arising in the father's germline. Liveborn males with *MECP2* mutations typically have an encephalopathy with progressive spasticity and early lethality.

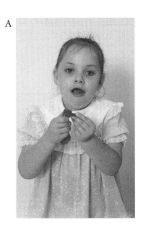
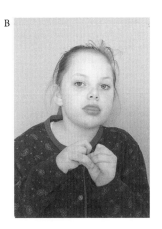
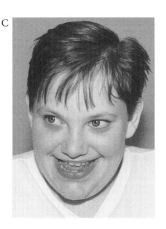

A   B   C

Rett Syndrome. Microcephaly and hand-wringing activity in a girl at ages 5, 7, and 14 years.

Mutations in *MECP2* have also been described in the PPM-X syndrome and three nonsyndromal XLID families (MRX 16, 64, and 79), indicating that not all mutations are lethal in males. Duplications of *MECP2* and adjacent genes in Xq28 have been found in XLID-Hypotonia-Recurrent Infections syndrome.

REFERENCES

Amir RE, Van den Veyver IB, Wan M, et al.: Rett syndrome is caused by mutations in X-linked MECP2, encoding methyl-CpG-binding protein 2. Nat Genet 23:185, 1999.

Couvert P, Bienvenu T, Aquaviva C, et al.: MECP2 is highly mutated in X-linked mental retardation. Hum Mol Genet 10:941, 2001.

Friez MJ, Jones JR, Clarkson K, et al.: Recurrent infections, hypotonia, and mental retardation caused by duplication of MECP2 and adjacent region in Xq28. Pediatrics 118:e1687, 2006.

Hagberg B, Aicardi J, Dias K, et al.: A progressive syndrome of autism, dementia, ataxia, and loss of purposeful hand use in girls: Rett's syndrome: report of 35 cases. Ann Neurol 14:471, 1983.

Klauck SM, Lindsay S, Beyer KS, et al.: A mutation hot spot for nonspecific X-linked mental retardation in the MECP2 gene causes the PPM-X syndrome. Am J Hum Genet 70:1034, 2002.

Meloni I, Bruttini M, Longo I, et al.: A mutation in the Rett syndrome gene, MECP2, causes X-linked mental retardation and progressive spasticity in males. Am J Hum Genet 67:982, 2000.

Moeschler JB, Charman CE, Berg SZ, et al.: Rett syndrome: natural history and management. Pediatrics 82:1, 1988.

Naidu S, Murphy M, Moser HW: Rett syndrome - natural history in 70 cases. Am J Med Genet 24 (Suppl 1):61, 1983.

Orrico A, Lam C, Galli L, et al.: MECP2 mutation in male patients with non-specific X-linked mental retardation. FEBS Lett 481:285, 2000.

Philippe C, Villard L, De Roux N, et al.: Spectrum and distribution of MECP2 mutations in 424 Rett syndrome patients: a molecular update. Eur J Med Genet 49:9, 2006.

Rett A: Uber ein eigenartiges hirnatrophisches syndrom bei hyperammonämie im kindesalter. Wien Med Woch 116:723, 1966.

Van Esch H, Bauters M, Ignatius J, et al.: Duplication of the MECP2 region is a frequent cause of severe mental retardation and progressive neurological symptoms in males. Am J Hum Genet 77:442, 2005.

Xiang F, Zhang Z, Clarke A, et al.: Chromosome mapping of Rett syndrome: a likely candidate region on the telomere of Xq. J Med Genet 35:297, 1998.

Yntema HG, Oudakker AR, Kleefstra T, et al.: In-frame deletion in MECP2 causes mild nonspecific mental retardation. Am J Med Genet 107:81, 2001.

DIFFERENTIAL MATRIX

Syndrome	Developmental Regression	Stereotypical Movements	Seizures	Comments
Rett	+	+	+	Acquired microcephaly, truncal ataxia, autistic features
XLID-Epilepsy	+	+	+	Hyporeflexia
Rett-Like Seizures-Hypotonia	+	0	+	Affects females predominantly, hypotonia
Bertini	+	0	+	Developmental delays, postnatal growth impairment, macular degeneration, ataxia, cerebellar hypoplasia, hypotonia
Pelizaeus-Merzbacher	+	0	+	Optic atrophy, dystonia, CNS dysmyelination, hypotonia
Pyruvate Dehydrogenase Deficiency	+	0	+	Microcephaly, ataxia, dysarthria, structural brain anomalies, lactic acidosis, hypotonia
XLID-Infantile Spasms (*ARX*-Associated XLID)	+	0	+	Early childhood death, EEG hypsarrhythmia pattern, hypotonia
Epilepsy-Intellectual Disability in Females	+	0	+	Affects only females

RETT-LIKE SEIZURES-HYPOTONIA

(EARLY ONSET SEIZURES-HYPOTONIA, EARLY INFANTILE EPILEPTIC ENCEPHALOPATHY)

OMIM 300672

Xp22

CDKL5 (STK9)

Definition. XLID with early onset and refractory seizures, hypotonia, and developmental regression, predominantly in females.

Somatic Features. Malformations are not a manifestation of this XLID syndrome. The face appears hypotonic with tented upper lip and open mouth. Microcephaly, usually postnatally acquired, is present in half of patients.

Growth and Development. Intrauterine growth is normal. Postnatally, head growth is variable, usually below average, and in the microcephalic range in about half of patients. Developmental progress may appear normal prior to the onset of seizures but thereafter stagnates and may regress.

Neurological Findings. Seizures usually begin in the first few months of life. Infantile spasms are typical, but a generalized tonic-clonic, myoclonic absence, and focal seizures also occur. Some girls progress through a regression pattern similar to Rett syndrome, but others are atypical in that they retain speech and purposeful hand movements and may not exhibit stereotypical movements or respiratory irregularity. Muscle tone is typically decreased, especially in the early years, but may increase with age, eventually resulting in spasticity.

Imaging. In most cases, brain imaging is normal except for small brain size.

Comment. Rett-Like Seizures-Hypotonia syndrome is one of three X-linked seizure disorders that predominantly affect females. Epilepsy-intellectual disability in females is caused by mutations in *PCDH19*, and males with mutations in this gene typically do not have seizures, intellectual disability, or other manifestations. Rett syndrome is caused by mutations in *MECP2*, and males with these mutations may have a progressive and lethal encephalopathy in infancy. *MECP2* mutations have also been found in males with PPM-X syndrome and nonsyndromal XLID (MRX 16, 64, 79). Males with mutations in *CDKL5* typically have early onset intractable epilepsy and intellectual disability comparable to or more severe than females. Several males with missense mutations or mutations near the 3' end of the gene have had milder and later onset encephalopathy.

REFERENCES

Bahi-Buisson N, Nectoux J, Rosas-Vargas H, et al.: Key clinical features to identify girls with CDKL5 mutations. Brain 131:2647, 2008.

Evans JC, Archer HL, Colley JP, et al.: Early onset seizures and Rett-like features associated with mutations in CDKL5. Eur J Hum Genet 13:1113, 2005.

Kalscheuer VM, Tao J, Donnelly A, et al.: Disruption of the serine/threonine kinase 09 gene causes severe X-linked infantile spasms and mental retardation. Am J Hum Genet 72:1401, 2003.

Mei D, Marini C, Novara F, et al.: Xp22.3 genomic deletions involving the CDKL5 gene in girls with early onset epileptic encephalopathy. Epilepsia 51:647, 2010.

Nemos C, Lambert L, Giuliano F, et al.: Mutations spectrum of CDKL5 in early-onset encephalopathies: a study of a large collection of French patients and review of the literature. Clin Genet 76:357, 2009.

Psoni S, Willems PJ, Kanavakis E, et al.: A novel p.Arg970X mutation in the last exon of the CDKL5 gene resulting in late-onset seizure disorder. Eur J Paediatr Neurol 14:188, 2010.

Scala E, Ariani F, Mari F, et al.: CDKL5/STK9 is mutated in Rett syndrome variant with infantile spasms. J Med Genet 42:103, 2005.

Tao J, Van Esch H, Hagedorn-Greiwe M, et al.: Mutations in the X-linked cyclin-dependent kinase-like 5 (CDKL5/STK9) gene are associated with severe neurodevelopmental retardation. Am J Hum Genet 75:1149, 2004.

Weaving LS, Christodoulou J, Williamson SL, et al.: Mutations of CDKL5 cause a severe neurodevelopmental disorder with infantile spasms and mental retardation. Am J Hum Genet 75:1079, 2004.

White R, Ho G, Schmidt S, et al.: Cyclin-dependent kinase-like 5 (CDKL5) mutation screening in Rett syndrome and related disorders. Twin Res Hum Genet 13:168, 2010.

Syndrome	Seizures	Hypotonia	Developmental Regression	Comments
Rett-Like Seizures-Hypotonia	+	+	+	Affects females predominantly
Bertini	+	+	+	Developmental delays, postnatal growth impairment, macular degeneration, ataxia, cerebellar hypoplasia
Pelizaeus-Merzbacher	+	+	+	Optic atrophy, dystonia, CNS dysmyelination
Pyruvate Dehydrogenase Deficiency	+	+	+	Microcephaly, ataxia, dysarthria, structural brain anomalies, lactic acidosis
Rett	+	+	+	Acquired microcephaly, truncal ataxia, autistic features, repetitive stereotypic hand movements
XLID-Infantile Spasms (*ARX*-Associated XLID)	+	+	+	Early childhood death, EEG hypsarrhythmia pattern
Epilepsy-Intellectual Disability in Females	+	0	+	Affects only females
Menkes	+	0	+	Growth deficiency, hypothermia, pallor, limited movement, hypertonicity, metaphyseal widening and spurs, arterial tortuosity, childhood death, hair abnormality, skeletal changes
Ornithine Transcarbamoylase Deficiency	+	0	+	Chronic or intermittent hyperammonemia, microcephaly, protein-induced vomiting and lethargy, metabolic disturbance, sensorium change, ataxia
XLID-Epilepsy	+	0	+	Repetitive stereotypical hand movements

ROIFMAN SYNDROME

(SPONDYLOEPIPHYSEAL DYSPLASIA, RETINAL DYSTROPHY AND ANTIBODY DEFICIENCY)

OMIM 300258

Definition. XLID with microcephaly, short stature, spondyloepiphyseal dysplasia, retinal pigmentary deposits, antibody deficiency, eczema, and hypotonia. The gene has not been mapped.

Somatic Features. Microcephaly with downslanting palpebral fissures, long eyelashes, long philtrum, and thin upper lip are typical craniofacial features. These manifestations may be accompanied by epicanthal folds, small anteverted nose, and midface hypoplasia. A pigmentary retinopathy occurs in some patients. Short and tapered digits with fifth-finger clinodactyly, convex nails, and horizontal palmar crease are common. Epiphyseal changes are present in multiple joints and the vertebral endplates are wavy and irregular.

Immunodeficiency becomes manifest by frequent infections, eczema, asthma, lymphadenopathy, and hepatosplenomegaly. Serum immunoglobulins are typically normal, but an eosinophilia and low antibody levels occur.

Growth and Development. Prenatal and postnatal growth impairment occurs. The head circumference measures at or below the 3rd centile. Global developmental delay is typical and cognitive performance is mildly to moderately impaired.

Neurological Findings. None

Heterozygote Expression. None

Comment. Several XLID syndromes have immunological impairment: XLID-Hypotonia-Recurrent Infections caused by *MECP2* duplication and XLID-Hypogammaglobulinema. Other XLID syndromes have spondyloepiphyseal or spondyloepimetaphyseal findings. The possibility that Roifman syndrome is allelic to one of these XLID syndromes has not been excluded.

REFERENCES

De Vries PJ, McCartney DL, McCartney E, et al.: The cognitive and behavioural phenotype of Roifman syndrome. J Intellect Disabil Res 50:690, 2006.

Roifman CM: Antibody deficiency, growth retardation, spondyloepiphyseal dysplasia and retinal dystrophy: a novel syndrome. Clin Genet 55:103, 1999.

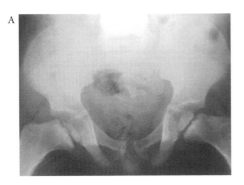
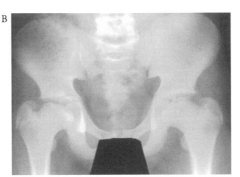

Roifman Syndrome. Radiographs of pelvis in two siblings at ages 12 and 19 years **(A, B)**, showing irregular epiphysial ossification of the femoral head and broad femoral neck.   Courtesy of Clinical Genetics. Copyright 1999. Munksgaard, Copenhagen.

Syndrome	Microcephaly	Skeletal Abnormalities	Hypotonia	Comments
Roifman	+	+	+	Short stature, spondyloepiphyseal dysplasia, retinal pigmentary deposits, antibody deficiency, eczema
Coffin-Lowry	+	+	+	Short stature, anteverted nares, tented upper lip, prominent lips and large mouth, large ears, soft hands with tapered digits, pectus carinatum, hypotonic facies, hypertelorism, arch fingerprints/low ridge count

SAY-MEYER SYNDROME

(TRIGONOCEPHALY WITH SHORT STATURE AND DEVELOPMENTAL DELAY)

OMIM 314320

Definition. XLID with short stature, microcephaly, hypotelorism, and craniosynostosis. The gene has not been mapped.

Somatic Features. Microcephaly with metopic ridging caused by synostosis of the metopic suture, synostosis affecting other cranial sutures, narrow frontal diameter, hypotelorism, and small fontanels are the major features. Low-set or retroverted ears and high palate may be present.

Growth and Development. Global growth retardation dates from the intrauterine period. Although long-term developmental outcome is not known, early childhood development is moderately delayed.

Neurological Findings. Seizures

Heterozygote Expression. None

Comment. The phenotype is based on a single family with three affected males in two generations. Craniosynostosis is rare among the XLID syndromes and, when present, it usually affects the metopic suture.

REFERENCE

Say B, Meyer J: Familial trigonocephaly associated with short stature and developmental delay. Am J Dis Child 135:711, 1981.

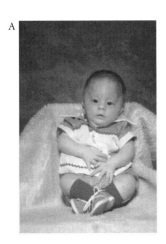 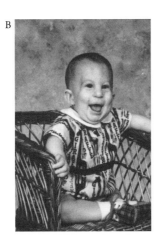 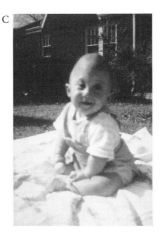

Say-Meyer Syndrome. Infant with microcephaly, bifrontal narrowing, prominent metopic ridging, and hypotelorism **(A)**; cousin with microcephaly, trigonencephaly, prominent metopic ridging, epicanthal folds, and hypotelorism **(B)**; maternal uncle with microcephaly trigonencephaly, narrow forehead with metopic ridge, and hypotelorism **(C)**.   Courtesy of Dr. Burhan Say, Tulsa Medical College, Tulsa, Oklahoma.

Syndrome	Microcephaly	Metopic Ridging or Synostosis	Hypotelorism	Comments
Say-Meyer	+	+	+	Short stature, craniosynostosis
Golabi-Ito-Hall (Renpenning)	+	+	0	Short stature, telecanthus, high nasal root, cupped ears, cardiac malformations, thoracic asymmetry, sacral dimple, dry/brittle/sparse hair, cutis marmorata, nail hypoplasia
XLID-Hypospadias	+	+	0	Trigonocephaly, synophrys, beaked nose, hypospadias
Juberg-Marsidi-Brooks	+	0	+	Short stature, dysgenesis of corpus callosum, deep-set eyes, blepharophimosis, cupped ears, bulbous nose, small mouth, thin upper lip, pectus excavatum, flexion contractures
Schimke	+	0	+	Sunken eyes, downslanting palpebral fissures, narrow nose, wide spacing of teeth, cupped ears, hypotonia, abducens palsy, hearing loss, vision loss, spasticity, choreoathetosis, contractures
Christian	0	+	+	Vertebral anomalies, abducens palsy

SCHIMKE SYNDROME

(SCHIMKE XLID SYNDROME, XLID-CHOREOATHETOSIS)

OMIM 312840

Definition. XLID with short stature, microcephaly, strabismus, sunken eyes, thin nose, impaired vision and hearing, abducens palsy, choreoathetosis, and spasticity. The gene has not been localized.

Somatic Features. Sunken eyes, downslanting palpebral fissures, apparent hypotelorism, narrow nose and alae nasi, strabismus, spacing of the teeth, and cupped ears give the distinctive facial appearance. Major malformations do not occur. In infancy they are hypotonic and feed poorly. This gives way to spasticity with increased deep tendon reflexes and Babinski signs. Microcephaly, spasticity, and involuntary limb movements become obvious during the first year. Hearing and vision are impaired, and esotropia occurs secondary to abducens palsy. The spasticity progressively worsens with age, eventually leading to rigidity and joint contractures, muscle atrophy, and loss of spontaneous movement.

Growth and Development. Prenatal growth is impaired, although the head circumference may be normal at birth. Microcephaly and short stature become obvious during the first year.

Cognitive Function. Not available

Neurological Findings. By early childhood, spasticity and choreoathetosis replaces hypotonia. The spasticity is reflected in increased deep tendon reflexes and Babinski signs and leads to widespread muscle wasting and joint contractures.

Heterozygote Expression. Mild congenital hearing loss was described in one carrier female and facial characteristics similar to affected males in another carrier female. No cognitive deficit has been reported.

Neuropathology. One case, who died at age 4 years of pneumonia, had postmortem examination. The brain was small with hypoplastic cerebellum, cystic changes in the globus pallidus, calcification of the basal ganglia, gliosis of the thalamus, and loss of Purkinje cells.

Comment. Schimke et al. reported this syndrome in three males in one family and one male in a second family. Linkage analysis was not possible. Abducens palsy has been described in only two other XLID syndromes (Christian and Christianson syndrome). In other clinical aspects, Schimke syndrome is also similar to Mohr-Tranebjaerg and Goldblatt Spastic Paraplegia syndromes.

REFERENCE

Schimke RN, Horton WA, Collins DL, et al.: A new X-linked syndrome comprising progressive basal ganglion dysfunction, mental and growth retardation, external ophthalmoplegia, postnatal microcephaly and deafness. Am J Med Genet 17:323, 1984.

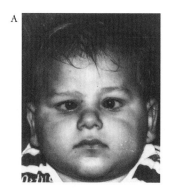
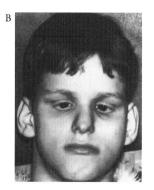
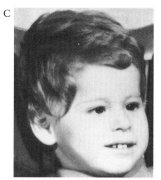
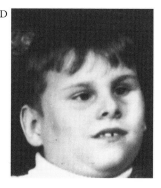

Schimke Syndrome. Cousins (**A, C**), maternal uncle (**B**), and sporcadic case (**D**) showing microcephaly, hypotelorism, deep-set eyes, downslanting palpebral fissures, strabismus, narrow nose and alae nasi, cupped ears, and spacing of the teeth.   Courtesy of Dr. Neil Schimke, Kansas University College of Health Sciences, Kansas City.

DIFFERENTIAL MATRIX

Syndrome	Impaired Vision and/or Hearing	Abducens Palsy	Spasticity or Ataxia	Comments
Schimke	+	+	+	Microcephaly, sunken eyes, downslanting palpebral fissures, narrow nose, wide spacing of teeth, cupped ears, hypotonia, choreoathetosis, contractures
Cerebro-Oculo-Genital	+	0	+	Microcephaly, hydrocephaly, short stature, agenesis of corpus callosum, microphthalmia, ptosis, hypospadias, cryptorchidism, clubfoot
Goldblatt Spastic Paraplegia	+	0	+	Nystagmus, optic atrophy, exotropia, muscle hypoplasia, spastic paraplegia, contractures
Mohr-Tranebjaerg	+	0	+	Neurological deterioration with childhood onset, dystonia
Proud (*ARX*-Associated XLID)	+	0	+	Seizures, short stature, microcephaly, agenesis of corpus callosum, cryptorchidism, inguinal hernias
Christianson	0	+	+	Short stature, microcephaly, general asthenia, contractures, seizures, ophthalmoplegia

SHASHI SYNDROME

(XLID-COARSE FACIES)

OMIM 300238

Xq26-q27

Definition. XLID with coarse facies, obesity, and macroorchidism.

Somatic Features. The face is described as coarse, specifically showing prominent supraorbital ridges, periorbital puffiness, narrow palpebral fissures, large ears, bulbous nose, and prominent lower lip. The head measured in the lower centiles. Obesity and macroorchidism were additional prominent findings. Cataracts occurred in the fourth decade.

Growth and Development. Postnatal growth appears variable with height from less than 3rd to the 90th centile. In the original family (Shashi et al., 2000), the head circumference varied from less than 3rd to the 50th centile. In a second family (Castro et al., 2003), the head size was greater than 97th centile.

Cognitive Function. IQs in the mildly to moderately impaired range.

Neurological Findings. Seizures occurred in affected males and carrier mothers reported by Castro et al. (2003).

Heterozygote Expression. Carriers have normal intelligence, although subtle craniofacial findings may be present.

Comment. The two families differ in that macrocephaly and seizures are present in one (Castro et al., 2003). Although the two families map to Xq26-q27, they may be different XLID entities. Two other XLID syndromes, both unmapped, share features with Shashi syndrome. Atkin-Flaitz syndrome has macrocephaly, hypertelorism, short stature, broad short hands, diastema, and microdontia as features different from Shashi syndrome. Clark-Baraitser syndrome differs in having macrocephaly but is similar in other respects. The possibility of allelism between two more of these conditions must await gene identification.

REFERENCES

Atkin JF, Flaitz K, Patil S, et al.: A new X-linked mental retardation syndrome. Am J Med Genet 21:697, 1985.

Castro NHC, Stocco dos Santos RC, Nelson R, et al.: Shashi XLMR syndrome: report of a second family. Am J Med Genet 118A:49, 2003.

Clark RD, Baraitser M: A new X-linked mental retardation syndrome. Am J Med Genet 26:13, 1987.

Shashi V, Berry MN, Shoaf S, et al.: A unique form of mental retardation with a distinctive phenotype maps to Xq26-q27. Am J Hum Genet 66:469, 2000.

A   B   C

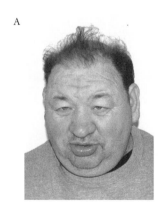 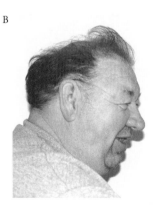 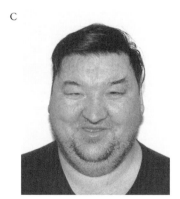

Shashi Syndrome. Adult brothers with coarse facies, short eyebrows, puffy eyelids, narrow palpebral fissures, bulbous nose, large ears, prominent lower lips, and obesity (**A-C**).   Courtesy of Dr. Vandana Shashi, Wake Forest University School of Medicine, Winston-Salem, NC.

DIFFERENTIAL MATRIX

Syndrome	Coarse Facies	Macroorchidism	Obesity	Comments
Shashi	+	+	+	Adult onset cataracts
Atkin-Flaitz	+	+	+	Macrocephaly, hypertelorism, downslanting palpebral fissures, broad nasal tip, thick lower lip, brachydactyly, seizures, short stature, features
Clark-Baraitser	+	+	+	Large stature, dental abnormalities, broad nasal tip, thick lower lip, macrocephaly
XLID-Hypogonadism-Tremor	+	0	+	Short stature, prominent lower lip, muscle wasting of legs, abnormal gait, hypogonadism, seizures, tremor

SHRIMPTON SYNDROME

(MRXS9)

OMIM 300709

Xq12-q21.31

Definition. XLID with microcephaly.

Somatic Features. Microcephaly, postnatally acquired, has been the only consistent finding. Short stature, although present, was also present in nonaffected males. Several affected males had strabismus, and one had spastic diplegia. Published photographs show almond-shaped eyes in childhood and prominent nose, overhanging columella, short philtrum, and prominent lower lip in adulthood.

Growth and Development. Prenatal growth appeared normal, with slowing of head growth in infancy.

Cognitive Function. Motor and speech development was globally delayed, with speech delay being more severe. Cognitive function was severely impaired.

Behavior. Behavior was not problematic and patients were generally friendly, although one male had occasional bouts of self-injury.

Heterozygote Expression. Some carrier females had learning difficulty in school.

Neurological Findings. Spastic diplegia in one case

Comment. The small head size, facial appearance, and short stature are reminiscent of Renpenning syndrome; however, the testes are normal size and the linkage limits are exclusive. XLID syndromes that map to this region appear to be distinct clinically from Shrimpton syndrome.

REFERENCES

Shrimpton AE, Braddock BR, Hoo JJ: Narrowing the map of a gene (MRXS9) for X-linked mental retardation, microcephaly, and variably short stature at Xq12-q21.31. Am J Med Genet 92:155, 2000.

Shrimpton AE, Daly KM, Hoo JJ: Mapping of a gene (MRXS9) for X-linked mental retardation, microcephaly, and variably short stature to Xq12-q21.31. Am J Med Genet 84:293, 1999.

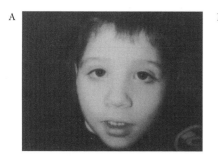
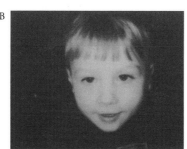
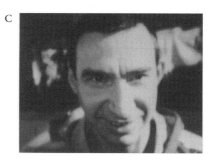

Shrimpton Syndrome. Brothers aged 3 1/2 years (A) and 5 1/2 years (B) with microcephaly, almond-shaped eyes, prominent midface and small jaw. Adult uncle (C) with microcephaly, overhanging columella and small jaw. Courtesy of Dr. Joe Hoo, Syracuse, New York and the American Journal of Medical Genetics. Copyright 1999, Wiley-Liss, Inc.

Syndrome	Microcephaly	Distinctive Facies	Short Stature	Comments
Shrimpton	+	+	+	Almond-shaped eyes, prominent nose with overhanging columella, short philtrum, prominent lower lip
ATRX-Associated XLID	+	+	+	Telecanthus/hypertelorism, small triangular nose, tented upper lip, open mouth, wide spacing of teeth, abnormal genitalia, minor musculoskeletal anomalies, hypotonia, erythrocyte HbH inclusions in some
Börjeson-Forssman-Lehmann	+	+	+	Coarse face, large ears, gynecomastia, narrow sloped shoulders, visual impairment, tapered digits, hypotonia, hypogonadism, obesity
Coffin-Lowry	+	+	+	Anteverted nares, tented upper lip, prominent lips and large mouth, large ears, soft hands with tapered digits, pectus carinatum, hypotonic facies, hypertelorism, arch fingerprints/low ridge count
Cornelia de Lange Syndrome, X-linked	+	+	+	Arched eyebrows, synophrys, long philtrum, thin lips, cutis marmorata, small hands and feet, hirsutism, enlarged cerebral ventricles, proximal thumbs, elbow restriction
Craniofacioskeletal	+	+	+	Mild cognitive impairment, craniofacial distinctiveness, small hands and feet, excessive fingerprint arches in females. Males die in early infancy with craniofacial, cardiac, skeletal, and genital abnormalities
Miles-Carpenter	+	+	+	Ptosis, small palpebral fissures, open mouth, pectus excavatum, scoliosis, long hands, camptodactyly, rockerbottom feet, arch fingerprints, unsteady gait, skeletal abnormality, spasticity
XLID-Microcephaly-Testicular Failure	+	+	+	Prominent supraorbital ridges, high nasal bridge, prominent nose, macrostomia, hypogonadism
CK	+	+	O	Asthenic build, neuronal migration disturbance, seizures, hypotonia, long thin face, scoliosis, behavior problems
Turner XLID (*AP1S2*-Associated XLID)	+	+	O	Hydrocephaly, long face with high forehead, long nose, prominent ears, basal ganglia calcifications, hypotonia, aggressive adult behavior

SIMPSON-GOLABI-BEHMEL SYNDROME

(SIMPSON DYSMORPHIA SYNDROME)

OMIM 312870

Xq26.2

GPC3

Definition. XLID with generalized overgrowth, prominent glabella, full midface, large mouth, prominent mandible, supernumerary nipples, cardiac defects, short hands and feet, and postaxial polydactyly. The responsible gene, *GPC3*, codes for an extracellular proteoglycan.

Somatic Features. Structural features are quite variable but more consistent than cognitive impairment. Generalized overgrowth is typical although the head may be large and stature normal. The facies appear coarse and often are misinterpreted in early childhood as representing Beckwith-Wiedemann syndrome, Hurler syndrome, or another storage disorder. The glabella is full, metopic ridging may occur, the eyes are widely set, the palpebral fissures often slant downward, the nasal bridge may be broad and flat with the nasal tip broad and upturned, the maxilla and mandible are prominent, and the mouth and tongue are large. The palate may be tall but only uncommonly is cleft. The lips are thick, and there may be a midline indentation of the lower lip. The neck may appear broad but not webbed. The ears usually have normal architecture. Supernumerary nipples are common. Perioral and palatal pigmentation have been reported. Heart defects in the form of structural anomalies and conduction defects have been present in some affected individuals.

The hands are broad and short with blunting of the distal phalanges. Postaxial polydactyly of the hands is typical, but broad thumbs and halluces and preaxial polysyndactyly of the halluces may occur as well. Hypoplasia or ridging of the index fingernails have been seen. Feet are likewise short. Inguinal hernias often occur in infancy. Large lobated or cystic kidneys with duplication of the collecting system and mild hydronephrosis have occurred. Cryptorchidism is common. Radiographs show advanced bone age, furrow of C2–3, cervical ribs, six lumbar vertebrae, and variable sacrococcygeal defects. A variety of other malformations, including diaphragmatic defects, have been occasionally noted.

Growth and Development. Prenatal and postnatal overgrowth occurs. Large head circumference is more consistent than excessive statural growth. Mild obesity may occur, and the liver and spleen may be enlarged.

Cognitive Function. Although most patients will have normal cognitive function, the IQ is less than in nonaffected individuals in the family. Less commonly, mild to moderate cognitive impairment is present; severe impairment is uncommon. The unusual facial appearance and clumsy motor function may contribute to the appearance of intellectual disability.

Neurological Findings. Hypotonia of variable degree commonly occurs in early life. Winging of the scapula, midchest depression, and wasting of the calf muscles may be manifestations of the hypotonia. There is a tendency to appear clumsy with stiff and wide-based gait. Seizures occur in a minority.

Heterozygote Expression. Carrier females are usually larger than noncarrier sisters and tend to have large face, large mouth, and supernumerary nipples. Cognitive function is usually normal, but some carrier females have had mild impairment.

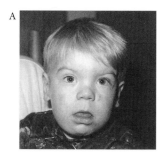
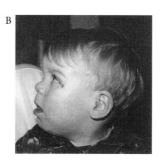
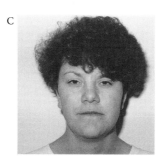

Simpson-Golabi-Behmel Syndrome. Male, age 20 months, with prominent forehead and depressed nasal bridge, short nose, long philtrum, and full lower lip (**A, B**); mother with macrocephaly, prominent forehead, flat midface, and prominent mandible (**C**).

Comment. Simpson-Golabi-Behmel syndrome shares with other overgrowth syndromes a predisposition to development of malignant tumors. Only intraabdominal tumors, including hepatocellular carcinoma, Wilms tumor, and neuroblastoma, have been described. A more severe disorder (OMIM 300209) with microcephaly; dysmorphic facies; and gastrointestinal, genitourinary, and skeletal anomalies has been termed Simpson-Golabi-Behmel syndrome, Type 2. Hydrops and early infancy deaths are common. A duplication of *CXORF5* (Xp22.2), the gene responsible for Oral-Facial-Digital I syndrome, was found in one family.

REFERENCES

Behmel A, Plöchl E, Rosenkranz W: A new X-linked dysplasia gigantism syndrome: Identical with the Simpson dysplasia syndrome? Hum Genet 67:409, 1984.

Brzustowicz LM, Farrell S, Khan MB, et al.: Mapping of a new SGBS locus to chromosome Xp22 in a family with a severe form of Simpson-Golabi-Behmel syndrome. Am J Hum Genet 65:779, 1999.

Budny B, Chen W, Omran H, et al.: A novel X-linked recessive mental retardation syndrome comprising macrocephaly and ciliary dysfunction is allelic to oral-facial-digital type I syndrome. Hum Genet 120:171, 2006.

Garganta CL, Bodurtha JN: Report of another family with Simpson-Golabi-Behmel syndrome and a review of the literature. Am J Med Genet 44:129, 1992.

Golabi M, Rosen L: A new X-linked mental retardation-overgrowth syndrome. Am J Med Genet 17:345, 1984.

Gurrieri F, Cappa M, Neri G: Further delineation of the Simpson-Golabi-Behmel (SGB) Syndrome. Am J Med Genet 44:136, 1992.

Neri G, Gurrieri F, Zanni G, et al.: Clinical and molecular aspects of the Simpson-Golabi-Behmel syndrome. Am J Med Genet 79:279, 1998.

Pilia G, Hughes-Benzie RM, MacKenzie A, et al.: Mutations in GPC3, a glypican gene, cause the Simpson-Golabi-Behmel overgrowth syndrome. Nat Genet 12:241, 1996.

Simpson JL, Landey S, New M, et al.: A previously unrecognized X-linked syndrome of dysmorphia. Birth Defects Orig Art Ser XI(2):18, 1975.

Terespolsky D, Farrell SA, Siegel-Bartelt J, et al.: Infantile lethal variant of Simpson-Golabi-Behmel syndrome associated with hydrops fetalis. Am J Med Genet 59:329, 1995.

Xuan JY, Besner A, Ireland M, et al.: Mapping of Simpson-Golabi-Behmel syndrome to Xq25-q27. Hum Mol Genet 3:133, 1994.

DIFFERENTIAL MATRIX

Syndrome	Macrocephaly	Digital Anomalies	Hypotonia	Comments
Simpson-Golabi-Behmel	+	+	+	Somatic overgrowth, supernumerary nipples, polydactyly
Opitz FG	+	+	+	Broad forehead, downslanted palpebral fissures, everted lower lip, dysgenesis of corpus callosum, cardiac defects, imperforate anus, constipation, broad flat thumbs and great toes
Atkin-Flaitz	+	+	0	Short stature, hypertelorism, downslanting palpebral fissures, broad nasal tip, thick lower lip, brachydactyly, seizures
Mucopolysaccharidosis IIA	+	+	0	Short stature, coarse facies, hepatosplenomegaly, hernias, joint stiffness, thick skin, hirsutism, behavioral disturbance
Coffin-Lowry	0	+	+	Microcephaly, short stature, hypertelorism, anteverted nares, tented upper lip, prominent lips and large mouth, large ears, soft hands with tapered digits, pectus carinatum
Miles-Carpenter	0	+	+	Microcephaly, short stature, ptosis, small palpebral fissures, open mouth, pectus excavatum, scoliosis, long hands, camptodactyly, rockerbottom feet, arch fingerprints, spasticity, unsteady gait

SMITH-FINEMAN-MYERS SYNDROME

Three reports have detailed the phenotypic manifestations of Smith-Fineman-Myers syndrome. Brothers were described in two reports and an isolated case in the third report. Phenotypic differences in the two sets of brothers introduce doubt that they have the same syndrome.

Smith, Fineman, and Myers (1980) reported two brothers with microdolichocephaly, upslanting palpebral fissures, ptosis, strabismus, cupped ears, flat philtrum, maxillary overbite, thin upper lip, scoliosis, bridged palmar creases, and long narrow feet with midfoot varus. There was diffuse hypotonia and severe developmental impairment. Both boys had low birth weight and short stature, the older brother had generalized seizures, the younger had minor motor seizures. Findings found in one brother, but not the other, included short sternum with flaring of the ribcage, femoral anteversion, hyperconvex and short fingernails, and double hair whorl. Both exhibited poor social skills and repetitive movements of the upper limbs. Pneumoencephalogram showed cortical atrophy.

Stephenson and Johnson (1985) reported a third unrelated case and follow-up of the original cases. They considered the boys to have similar craniofacial findings with microdolichocephaly, narrow face, decreased frontonasal angle, decreased nasolabial folds, smooth philtrum, prominent maxilla with overbite, prominent upper central incisors, patulous lower lip, and micrognathia. They also had short stature, thin habitus, pectus excavatum, bridged palmar creases, foot deformities, light pigmentation with freckles, and seizures. Although initially the brothers had hypotonia, they became mildly spastic with hypertonia and hyper-reflexia during childhood. The isolated case lacked midfoot varus and upslanted palpebral fissures and had optic nerve hypoplasia and bifid uvula.

Adès and colleagues (1991) reported two brothers that they considered had the same syndrome. Their patients had frontal hair upsweep, hypertelorism, downslanting palpebral fissures, short nose, short philtrum with tented upper lip, prominent lower lip, open mouth, small hands with short tapered fingers, and cryptorchidism. Hall (1992) has pointed out the resemblance of these brothers to Alpha-Thalassemia Intellectual Disability Syndrome. They lacked hemoglobin H inclusions seen in some cases with Alpha-Thalassemia Intellectual Disability Syndrome, but mutational analysis of the *ATRX* gene has not been reported.

REFERENCES

Adès LC, Kerr B, Turner G, et al.: Smith-Fineman-Myers syndrome in two brothers. Am J Med Genet 40:467, 1991. (Also see letter by Hall: Am J Med Genet 44:250, 1992 and response by Adès: Am J Med Genet 44:251, 1992.)

Smith RD, Fineman RM, Myers GG: Short stature, psychomotor retardation, and unusual facial appearance in two brothers. Am J Med Genet 7:5, 1980.

Stephenson LD, Johnson JP: Smith-Fineman-Myers syndrome: Report of a third case. Am J Med Genet 22:301, 1985.

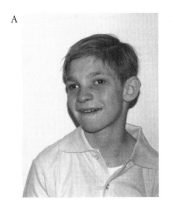
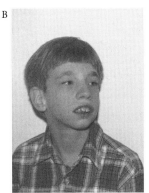
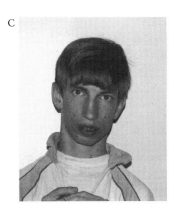

Smith-Fineman-Myers Syndrome. Microdolichocephaly, upslanting palpebral fissures, ptosis, strabismus, cupped ears, flat philtrum, maxillary overbite, and thin upper lip in two brothers ages 13 years and 15 years (**A, B**); microdolichocephaly, narrow face, decreased nasolabial folds, smooth philtrum, maxillary overbite, patulous lower lip, and micrognathia in a sporadic case at age 22 years (**C**). Courtesy of Dr. John Johnson, Shodair Hospital, Helena, Montana.

SNYDER-ROBINSON SYNDROME

OMIM 309583

Xp22.11

SMS

Definition. XLID with prominent lower lip, high/cleft palate, asthenic build, kyphoscoliosis, long hands and fingers, seizures, and nasal speech.

Somatic Features. Facial characteristics include asymmetry, high or cleft palate, and prominent lower lip. Midface flatness or retraction may occur. General asthenic build may be accompanied by narrow thorax, pectus excavatum, kyphoscoliosis, long thin hands with hyperextensible digits, long great toes, and osteoporosis.

Growth and Development. Birth weight is low in some individuals. Adult stature has been variable, ranging from below the 3rd centile to above the 97th centile. Head circumference tends to be above average. Motor and language milestones are moderately delayed.

Cognitive Function. Mild cognitive impairment was the rule in the first family reported, but more severely impaired individuals have been subsequently identified.

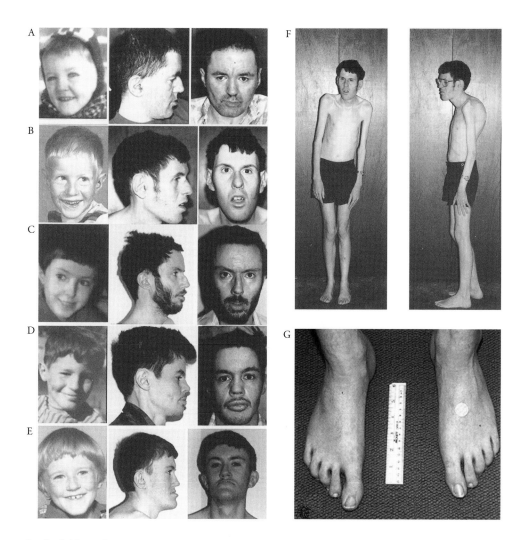

Snyder-Robinson Syndrome. Facial appearance in childhood and adult life **(A–E)**. Facial asymmetry and prominent lower lip become apparent with age. Asthenic build with decreased musculature and kyphoscoliosis in adult **(F)**; long halluces in adult **(G)**.

Neurological Findings. Hypotonia occurs especially during early childhood. Asymmetric facial movement, spasticity, and seizures have been noted in one or more males.

Imaging. Decreased volume of cerebellum, hippocampus, and red nucleus.

Heterozygote Expression. Carrier females have no cognitive impairment or somatic manifestation.

Comment. Initially reported as nonsyndromal XLID with hypotonia, the Snyder-Robinson syndrome is now defined primarily by facial and skeletal manifestations. The spermine synthase gene, *SMS*, converts spermidine to spermine. Mutations lead to intracellular deficiency of spermine, an essential polyamine.

REFERENCES

Arena JF, Schwartz C, Ouzts L, et al.: X-linked mental retardation with thin habitus, osteoporosis, and kyphoscoliosis: linkage to Xp21.3-p22.12. Am J Med Genet 64:50, 1996.

Cason AL, Ikeguchi Y, Skinner C, et al.: X-linked spermine synthase gene (SMS) defect: the first polyamine deficiency syndrome. Eur J Hum Genet 11:937, 2003.

de Alencastro G, McCloskey DE, Kliemann SE, et al.: New SMS mutation leads to a striking reduction in spermine synthase protein function and a severe form of Snyder-Robinson X-linked recessive mental retardation syndrome. J Med Genet 45:539, 2008.

Kesler SR, Schwartz C, Stevenson RE, Reiss AL: The impact of spermine synthase (SMS) mutations on brain morphology. Neurogenetics.10:299, 2009.

Snyder RD, Robinson A: Recessive sex-linked mental retardation in the absence of other recognizable abnormalities: Report of a family. Clin Pediatr 8:669, 1969.

DIFFERENTIAL MATRIX

Syndrome	Tall Stature	Asthenic Build	Hypotonia	Comments
Snyder-Robinson	+	+	+	High or cleft palate, prominent lower lip, kyphoscoliosis, long great toes, nasal speech, hypotonia in childhood
Lujan	+	+	0	Marfanoid habitus, long face, prominent forehead, high palate, micrognathia, long digits, pectus excavatum, joint hyperextensibility, seizures, hyperactivity
Simpson-Golabi-Behmel	+	0	+	Somatic overgrowth, supernumerary nipples, polydactyly
Allan-Herndon-Dudley	0	+	+	Large ears with cupping or abnormal architecture, muscle hypoplasia, contractures, dysarthria, athetosis, ataxia, spastic paraplegia
Arts	0	+	+	Growth deficiency, poor muscle development, areflexia, ataxia, deafness, vision loss, seizures, childhood death
CK	0	+	+	Microcephaly, neuronal migration disturbance, seizures, long thin face, scoliosis, behavior problems

STOCCO DOS SANTOS SYNDROME

OMIM 300434

Xp11.2

SHROOM4 (KIAA1202)

Definition. XLID with low birth weight, short stature, hypertelorism, epicanthus, strabismus, hip dislocation, hirsutism, recurrent infections, and precocious puberty.

Somatic Features. A clear facial phenotype has not been described, although photographs and clinical reports describe hypertelorism, heavy eyebrows, epicanthus, strabismus, short palpebral fissures, short philtrum, thin upper lip, and prominent nasal tip. All affected males have congenital hip dislocation, kyphosis, hirsutism, and precocious puberty and experience recurrent respiratory infections in childhood. Clubfoot has occurred in some cases.

Growth and Development. Low birth weight is described. Postnatally, short stature continues, but head growth is normal. Precocious puberty has occurred at ages 7 to 8 years. Details of developmental progress in early childhood have not been described. Speech has been absent in some cases.

Cognitive Function. Severe impairment

Heterozygote Expression. None

Comment. Although precocious puberty occurs with increased frequency among individuals with intellectual disability, among the XLID syndromes, it is reported only in Stocco dos Santos and XLID-Precocious Puberty syndromes.

REFERENCES

Hagens O, Dubos A, Abidi F, et al.: Disruptions of the novel KIAA1202 gene are associated with X-linked mental retardation. Hum Genet 118:578, 2006.

Hockey A: X-linked intellectual handicap and precocious puberty with obesity in carrier females. Am J Med Genet 23:127, 1986.

Stocco dos Santos RC, Barretto OCO, Nonoyama K, et al.: X-linked syndrome: Mental retardation, hip luxation, and G6PD variant [Gd(+) Butantan]. Am J Med Genet 39:133, 1991.

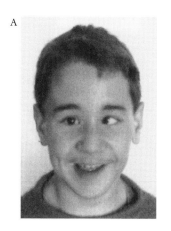 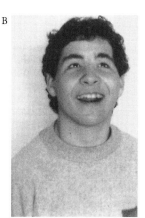 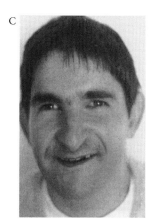 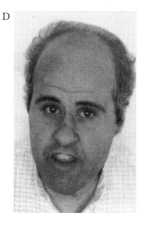

Stocco dos Santos Syndrome. Ten-year-old male with strabismus, epicanthus, hypertelorism, cataract of the right eye, long straight nose with overhanging tip, and flared alae nasi **(A)**; cousins with similar facial manifestations but without cataract at ages 16 years **(B)**; 28 years **(C)**; and 30 years **(D)**.   Courtesy of Dr. Rita Stocco dos Santos, Instituto Butantan, São Paulo, Brasil.

Syndrome	Short Stature	Congenital Hip Dislocation	Recurrent Infections	Comments
Stocco dos Santos	+	+	+	Heavy eyebrows, strabismus, short palpebral fissures, short philtrum, thin upper lip, prominent nasal tip, hirsutism, kyphosis, precocious puberty
Hereditary Bullous Dystrophy, X-linked	+	0	+	Microcephaly, upslanting palpebral fissures, protruding ears, digits short and tapered, cardiac defects, bullous dystrophy, small testes, early death from pulmonary infection
XLID-Hypotonia-Recurrent Infections	+	0	+	Hypertelorism, downslanting palpebral fissures, gastroesophageal reflux, hypotonic facies, developmental regression, seizures, childhood death

STOLL SYNDROME
(XLID-SHORT STATURE-HYPERTELORISM-HYPOTONIA)

Definition. XLID with short stature, prominent forehead, broad nasal tip with anteverted nares, and hypotonia. The gene has not been mapped.

Somatic Features. Short stature and craniofacial features predominate. In addition to frontal prominence or bossing, facial characteristics include ocular hypertelorism, depressed bridge of nose, anteverted nares, and flattening of the malar area. Published photographs suggest some tenting of the upper lip. Hypotonia was evident but only during early childhood.

Growth and Development. Although prenatal growth is normal, postnatal growth slows with short stature dating from childhood. Affected males are said to have large foreheads, but head circumference measurements have not been reported. Details of early childhood development are not available.

Cognitive Function. Mild impairment

Neurological Findings. Hypotonia, present in infancy and early childhood, resolves within a few years.

Heterozygote Expression. Two carrier females were reported to have the same facial appearance as affected males, but normal cognitive function.

Imaging. Normal cranial ultrasonography and tomography

Comment. The craniofacial phenotype, based on a single family, appears different from other XLID syndromes.

REFERENCE

Stoll C, Géraudel A, Chauvin A: New X-linked syndrome of mental retardation, short stature, and hypertelorism. Am J Med Genet 39:474, 1991.

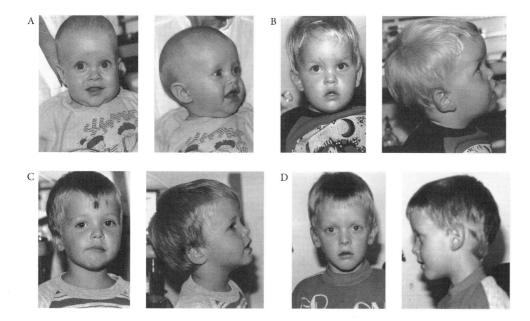

Stoll Syndrome. Brothers at ages 9 months **(A)** and 33 months **(B)** and at ages 4 years **(C)** and 6 years **(D)** showing macrocephaly, frontal bossing, hypertelorism, depressed nasal bridge, anteverted nostrils, and malar hypoplasia.   Courtesy of Dr. Claude Stoll, University of Strasbourg, Strasbourg, France.

DIFFERENTIAL MATRIX

Syndrome	Short Stature	Hypertelorism	Hypotonia	Comments
Stoll	+	+	+	Forehead prominence, depressed nasal root, anteverted nares
ATRX-Associated XLID	+	+	+	Microcephaly, small triangular nose, tented upper lip, open mouth, wide spacing of teeth, abnormal genitalia, minor musculoskeletal anomalieshypotonia, erythrocyte HbH inclusions in some
Coffin-Lowry	+	+	+	Microcephaly, anteverted nares, tented upper lip, prominent lips, large mouth, large ears, soft hands with tapered digits, pectus carinatum
Proud (*ARX*-Associated XLID)	+	+	+	Hearing loss, vision loss, agenesis of corpus callosum, cryptorchidism, inguinal hernias, ataxia, spasticity, seizures
Vasquez	+	+	+	Microcephaly, gynecomastia, obesity, hypogonadism
Aarskog	+	+	0	Downslanting palpebral fissures, ptosis, cupped ears, anteverted nares, brachydactyly, horizontal palmar crease, midfoot varus, joint laxity, shawl scrotum, cryptorchidism, inguinal hernias
Atkin-Flaitz	+	+	0	Macrocephaly, downslanting palpebral fissures, broad nasal tip, thick lower lip, brachydactyly, seizures
Otopalatodigital I (*FLNA*-Associated XLID)	+	+	0	Conductive hearing impairment, prominent brow, broad nasal root, downslanting palpebral fissures, cleft palate, blunted distal phalanges, irregular curvature and spacing of digits, limitation of elbow movement
Otopalatodigital II (*FLNA*-Associated XLID)	+	+	0	Hearing impairment, prominent forehead, flat/ broad nasal bridge, downslanting palpebral fissures, flat midface, cleft palate, blunted flexed overlapping fingers, rockerbottom feet, hypoplastic fibulae, subluxed/ dislocated joints
Miles-Carpenter	+	0	+	Microcephaly, ptosis, small palpebral fissures, open mouth, pectus excavatum, scoliosis, long hands, camptodactyly, rockerbottom feet, arch fingerprints, spasticity, unsteady gait
Smith-Fineman-Myers	+	0	+	Microcephaly, ptosis, flat philtrum, scoliosis, midfoot varus, narrow feet, seizures
Wittwer	+	0	+	Microcephaly, microphthalmia, hearing loss, vision loss, genitourinary anomalies, seizures
XLID-Psoriasis	0	+	+	Open mouth, large ears, seizures, psoriasis

SUTHERLAND-HAAN SYNDROME (*SEE ALSO* RENPENNING SYNDROME)

(MRXS3, SUTHERLAND SYNDROME)

OMIM 309470

Xp11.23

PQBP1

Definition. XLID with short stature, microcephaly, small testes, and spastic diplegia. A mutation has been found in *PQBP1*, making Sutherland-Haan syndrome allelic with Renpenning, Cerebro-Palato-Cardiac, Golabi-Ito-Hall, and Porteous syndromes.

Somatic Features. Short stature, microbrachycephaly, small testes, and spastic diplegia dominate the phenotype. Major malformations were exceptional, one male having imperforate anus and a second having anal stenosis. Facial manifestations include upslanted palpebral fissures, strabismus, maxillary hypoplasia, and, in some cases, large ears and mild prognathism. There was a tendency to lean body mass and pectus excavatum, scoliosis, stiffness of small joints, and pes cavus. Special senses appeared normal with

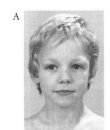
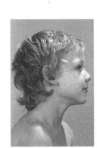
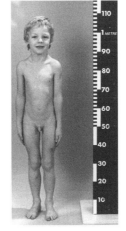
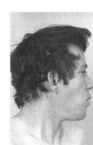
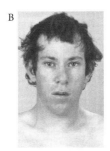
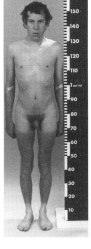
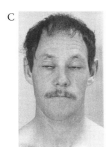
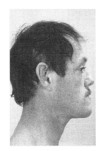
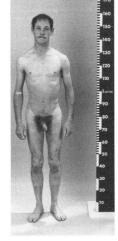

Sutherland-Haan Syndrome. Five-year-old male with microcephaly and normal facial appearance **(A)**. Twenty-eight-year-old with microbrachycephaly, short stature, asthenic body build, long face, and upslanting palpebral fissures **(B)**; 34-year-old with microbrachcephaly, maxillary hypoplasia, and asthenic body build **(C)**.   Courtesy of Dr. Grant Sutherland, Women's and Children's Hospital, Adelaide, Australia.

the exception of one case of deafness possibly related to recurrent otitis and mastoiditis.

Growth and Development. Intrauterine growth appears mildly impaired, with birth weights in the lower centiles. Postnatal growth is similarly slow with adult height and head circumference usually below -2SD. Testicular volume measures in the lower centiles and is possibly related to delay in puberty, decreased body hair, and early baldness. There is mild-to-moderate delay of speech and motor milestones.

Cognitive Function. Affected males exhibit a wide range of cognitive function from low-normal to moderate impairment.

Neurological Findings. Several males experience poor feeding during infancy. Increased muscle tone and hyperreflexia of lower limbs may be noted by early childhood, is of mild to moderate severity, and does not appear progressive.

Heterozygote Expression. Carrier females show no cognitive or somatic abnormalities.

Imaging. Prominent ventricles secondary to mild cerebral atrophy was found in one affected male on CT scan.

Comment. Only one family has been reported. Eight males were affected in three generations. The major features – short stature, microcephaly and small testes – are found in Renpenning syndrome with which Sutherland-Haan syndrome is now known to be allelic. The index family with Renpenning syndrome lacked the musculoskeletal features and spastic diplegia reported in Sutherland-Haan syndrome. Hamel Cerebro-Palato-Cardiac, Porteous, and Golabi-Ito-Hall syndromes are also allelic XLID entities.

REFERENCES

Gedeon A, Haan E, Mulley J: Gene localization for Sutherland-Haan syndrome (SHS:MIM 309470). Am J Med Genet 64:78, 1996.

Kalscheuer VM, Freude K, Musante L, et al.: Mutations in the polyglutamine binding protein 1 gene cause X-linked mental retardation. Nat Genet 35:313, 2003.

Lubs H, Abidi FE, Echeverri R, et al.: Golabi-Ito-Hall syndrome results from a missense mutation in the WW domain of the PQBP1 gene. J Med Genet 43:e30, 2006.

Stevenson RE, Bennett CW, Abidi F, et al.: Renpenning syndrome comes into focus. Am J Med Genet A 134:415, 2005.

Sutherland GR, Gedeon AK, Haan EA, et al.: Linkage studies with the gene for an X-linked syndrome of mental retardation, microcephaly and spastic diplegia. Am J Med Genet 30:493, 1988.

DIFFERENTIAL MATRIX

Syndrome	Microcephaly	Short Stature	Small Testes	Comments
Sutherland-Haan (Renpenning)	+	+	+	Upslanting palpebral fissures, asthenic habitus, pectus excavatum, scoliosis, stiff joints, pes cavus, spasticity
Abidi	+	+	+	Sloping forehead, cupped ears
ATRX-Associated XLID	+	+	+	Telecanthus/hypertelorism, small triangular nose, tented upper lip, open mouth, wide spacing of teeth, minor musculoskeletal anomalies, hypotonia, erythrocyte HbH inclusions in some
Hereditary Bullous Dystrophy, X-linked	+	+	+	Upslanting palpebral fissures, protruding ears, digits short and tapered, cardiac defects, bullous dystrophy, early death from pulmonary infection
XLID-Hypogonadism-Tremor	+	+	+	Prominent lower lip, muscle wasting of legs, abnormal gait, hypogonadism, obesity, seizures, tremor
XLID-Microcephaly-Testicular Failure	+	+	+	Prominent supra-orbital ridges, high nasal bridge, prominent nose, macrostomia, hypogonadism
Miles-Carpenter	+	+	0	Ptosis, small palpebral fissures, open mouth, pectus excavatum, scoliosis, long hands, camptodactyly, rockerbottom feet, arch fingerprints, spasticity, unsteady gait
Pettigrew	+	0	+	Microcephaly or hydrocephaly, long face with macrostomia and prognathism, Dandy-Walker malformation, spasticity, contractures, choreoathetosis, iron deposits in basal ganglia, seizures

TARP SYNDROME

(TALIPES EQUINOVARUS-ATRIAL SEPTAL DEFECT-ROBIN SEQUENCE-PERSISTENCE
OF LEFT SUPERIOR VENA CAVA, X-LINKED ROBIN SYNDROME)

OMIM 311900

Xp11.23

RBM10

Definition. XLID with talipes equinovarus, atrial septal defects, persistence of the left superior vena cava, optic atrophy, hearing loss, structural brain anomalies, cardiac rhythm disturbance, hypotonia and early lethality. Mutations have been found in *RBM10* which encodes an RNA binding motif protein.

Somatic Features. Structural changes are widespread involving the brain, face, heart, great vessels, and limbs. Facial manifestations include optic atrophy, upslanted palpebral fissures, low-set and retroverted ears, micrognathia, and cleft palate. Dysgenesis of the corpus callosum and caudate, cerebellar hypoplasia, and megacisterna magna have been described. Atrial septal defect is the usual cardiac malformation and may be linked functionally with cardiac arrhythmias. Persistence of the left superior vena cava, talipes equinovarus, and cryptorchidism occur in the majority of cases. Early lethality is typical, although survival to age 3 years in a ventilator-dependent state has been described in one case.

Growth and Development. Prenatal growth is normal. Early lethality has precluded observation of postnatal growth and developmental progress. The single male that survived past infancy had hearing loss and vision impairment, was noncommunicative, and remained ventilator-dependent at night.

Cognitive Function. Presumed to be severely impaired.

Natural History. Death during infancy is the rule. An increase in fetal wastage suggests prenatal lethality may occur as well.

Comment. Although three families have been reported, observations are limited by early lethality. Nonsense or frameshift mutations have been reported in all three families.

REFERENCES

Gorlin RJ, Cervenka J, Anderson RC, et al.: Robin's syndrome. A probably X-linked recessive subvariety exhibiting persistence of left superior vena cava and atrial septal defect. Am J Dis Child 119:176, 1970.

Gripp KW, Hopkins E, Johnston JJ, et al.: Long term survival in TARP syndrome and confirmation of RBM10 as the disease causing gene. David W. Smith Workshop on Malformations and Morphogenesis, Lake Arrowhead, CA, September 9-14, 2011.

Johnston JJ, Tear JK, Cherukuri PF, et al.: Massively parallel sequencing of exons on the X chromosome identifies RBM10 as the gene that causes a syndromic form of cleft Palate. Am J Hum Genet 86:743, 2010.

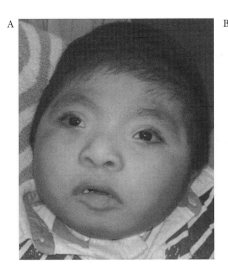
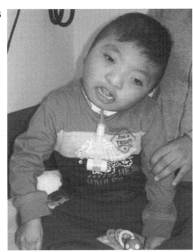
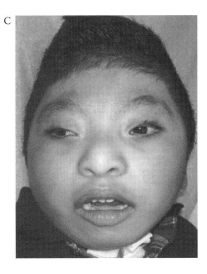

TARP Syndrome. Microcephaly, round face, arched eye brows, upslanting palpebral fissures, short nasal tip, downturned corners of the mouth and everted lower lip at age 26 (A), 37 (B) and 43 (C) months. At age 37 months, he required assistance sitting and had a tracheostomy. Courtesy of Dr. Karen Gripp, A.I. DuPont Hospital for Children, Wilmington, DE.

DIFFERENTIAL MATRIX

Syndrome	Cardiac Malformation/ Cardiomyopathy	Brain Malformation	Facial Clefting	Comments
TARP	+	+	+	Micrognathia, talipes equinovarus, atrial septal defect, persistence of left superior vena cava, hearing loss, visual impairment, arrhythmia, hypotonia, early childhood death
MIDAS	+	+	0	Ectodermal dysplasia, ocular anomaly, microphthalmia, ocular dysgenesis, corneal opacification, dermal aplasia
Optiz FG	+	+	0	Macrocephaly, digital anomalies, hypotonia broad forehead, downslanted palpebral fissures, everted lower lip, imperforate anus, constipation, broad flat thumbs and great toes
Cerebro-Palato-Cardiac	+	0	+	Distinctive facial features, microcephaly, short stature, cupped ears, bulbous nose, short philtrum, tented upper lip, childhood death
Lenz Microphthalmia	+	0	+	Ocular anomaly, limb anomaly, urogenital anomaly, microcephaly, malformed ears, thumb duplication or hypoplasia, narrow shoulders
Simpson-Golabi-Behmel	+	0	+	Macrocephaly, digital anomalies, hypotonia, somatic overgrowth, supernumerary nipples, polydactyly
Telecanthus-Hypospadias	+	0	+	Telecanthus, urogenital anomalies, high broad nasal root, dysplastic ears, abnormal cranial contour or symmetry
Oral-Facial-Digital I	0	+	+	Oral frenula/tongue hamartomas, brachydactyly, sparse scalp hair, dystopia canthorum, flat midface, hypoplastic alae nasi, syndactyly, clinodactyly, polycystic kidneys

TELECANTHUS-HYPOSPADIAS SYNDROME

(HYPERTELORISM-HYPOSPADIAS SYNDROME, OPITZ BBB SYNDROME,

OPITZ G SYNDROME)

OMIM 300000

Xp.2

MID1

Definition. XLID with telecanthus, high broad nasal root, and hypospadias.

Somatic Features. Structural anomalies of the midline dominate the somatic phenotype. Telecanthus, broad and high nasal root, dysplastic or posteriorly rotated ears, and cleft lip and palate are placed on an oval facial background with narrow forehead. Epicanthus, bifid uvula, high palate, micrognathia and clefts, or other anomalies of the pharynx, larynx, and trachea may occur. The cranium may be marked by a metopic ridge, scaphocephaly, brachycephaly, oxycephaly, or asymmetry. Cardiac malformations (including septal defects, patent ductus arteriosus, coarctation, and pulmonary valve incompetence) occur in a minority. Hypospadias occurs in almost all males but with variable meatal placement. Cryptorchidism, hypoplastic or cleft scrotum, inguinal hernias, and imperforate anus also occur. Stridor, dysphagia, gastroesophageal reflux, aspiration, and hoarse/weak cry may complicate the early course. Early death has occurred.

Growth and Development. About one-third have microcephaly and short stature.

Cognitive Function. Most males have developmental delay, poor school performance, or mild cognitive deficits by testing.

Heterozygote Expression. Carrier females typically have telecanthus but uncommonly have other facial features. Cognitive function is normal.

Imaging. None

Comment. Heterogeneity with at least two gene loci, one autosomal (22q11.2) and one X chromosomal (Xp22), has resolved the controversy regarding the genetic basis of the Telecanthus-Hypospadias syndrome.

REFERENCES

Christian JC, Bixler D, Blythe SC, et al.: Familial telecanthus with associated congenital anomalies. In Bergsma D, ed, The Clinical Delineation of Birth Defects. II. Malformation Syndromes. New York: The National Foundation-March of Dimes. Birth Defects: Orig Art Ser V(2):82, 1969.

May M, Huston S, Wilroy S, et al.: Linkage analysis in a family with Opitz GBBB syndrome refines the location of the gene to a 4 cM region. Am J Med Genet 68:244, 1997.

Opitz JM, Summitt RL, Smith DWG: The BBB syndrome. Familial telecanthus with associated congenital anomalies. In Bergsma D, ed, The Clinical Delineation of Birth Defects. II. Malformation Syndromes. New York: The National Foundation-March of Dimes. Birth Defects: Orig Art Ser V(2):86, 1969.

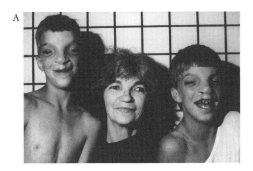
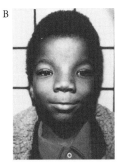
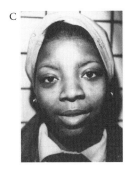

Telecanthus-Hypospadias Syndrome. Twin brothers at age 8 years showing telecanthus and bilateral cleft lip and palate, and their mother with telecanthus and a broad nasal tip **(A)**; 8-year-old male with telecanthus and high broad nasal bridge **(B)**; mother of boy in **B** with telecanthus **(C)**. Courtesy of Dr. Cathy Stevens, T.C. Thompson Children's Hospital, Chattanooga, TN.

Quaderi NA, Schweiger S, Gaudenz K, et al.: Opitz G/BBB syndrome, a defect of midline development, is due to mutations in a new RING finger gene on Xp22. Nat Genet 17:285, 1997.

Robin NH, Feldman GJ, Aronson AL, et al.: Opitz syndrome is genetically heterogeneous, with one locus on Xp22, and a second locus on 22q11.2. Nat Genet 11:459, 1995.

Robin NH, Opitz JM, Meunke M: Opitz G/BBB syndrome: Clinical comparisons of families linked to Xp22 and 22q, and a review of the literature. Am J Med Genet 62:305, 1996.

Stevens CA, Wilroy RS: The telecanthus-hypospadias syndrome. J Med Genet 25:536, 1988.

Winter J, Lehmann T, Suckow V, et al.: Duplication of the MID1 first exon in a patient with Opitz G/BBB syndrome. Hum Genet 112:249, 2003.

DIFFERENTIAL MATRIX

Syndrome	Telecanthus	Cardiac Defects	Urogenital Anomalies	Comments
Telecanthus-Hypospadias	+	+	+	High broad nasal root, dysplastic ears, cleft lip/palate, abnormal cranial contour or symmetry
ATRX-Associated XLID	+	+	+	Microcephaly, short stature, small testes, small triangular nose, tented upper lip, open mouth, wide spacing of teeth, genital anomalies, musculoskeletal anomalies, hemoglobin H inclusions in erythrocytes
Golabi-Ito-Hall (Renpenning)	+	+	0	Microcephaly, short stature, high nasal root, cupped ears, thoracic asymmetry, sacral dimple, dry/brittle/sparse hair, cutis marmorata, nail hypoplasia
MIDAS	+	+	0	Microphthalmia, ocular dysgenesis, corneal opacification, dermal aplasia, dysgenesis of corpus callosum, cardiomyopathy
Simpson-Golabi-Behmel	+	+	0	Somatic overgrowth, supernumerary nipples, polydactyly
Hall Orofacial	+	0	+	Normal growth, upslanted and short palpebral fissures, prominent nasal tip, hypertelorism, high nasal bridge, inguinal hernia
Proud (*ARX*-Associated XLID)	+	0	+	Microcephaly, hearing loss, vision loss, agenesis of corpus callosum, cryptorchidism, inguinal hernias, ataxia, spasticity, seizures
XLID-Psoriasis	+	0	+	Hypertelorism, open mouth, large ears, hypotonia, seizures, psoriasis
Lenz Microphthalmia	0	+	+	Microcephaly, microphthalmia, ocular dysgenesis, malformed ears, cleft lip/palate, thumb duplication or hypoplasia, narrow shoulders
XLID-Hereditary Bullous Dystrophy	0	+	+	Microcephaly, short stature, upslanting palpebral fissures, protruding ears, short and tapered digits, bullous dystrophy, small testes, early death from pulmonary infection

TURNER XLID (*SEE ALSO AP1S2*-ASSOCIATED XLID)

(MRX59, FRIED SYNDROME, XLID-HYDROCEPHALY-BASAL GANGLIA CALCIFICATION)

OMIM 300630

Xp22.2

AP1S2

Definition. XLID with microcephaly, hydrocephaly, basal ganglia calcifications, hypotonia, and aggressive adult behavior. The responsible gene is involved in the formation and processing of endocytic vesicles.

Somatic Features. Turner XLID is characterized by childhood hypotonia, microcephaly, variable stature, and aggressive behavior in adulthood. The face was long with high forehead, long nose, prominent ears, and small jaw. Two characteristic findings were marked delay in walking and difficult behavior. Fried syndrome (hydrocephaly with basal ganglia calcification) and MRX59 have been found to be allelic conditions.

Growth and Development. Prenatal growth is reported to be normal in some affected males. Microcephaly is noted in early childhood in most and short stature less frequently so. Development is globally delayed, with delay in walking particularly notable.

Cognitive Function. Intelligence is variably impaired, ranging from mild to severe. Problem behavior is particularly notable, especially in adulthood.

Behavior. Typically, affected males are agitated and aggressive, self-abusive, and destructive.

Neurological Findings. Marked hypotonia occurs in childhood, spasticity occasionally in adulthood.

Heterozygote Expression. No manifestation

Imaging. Brain imaging shows enlargement of the cerebral ventricles and calcifications of the basal ganglia.

Comment. The presence of hydrocephaly and spasticity may cause confusion with Hydrocephaly-MASA Spectrum, but the presence of basal ganglia calcifications in Turner

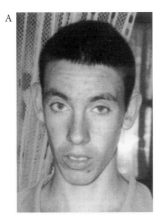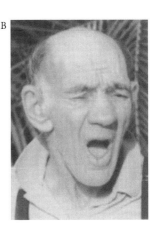

Turner XLID Syndrome. Prominent forehead, long face and nose, large ears, and small pointed jaw in 15-year-old male and 70-year-old great uncle (**A, B**).   Courtesy of Dr. Gillian Turner, New South Wales, Australia.

XLID allows clinical differentiation, and gene analysis for both syndromes permits molecular confirmation.

REFERENCES

Borck G, Mollà-Herman A, Boddaert N, et al.: Clinical, cellular, and neuropathological consequences of AP1S2 mutations: further delineation of a recognizable X-linked mental retardation syndrome. Hum Mutat 29:966–974, 2008.

Fried K: X-linked mental retardation and/or hydrocephalus. J Med Genet 10:17, 1973.

Saillour Y, Zanni G, Des Portes V, et al.: Mutations in the AP1S2 gene encoding the sigma 2 subunit of the adaptor protein 1 complex are associated with syndromic X-linked mental retardation with hydrocephalus and calcifications in basal ganglia. J Med Genet 44:739, 2007.

Strain L, Wright AF, Bonthron DT: Fried syndrome is a distinct X linked mental retardation syndrome mapping to Xp22. J Med Genet 34:535, 1977.

Tarpey PS, Stevens C, Teague J, et al.: Mutations in the gene encoding the sigma 2 subunit of the adaptor protein 1 complex (AP1S2), cause X-linked mental retardation. Am J Hum Genet 79:1119, 2006.

Turner G, Gedeon A, Kerr B, et al.: Syndromic form of X-linked mental retardation with marked hypotonia in early life, severe mental handicap, and difficult adult behavior maps to Xp22. Am J Med Genet 117A:245, 2003.

Syndrome	Microcephaly	Basal Ganglia Calcification or Deposits	Hypotonia	Comments
Turner XLID (*AP1S2*-Associated XLID)	+	+	+	Hydrocephaly, long face with high forehead, long nose, prominent ears, aggressive adult behavior
Pettigrew	+	+	+	Dandy-Walker malformation, hydrocephaly, long face with macrostomia, small testes, contractures, choreoathetosis, cerebellar hypoplasia, spastic paraplegia, seizures
Schimke	+	+	+	Sunken eyes, downslanting palpebral fissures, narrow nose, wide spacing of teeth, cupped ears, choreoathetosis, contractures, impaired vision and/or hearing, abducens palsy, spasticity or ataxia
Christianson	+	+	0	Short stature, general asthenia, contractures, seizures, ophthalmoplegia, absent speech, ambulation and continence, truncal ataxia, cerebellar and brainstem hypoplasia
Gustavson	+	+	0	Short stature, optic atrophy with blindness, large ears, deafness, joint contractures, rockerbottom feet, brain undergrowth, hydrocephaly, cerebellar hypoplasia, seizures, spasticity
ATRX-Associated XLID	+	0	+	Short stature, telecanthus/hypertelorism, small triangular nose, tented upper lip, open mouth, wide spacing of teeth, abnormal genitalia, minor musculoskeletal anomalies, erythrocyte HbH inclusions in some
CK	+	0	+	Asthenic build, long thin face, scoliosis, behavior problems, neuronal migration disturbance, seizures
Roifman	+	0	+	Short stature, spondyloepiphyseal dysplasia, retinal pigmentary deposits, antibody deficiency, eczema
Pelizaeus-Merzbacher	0	+	+	Optic atrophy, dystonia, CNS dysmyelination, ataxia, spastic paraplegia, nystagmus

URBAN SYNDROME

Assignment of XLID syndrome status is tentative, based on the clinical report of two brothers with short stature, small hands and feet with digital contractures, osteoporosis, obesity, and genital anomalies. Both had low birth weight at term gestation. Craniofacial manifestations were upslanting palpebral fissures, lateral extension of the eyebrows, and tented upper lip. One brother had strabismus and small optic discs. Both had abnormalities of eye movement. Skeletal manifestations included wormian bones in the lambdoid sutures, small hands and feet with wasting of the intrinsic muscles and finger contractures, narrow iliac wings, osteoporosis, and fractures with inadequate provocation. The body acquired eunuchoid shape and truncal obesity. At age 20 years, the older brother had moderate facial, axillary, and body hair; small penis; and large testes (4.5 x 5 cm). The younger brother had small penis, scant pubic hair, and undescended testes.

Speech and motor milestones were moderately delayed. IQ measurements were 67 and 71 during teenage years.

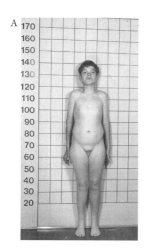
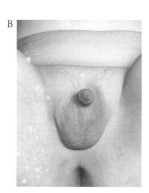
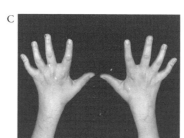

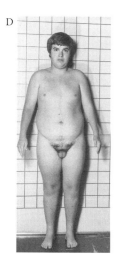
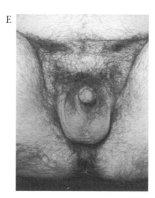
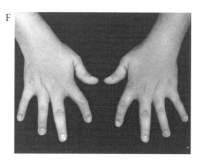

Urban Syndrome. Seventeen-year-old with short stature, truncal obesity, eunuchoid habitus, small phallus, and small hands with digital contractures (A–C); short stature, truncal obesity, small phallus, and small hands with digital contractures in a 20-year-old brother (D–F). Courtesy of Dr. Walter Meyer, III, University of Texas Medical Branch at Galveston, Galveston.

During childhood, both brothers had chronic constipation. They had low serum thyroxine and T$_3$ resin uptake.

The findings in these two males are suggestive of those in XLID syndromes with obesity, hypotonia, and hypogonadism (e.g., Börjeson-Forssman-Lehmann, Vasquez, and Wilson-Turner syndromes). Hypotonia was never noted in these brothers, however, and the oldest appears moderately masculinized and has normal gonadotropins.

REFERENCE

Urban MD, Rogers JG, Meyer WJ: Familial syndrome of mental retardation, short stature, contractures of the hands, and genital anomalies. J Pediatr 94:52, 1979.

VACTERL-HYDROCEPHALUS SYNDROME

(HUNTER-MACMURRAY SYNDROME, VACTERL-H SYNDROME)

OMIM 314390

Xp22.2

FANCB

Definition. XLID with hydrocephaly and vertebral, tracheoesophageal, renal, and limb malformations.

Somatic Features. A wide array of malformations affecting nearly all systems contributes to the seriousness and early lethality in this entity. Only the heart appears to be exempt. Hydrocephaly, the manifestation that distinguishes the syndrome from sporadic VACTERL association, is caused by aqueductal stenosis. Microphthalmia, cleft palate, and apparently low-set ears may be the only other craniofacial features. Radial deficiency with club hands and absent thumbs is the typical limb anomaly. Genitalia may be hypoplastic or abnormally formed. Imperforate anus and a number of internal malformations (tracheoesophageal fissure, abnormal lung lobation, accessory spleens, intestinal atresia, and ectopic or horseshoe kidney malformations) complete the phenotype. Most infants die in the neonatal period.

Growth and Development. Intrauterine growth retardation and hydrocephaly combine to give the appearance of marked craniotruncal disproportion.

Cognitive Function. Early lethality precludes definitive assessment of cognitive abilities, but severe impairment is presumed based on the marked hydrocephaly and the developmental course of the few survivors.

Heterozygote Expression. None reported

Imaging. Prenatal ultrasound has documented hydrocephaly and upper limb anomalies in most cases.

Neuropathology. Although hydrocephaly resulting from stenosis or other anomaly of the aqueduct of Sylvius is the usual postmortem finding, other structural defects of the brain have been reported.

Comment. Only a minority of cases of concurrence of hydrocephaly and VACTERL anomalies can be accounted for by this X-linked syndrome. Most patients represent cases with autosomal recessive syndrome and sporadic cases in which causation is not understood.

REFERENCES

Evans JA, Stranc LC, Kaplan P, et al.: VACTERL with hydrocephalus: Further delineation of the syndrome(s). Am J Med Genet 34:177, 1989.

Froster UG, Wallner SJ, Reusche E, et al.: VACTERL with hydrocephalus; and branchial arch defects: Prenatal, clinical, and autopsy findings in two brothers. Am J Med Genet 62:169, 1996.

Holden ST, Cox JJ, Kesterton I, et al.: Fanconi anaemia complementation group B presenting as X linked VACTERL with hydrocephalus syndrome. J Med Genet 43:750, 2006.

Hunter AGW, MacMurray B: Malformations of the VATER association plus hydrocephalus in a male infant and his maternal uncle. Proc Greenwood Genet Center 6:146, 1987.

Lurie IW, Ferencz C: VACTERL-Hydrocephaly, DK-Phocomelia, and Cerebro-Cardio-Radio-Reno-Rectal Community. Am J Med Genet 70:144, 1997.

Vandenborne K, Beemer F, Fryns JP, et al.: VACTERL with hydrocephalus. A distinct entity with a variable spectrum of multiple congenital anomalies. Genet Couns 4:199, 1993.

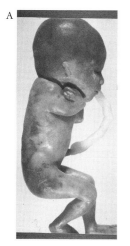

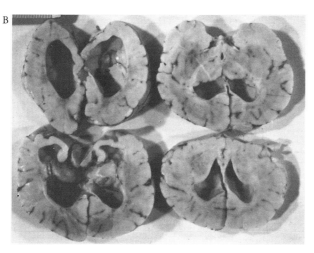

VACTERL-Hydrocephalus Syndrome. Newborn infant with hydrocephaly, small ears, and radial aplasia (A). Hydrocephaly on cut brain sections (B).   Courtesy of Dr. Ursula Froster, University of Leipzig, Germany.

DIFFERENTIAL MATRIX

Syndrome	Hydrocephaly	Limb Anomalies	Early Lethality	Comments
VACTERL-Hydrocephalus	+	+	+	Vertebral anomalies, radial limb defects, tracheal and esophageal anomalies, renal malformations, anal anomalies
Hydrocephaly-MASA Spectrum	+	+	+	Adducted thumbs, spastic paraplegia, dysgenesis of corpus callosum
Hydrocephly-Cerebellar Agenesis	+	0	+	Absent cerebellar hemispheres, hypotonia, seizures

VASQUEZ SYNDROME

Definition. XLID with short stature, microcephaly, hypotonia, obesity, hypogonadism, and gynecomastia. The gene has not been localized.

Somatic Features. Craniofacial manifestations include microbrachycephaly, narrow bifrontal diameter, small eyes and upslanting palpebral fissures. Cleft soft palate was present in one case. Truncal obesity and eunuchoid habitus with cubitus valgus and genu valgum becomes obvious with age. Hands and feet are normal size, but the hands have ulnar deviation, and fifth-finger clinodactyly and camptodactyly may be present. One patient had thoracolumbar kyphoscoliosis. The genitalia are underdeveloped, and evidence of hypogonadism with gynecomastia, incomplete virilization, and high-pitched voice are obvious. Hypotonia, obvious prenatally by decreased fetal movement, persists into adult life.

Growth and Development. Only limited information is available on growth. Birth weight was reduced in one infant. Short stature appears consistent and head circumference has been small in all except one case.

Neurological Findings. Hypotonia is the major neuromuscular abnormality. Seizures occurred in one case.

Heterozygote Expression. None

Imaging. Not available

Laboratory. Low serum testosterone and low response to human chorionic gonadotropin are indicative of hypogonadotrophic hypogonadism. Testicular biopsy has shown abnormal lining of the seminiferous tubules, presence of mononuclear and inflammatory cells, and decreased Leydig cells, spermatogonia, and spermatids.

Comment. Hypotonia, hypogonadism, and obesity constitute a triad of clinical findings present in several XLID syndromes (*see* Differential Matrix). To date, only two separate linkage regions have been identified: the pericentromeric region encompassing loci for Alpha-Thalassemia Intellectual Disability and Wilson-Turner syndromes and Xq26 (Börjeson-Forssman-Lehmann syndrome).

REFERENCE

Vasquez SB, Hurst DL, Sotos JF: X-linked hypogonadism, gynecomastia, mental retardation, short stature, and obesity - a new syndrome. J Pediatr 94:56, 1979.

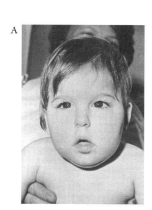
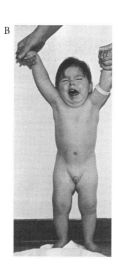
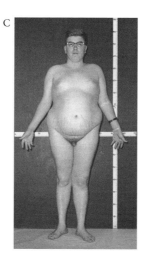
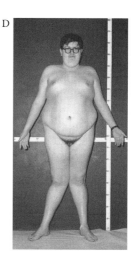

Vasquez Syndrome. Thirty-month-old with short stature, rounded face, and obesity (**A, B**); 18-year-old uncle with short stature, obesity, gynecomastia, eunuchoid habitus, cubitus valgum, and decreased virilization (**C**); 19-year-old uncle with short stature, obesity, gynecomastia, eunuchoid habitus, decreased virilization, and genu valgum (**D**). Courtesy of Dr. Juan Sotos, Children's Hospital, Columbus, OH.

DIFFERENTIAL MATRIX

Syndrome	Obesity	Hypotonia	Hypogonadism	Comments
Vasquez	+	+	+	Microcephaly, short stature, gynecomastia
Börjeson-Forssman-Lehmann	+	+	+	Short stature, microcephaly, coarse face, large ears, gynecomastia, narrow sloped shoulders, visual impairment, tapered digits
MEHMO	+	+	+	Short stature, microcephaly, edematous hands and feet, equinovarus deformity, seizures, early childhood death
Wilson-Turner	+	+	+	Normal growth, small hands and feet, tapered digits, gynecomastia, emotional lability
Urban	+	0	+	Short stature, small hands and feet, digital contractures, osteoporosis
XLID-Panhypopituitarism	+	0	+	Short stature, small sella turcica, deficiency of pituitary, thyroid, adrenal, and gonadal hormones
Young-Hughes	+	0	+	Short stature, small palpebral fissures, cupped ears, ichthyosiform scaling
ATRX-Associated XLID	0	+	+	Microcephaly, short stature, telecanthus/hypertelorism, small triangular nose, tented upper lip, open mouth, wide spacing of teeth, minor musculoskeletal anomalies, erythrocyte HbH inclusions in some
Pettigrew	0	+	+	Dandy-Walker malformation, spasticity, microcephaly or hydrocephaly, long face with macrostomia and prognathism, small testes, contractures, choreoathetosis, iron deposits in basal ganglia, seizures

WAISMAN-LAXOVA SYNDROME

(WAISMAN SYNDROME, XLID-PARKINSONISM)

OMIM 311510

Xq27.3-qter

Definition. XLID with macrocephaly, strabismus, Parkinsonian rigidity and tremors, and seizures. The gene has not been identified but is localized distal to DXS98 in Xq27.3.

Somatic Features. Although normal at birth, the head circumference increases thereafter and generally exceeds the 98th centile throughout childhood and adult life. Frontal prominence accompanies the macrocephaly. Otherwise, the craniofacial appearance is not distinctive, although high palate and crowded teeth occur in most and protruding ears in some. Multiple diffuse pigmented papules occur on the trunk in several cases.

Growth and Development. Intrauterine growth is normal. Postnatal height and weight are also normal, but macrocephaly with frontal bossing becomes apparent by early childhood. All developmental milestones are moderately delayed. Walking and first words begin by about age 2 years and use of sentences is delayed until after age 4 to 5 years.

Cognitive Function. IQ measurements range from below 30 to 70.

Neurological Findings. Neurological signs dominate the phenotype and have been documented as early as age 2 years. A general paucity of movement, tremors of the trunk and limbs, choreoathetoid movements, persistence of frontal lobe reflexes, cogwheel rigidity of the upper limbs, slow and shuffling gait, stooped posture, and hypokinetic dysarthria occur in most affected males. Seizures occur less often.

Imaging. Pneumoencephalography and cranial CT show brain enlargement with normal ventricles and no calcification.

A 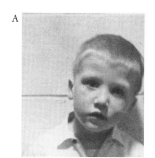 B 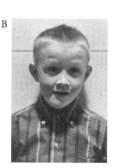 C 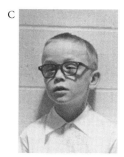 D 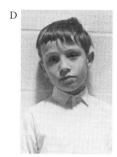 E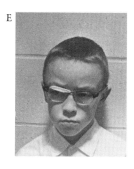

F 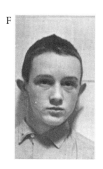 G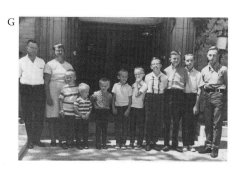

Waisman-Laxova Syndrome. Normal facial features in six affected males at ages 4, 6, 8, 9, 10 and 15 years **(A–F)**. Family group showing affected males; unaffected brothers are first, third, and fourth from right **(G)**.   Courtesy of Dr. Renata Laxova, University of Wisconsin-Madison, Madison.

Comment. In the absence of hydrocephaly, macrocephaly is an uncommon finding among the XLID syndromes. Fragile X, Mucopolysaccharidosis II, Atkin-Flaitz, Lujan, Opitz FG, Clark-Baraitser, and Simpson-Golabi-Behmel syndromes may have macrocephaly without hydrocephaly. The phenotypes of these XLID syndromes are sufficiently distinctive that they should not be confused with Waisman-Laxova syndrome.

REFERENCES

Gregg RG, Metzenberg AB, Hogan K, et al.: Waisman syndrome, a human X-linked recessive basal ganglia disorder with mental retardation: Localization to Xq27.3-qter. Genomics 9:701, 1991.

Laxova R, Brown ES, Hogan K, et al.: An X-linked recessive basal ganglia disorder with mental retardation. Am J Med Genet 21:681, 1985.

DIFFERENTIAL MATRIX

Syndrome	Spasticity	Choreoathetosis	Tremors or Rigidity	Comments
Waisman-Laxova	+	+	+	Macrocephaly, strabismus
Pettigrew	+	+	+	Dandy-Walker malformation, microcephaly or hydrocephaly, long face with macrostomia and prognathism, small testes, contractures, iron deposits in basal ganglia, seizures
Lesch-Nyhan	+	+	+	Self-mutilation, hyperuricemia
XLID-Spastic Paraplegia-Athetosis	+	+	+	Nystagmus, weakness, dysarthria, muscle wasting, contractures
AP1S2-Associated XLID	+	+	0	Hydrocephaly, calcifications of basal ganglia, muscle hypoplasia, sensory impairment
Schimke	+	+	0	Microcephaly, sunken eyes, downslanting palpebral fissures, narrow nose, wide spacing of teeth, cupped ears, hypotonia, abducens palsy, hearing loss, vision loss, contractures
Gustavson	+	0	+	Microcephaly, short stature, optic atrophy with blindness, large ears, deafness, joint contractures, rockerbottom feet, brain undergrowth, hydrocephaly, cerebellar hypoplasia, seizures
Pelizaeus-Merzbacher	+	0	+	Optic atrophy, nystagmus, hypotonia, ataxia, dystonia, CNS dysmyelination
PPM-X	+	0	+	Macroorchidism, psychosis, Parkinsonian features

WARKANY SYNDROME

(INTRAUTERINE GROWTH RETARDATION–MICROCEPHALY INTELLECTUAL DISABILITY SYNDROME)

The designation Warkany syndrome is based on a single family with six affected males in three generations. Limited details were provided on two brothers who had intrauterine growth retardation, short stature, and microcephaly. One brother had ptosis, cupped ears, thin neck, and flat chest. Developmental milestones were moderately delayed and IQ measurements were approximately 50. Carrier females had intrauterine growth retardation, but normal postnatal growth and development.

REFERENCES

Warkany J: Intrauterine growth retardation, in J Warkany: *Congenital Malformations. Notes and Comments.* Year Book Medical Publishers, Chicago, 1971, p.143.
Warkany J, Monroe BB, Sutherland BS: Intrauterine growth retardation. Am J Dis Child 102:249, 1961.

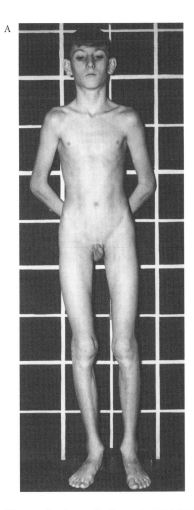
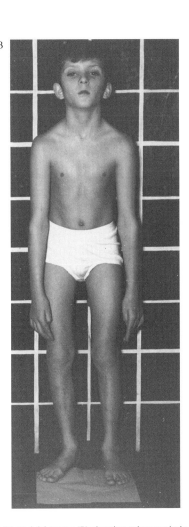

Warkany Syndrome. Brothers at ages 12 years **(A)** and 14 years **(B)** showing microcephaly, cupped ears, general asthenic habitus, and short stature.   Courtesy of Dr. Wladimir Wertelecki, University of South Alabama College of Medicine, Mobile.

WIEACKER-WOLFF SYNDROME

(XLID-MUSCLE ATROPHY-CONTRACTURES-OCULOMOTOR APRAXIA)

OMIM 314580

Xp11.3-q13

Definition. XLID with foot contractures, distal muscle atrophy, dysarthria, and oculomotor apraxia. The gene has not been identified but is linked to markers in the pericentromeric region of the X-chromosome.

Somatic Features. Musculoskeletal findings date from birth, appear slowly progressive, and are most striking in the lower limbs. Usually described as clubbed at birth, the feet are contracted at all joints with calcaneovalgus position and rockerbottom appearance being usual. The toes are crowded with flexion contractures. The legs taper distally, giving the appearance of muscle underdevelopment or wasting of the muscles, especially the peroneal muscles. The upper limbs are similarly involved, but to a less severe degree. Evidence that neuropathic involvement is widespread include generalized weakness, mild ptosis, sluggish reaction of the pupils to light and convergence, defective horizontal and vertical eye movement, strabismus, dysarthria, and kyphoscoliosis. Muscle biopsy shows muscle cell atrophy suggestive of a neuropathy. Sensation and nerve conduction appear normal.

Growth and Development. Details of growth are not available. Acquisition of motor skills and speech is moderately delayed.

Cognitive Function. Older individuals appear more severely impaired than those younger, perhaps reflecting less exposure to educational opportunities in times past. Alternatively, there may be progressive loss of cognitive abilities.

Neurological Findings. An underlying neuropathy best explains the generalized muscle weakness, distal muscle atrophy, and contractures.

Heterozygote Expression. None

Laboratory. Motor and sensory nerve conduction velocities, serum creatine kinase, and electroencephalography are normal. Muscle biopsy shows atrophic muscle cells dispersed in a neuropathogenic fashion.

Imaging. Normal

Comment. Although underdevelopment of the skeletal musculature and weakness may be present in several XLID syndromes, contractures at birth are described only in Wieacker-Wolff syndrome.

REFERENCES

Kloos DU, Jakubiczka S, Wienker T, et al.: Localization of the gene for Wieacker-Wolff syndrome in the pericentromeric region of the X chromosome. Hum Genet 100:426, 1997.

Wieacker P, Wolff G, Wienker TF, et al.: A new X-linked syndrome with muscle atrophy, congenital contractures, and oculomotor apraxia. Am J Med Genet 20:597, 1985.

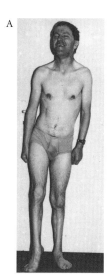
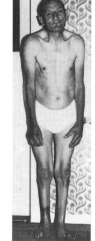
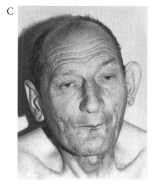
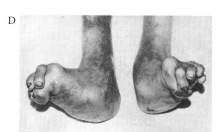

Wieacker-Wolff Syndrome. Scoliosis, muscle wasting of the distal limbs, and foots contractures in a 33-year-old (**A**) and his 63-year-old uncle (**B–D**). Courtesy of the *American Journal of Medical Genetics*, Copyright 1985, Alan R. Liss.

Syndrome	Muscle Hypoplasia or Atrophy	Contractures	Ocular Palsies	Comments
Wieacker-Wolff	+	+	+	Distal muscle atrophy, dysarthria, weakness
Christianson	+	+	+	Short stature, microcephaly, general asthenia, seizures, ophthalmoplegia
Allan-Herndon-Dudley	+	+	0	Large ears with cupping or abnormal architecture, childhood hypotonia, dysarthria, athetosis, ataxia, spastic paraplegia
Apak Ataxia-Spastic Diplegia	+	+	0	Short stature, clubfoot, ataxia, spastic paraplegia
Duchenne Muscular Dystrophy	+	+	0	Hypertrophy of calf muscle, elevated muscle enzymes, progressive weakness, loss of reflexes, muscle wasting
Goldblatt Spastic Paraplegia	+	+	0	Optic atrophy, exotropia, nystagmus, ataxia, spastic paraplegia, dysarthria
XLID-Spastic Paraplegia-Athetosis	+	+	0	Nystagmus, weakness, dysarthria, spastic paraplegia, muscle wasting
Schimke	0	+	+	Microcephaly, sunken eyes, downslanting palpebral fissures, narrow nose, wide spacing of teeth, cupped ears, hypotonia, abducens palsy, hearing loss, vision loss, spasticity, choreoathetosis

WILSON-TURNER SYNDROME

(MRXS6, WILSON SYNDROME)

OMIM 309585

Xq11.1

LAS1L

Definition. XLID with obesity, gynecomastia, tapered digits, small feet, and emotional lability. A mutation in *LAS1L* has been found in the original family.

Somatic Features. Patients lack distinctive facial features except for thick eyebrows. They have normal stature and cranial growth. The hands tend to be small and tapering, and the feet are small. Truncal obesity and gynecomastia or lipomastia become apparent at puberty. Genital development varies from normal to hypogenitalism, with small penis and small or undescended testes. Body hair tends to be scant and pubic hair varies with genital development. Some males have pes planus, others pes cavus.

Growth and Development. Normal pre- and postnatal growth is reported, with most males becoming obese and developing gynecomastia at puberty. Developmental milestones are globally delayed, with speech more severely impaired. Some males have little or no speech.

Cognitive Function. Variable, but usually mild-to-moderate, impairment of cognitive function occurs.

Behavior. In general, affected males are quiet with a cheerful temperament, although several have appeared easily upset, tearful, or aggressive.

Neurological Findings. Poor muscle tone and excessive drooling during infancy has been noted in some cases but not in others. Stuttering appears quite common.

Heterozygote Expression. None

Laboratory. A possible disturbance of hypothalamic-pituitary-gonadal axis has been suspected on the basis of decreased or low normal androgens with normal FSH and LH.

Comment. Wilson-Turner syndrome shares the phenotypic triad of hypotonia, hypogonadism, and obesity with other XLID syndromes (Börjeson-Forssman-Lehmann, MEHMO, and Vasquez syndromes). The responsible genes are known for all except Vasquez syndrome.

REFERENCES

Gedeon A, Mulley J, Turner G: Gene localisation for Wilson-Turner syndrome (WTS:MIM 309585). Am J Med Genet 64:80, 1994.

Wilson M, Mulley J, Gedeon A, et al.: New X-linked syndrome of mental retardation, gynecomastia, and obesity is linked to DXS255. Am J Med Genet 40:406, 1991.

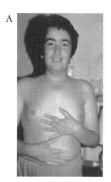 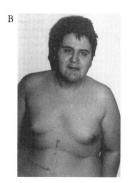 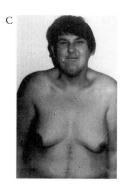 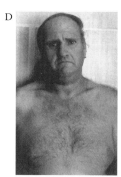

Wilson-Turner Syndrome. Heavy eyebrows, synophrys, gynecomastia, and obesity in affected males at ages 13 years **(A)**, 19 years **(B)**, 25 years **(C)**, and 48 years **(D)**.   Courtesy of the *American Journal of Medical Genetics*, Copyright 1991, Wiley-Liss, Inc.

DIFFERENTIAL MATRIX

Syndrome	Obesity	Hypogonadism	Hypotonia	Comments
Wilson-Turner	+	+	+	Normal growth, small hands and feet, tapered digits, gynecomastia, emotional lability
Börjeson-Forssman-Lehmann	+	+	+	Short stature, microcephaly, coarse facies, large ears, gynecomastia, narrow sloped shoulders, visual impairment, tapered digits
MEHMO	+	+	+	Short stature, microcephaly, edematous hands and feet, equinovarus deformity, seizures, early childhood death
Vasquez	+	+	+	Microcephaly, short stature, gynecomastia
Urban	+	+	0	Short stature, small hands and feet, digital contractures, osteoporosis
Young-Hughes	+	+	0	Short stature, small palpebral fissures, cupped ears, ichthyosiform scaling
XLID-Panhypopituitarism	+	+	0	Short stature, small sella turcica, deficiency of pituitary, thyroid, adrenal, and gonadal hormones
ATRX-Associated XLID	0	+	+	Microcephaly, short stature, telecanthus/hypertelorism, small triangular nose, tented upper lip, open mouth, wide spacing of teeth, minor musculoskeletal anomalies, erythrocyte HbH inclusions in some
Pettigrew	0	+	+	Dandy-Walker malformation, spasticity, microcephaly or hydrocephaly, long face with macrostomia, small testes, contractures, choreoathetosis, iron deposits in basal ganglia, seizures

WITTWER SYNDROME

OMIM 300421

Xp22.3

Definition. XLID with growth failure, microcephaly with large fontanels, frontal prominence, hypertelorism, long philtrum, thin upper lip, cupped ears, blindness, hearing loss, and seizures. The gene localization is based on concordance for markers in Xp22.3.

Somatic Features. Recessed eyes, bringing the forehead and cheeks into prominence, give the face a distinctive appearance. Craniofacial appearance is further characterized by large fontanels, downslanting palpebral fissures, hypertelorism, epicanthus, anteverted nares, long philtrum, thin upper lip, and cupped ears. One infant had microphthalmia and sclerocornea, and another had optic atrophy. Minor skeletal anomalies may include fifth-finger clinodactyly, single palmar creases, bell-shaped chest, clubfoot with camptodactyly, and delayed bone maturation.

Cryptorchidism, epispadias, vesicoureteral reflux, and hydronephrosis have been described. Blindness dates from birth and hearing loss is evident early in childhood.

Growth and Development. Intrauterine growth is impaired and all postnatal growth parameters fall far below the normal centiles. All developmental milestones lag markedly behind. Speech and independent ambulation are never achieved.

Cognitive Function. Severe impairment based on childhood developmental progress.

Neurological Findings. Generalized seizures develop during infancy. Weakness and poor muscle tone persist throughout childhood.

Heterozygote Expression. Mild intellectual disability was described in one mother.

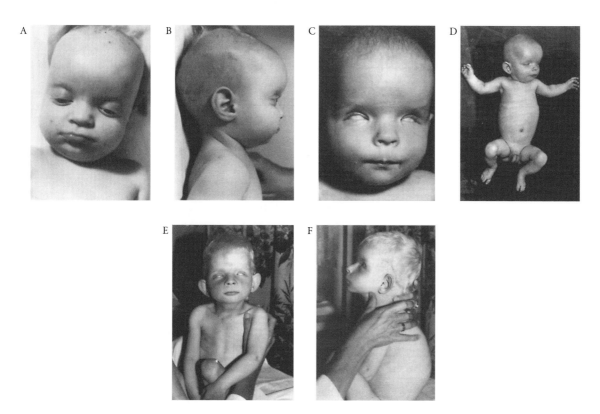

Wittwer Syndrome. Four-month-old male with prominent forehead, retracted midface, hypertelorism, downslanted palpebral fissures, and thin upper lip (A, B); prominent forehead, hypertelorism, epicanthal folds, downslanted palpebral fissures, retracted midface, long philtrum, thin upper lip, cupped ears, microphthalmia, and sclerocornea in a cousin at age 6 months (C, D); and 5 years (E, F).   Courtesy of the *American Journal of Medical Genetics*, Copyright 1995, Wiley-Liss, Inc.

Imaging. Cranial ultrasound and CT were normal in two infants. CT suggested dysgenesis of the corpus callosum in another infant, but this was not confirmed at autopsy.

Neuropathology. Postmortem examination on one infant showed cerebellar atrophy and hydrocephalus.

Comment. This entity is based on a description of three affected males in one family.

REFERENCES

Wieland I, Muschke P, Wieacker P: Further delineation of Wittwer syndrome and refinement of the mapping region. Am J Med Genet A, 116A:57, 2003.

Wittwer B, Kircheisen R, Leutelt J, et al.: New X-linked mental retardation syndrome with the gene mapped tentatively in Xp22.3. Am J Med Genet 64:42, 1996.

DIFFERENTIAL MATRIX

Syndrome	Blindness	Hearing Loss	Genitourinary Anomalies	Comments
Wittwer	+	+	+	Microcephaly, short stature, microphthalmia, hypertelorism, hypotonia, seizures
Proud (ARX-Associated XLID)	+	+	+	Microcephaly, agenesis of corpus callosum, cryptorchidism, inguinal hernias, ataxia, spasticity, seizures
Arts	+	+	0	Growth deficiency, poor muscle development, hypotonia, areflexia, ataxia, seizures, childhood death
Gustavson	+	+	0	Microcephaly, short stature, optic atrophy with blindness, large ears, joint contractures, rockerbottom feet, brain undergrowth, hydrocephaly, cerebellar hypoplasia, spasticity, seizures
Norrie	+	+	0	Ocular dysgenesis and degeneration, adult-onset hearing loss
Mohr-Tranebjaerg	+	+	0	Neurological deterioration with childhood onset, dystonia, spasticity
Paine	+	+	0	Microcephaly, short stature, optic atrophy, spasticity, seizures
Schimke	+	+	0	Microcephaly, sunken eyes, downslanting palpebral fissures, narrow nose, wide spacing of teeth, cupped ears, hypotonia, abducens palsy, spasticity, choreoathetosis, contractures
Ataxia-Deafness-Dementia, X-linked	+	+	0	Optic atrophy, spastic paraplegia, ataxia, hypotonia, seizures, childhood death
Cerebro-Oculo-Genital	+	0	+	Microcephaly, hydrocephaly, short stature, agenesis of corpus callosum, microphthalmia, ptosis, hypospadias, cryptorchidism, clubfoot, spasticity
Goltz	+	0	+	Cataracts, ocular dysgenesis, linear areas of dermal aplasia, cutaneous adipose herniations, dystrophic nails, abnormal teeth and hair, vertebral anomalies, limb reduction defects
Lenz Microphthalmia	+	0	+	Microcephaly, microphthalmia, ocular dysgenesis, malformed ears, cleft lip/palate, cardiac anomalies, thumb duplication or hypoplasia, narrow shoulders
Lowe	+	0	+	Short stature, cataracts, hypotonia, aminoaciduria, progressive renal disease

XLID-ARCH FINGERPRINTS-HYPOTONIA SYNDROME (*SEE ALSO ATRX*-ASSOCIATED XLID)

OMIM 309580

Xq21.1

ATRX (XNP)

Definition. XLID with distinctive facies, poor muscle tone, tapered fingers, arch fingerprints, genu valgum, and absent deep tendon reflexes. A mutation has been found in *ATRX*, making this syndrome allelic with Alpha-Thalassemia Intellectual Disability syndrome.

Somatic Features. The face appears large in relation to the cranium and has a squarish configuration. Subcutaneous tissues of the upper eyelids, helices of the ears, alae nasi, and columella are thickened. The upper lip is arched, especially during childhood, and permanent teeth appear small in two affected males.

Overall decreased muscle tone is reflected in persistent drooling, cupped ears, arched upper lip, genu valgum, absent reflexes, and perhaps in the tapered fingers and thickened soft tissues of the eyelids, ears, and nose. Presumably decreased muscle tone contributed, in part, to the delay in motor milestones. The cause for decreased muscle tone and absent deep tendon reflexes was not identified.

An excessive number of fingerprint arches and low loops were found in the three living males. The average ridge count was 28 in two affected males and 154 in five unaffected brothers. There was associated tapering of the digits and small distal phalanges. None of the five unaffected brothers or two obligate carrier females has excessive arches or low total ridge counts.

Growth and Development. Intrauterine and postnatal growth is comparable in affected and unaffected males,

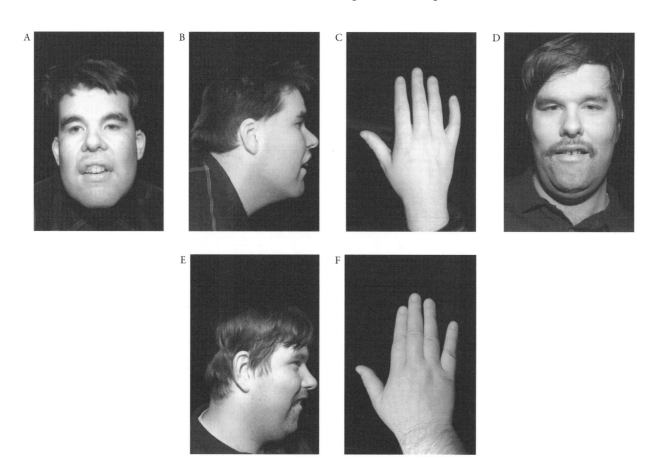

XLID-Arch Fingerprints-Hypotonia. Large, squarish face, heavy eyelids, thickened helices, thickened alae nasi, broad philtrum with tented upper lip, and tapered fingers in a 28-year-old male (**A–C**); similar features in 32-year-old brother (**D-F**).

with the exception that affected males are heavier. Sexual maturation occurs at the appropriate time.

Cognitive Function. Motor and language development is moderately delayed with adult IQs measuring between 40 and 50.

Neurological Findings. Deep tendon reflexes are absent.

Imaging. None

Neuropathology. None

Comment. This syndrome has certain manifestations (hypotonia, open mouth with arched upper lip, tapered digits) typically present in Alpha-Thalassemia Intellectual Disability syndrome but differs in many other manifestations (severity of intellectual disability, absent speech, seizures, lack of bowel or bladder control, constipation, telecanthus or hypertelorism, small triangular nose, spacing of teeth, small and simple ears, genital anomalies, short stature, brachydactyly, presence of hemoglobin H inclusions in erythrocytes) of that entity. The *ATRX* mutation in XLID-Arch Fingerprints-Hypotonia is near the 5' end of the gene and has been associated with milder expression.

Excessive fingerprint arches have been found in several chromosomal and single-gene disorders. Coffin-Lowry, Miles-Carpenter, and Chudley-Lowry syndromes are distinctive XLID syndromes in which excessive arches have been reported. Coffin-Lowry syndrome has distinctive facial and skeletal features, heterozygote manifestations,

and gene localization to Xp22. Miles-Carpenter syndrome maps close to the entity reported here but may be distinguished by microcephaly, facial asymmetry, rockerbottom feet, contractures, and spastic paraplegia. There are a number of similarities between XLID-Arch Fingerprints-Hypotonia and the condition reported by Chudley et al. (1988). That condition, characterized by moderate-severe intellectual disability, has bitemporal narrowing, almond-shaped eyes, small nose, open mouth with arched upper lip, short stature, low fingerprint ridge count, obesity, hypogonadism, genu valgum, and brachydactyly, has been found to have the same *ATRX* mutation as XLID-Arch Fingerprints-Hypotonia.

A number of X-linked entities with intellectual disability and obesity have been described. Often these entities are associated with hypotonia, hypogonadism, and short stature and may be distinguished from the syndrome reported here by the latter two manifestations.

REFERENCES

Abidi FE, Cardoso C, Lossi AM, et al.: Mutation in the 5' alternatively spliced region of the XNP/ATR-X gene causes Chudley-Lowry syndrome. Eur J Hum Genet 13:176, 2005.

Chudley AE, Lowry RB, Hoar DI: Mental retardation, distinct facial changes, short stature, obesity, and hypogonadism: a new X-linked mental retardation syndrome. Am J Med Genet 31:741, 1988.

Gibbons RJ, Wada T, Fisher CA, et al.: Mutations in the chromatin-associated protein ATRX. Hum Mutat 29:796, 2008.

Stevenson RE, Häne B, Arena JF, et al.: Arch fingerprints, hypotonia, and areflexia associated with X linked mental retardation. J Med Genet 34:465, 1997.

DIFFERENTIAL MATRIX

Syndrome	Hypotonic Facies	Tapered Digits	Excessive Fingerprint Arches	Comments
XLID-Arch Fingerprints-Hypotonia (*ATRX*-Associated XLID)	+	+	+	Genu valgum, areflexia, hypotonia
Coffin-Lowry	+	+	+	Microcephaly, short stature, hypertelorism, anteverted nares, tented upper lip, prominent lips and large mouth, large ears, soft hands, pectus carinatum
Wilson-Turner	+	+	0	Normal growth, small hands and feet, obesity, hypogonadism, gynecomastia, emotional lability

XLID-ATAXIA-APRAXIA

(TRANEBJAERG SYNDROME II)

Definition. XLID with ataxia and dyspraxia with variable cognitive function.

Somatic Features. Major malformations do not occur and craniofacial manifestations are incompletely described. Prominent high forehead, cupped ears, and thin upper lip are evident in the published photographs. Although the head circumference is said to be increased, the measurements provided are near the 50th centile. Clubfoot was noted in two boys.

Growth and Development. Pre- and postnatal growth is normal. Developmental milestones are mildly delayed.

Cognitive Function. Verbal and performance assessments showed considerable discordance, with verbal function measuring below average but within the normal range. In one family, performance measures were in the mildly impaired range; in the second family, measures were in the low-normal range.

Neurological Findings. Nonprogressive ataxia and dyspraxia manifest as inability to copy simple geometric figures, and incoordination of limbs, ocular, and tongue movements are noted from early childhood. Hypotonia, tremors, and seizures also occur.

Heterozygote Expression. One carrier female had mild constructional dyspraxia and dysgraphia but normal intellectual function.

Imaging. Brain atrophy was described in two individuals.

Comment. Tranebjaerg et al. (1992) reported two families, one with six affected males and the other with three affected males.

REFERENCE

Tranebjaerg L, Lou H, Andresen J: New X-linked syndrome with apraxia, ataxia, and mental deficiency: Clinical, cytogenetic and neuropsychological studies in two Danish families. Am J Med Genet 43:498, 1992.

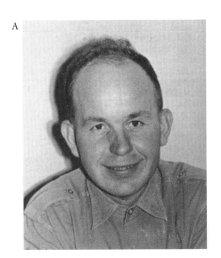
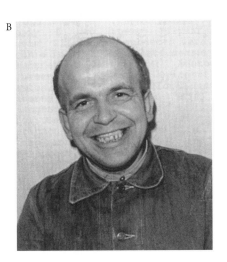
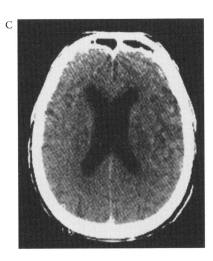

XLID-Ataxia-Apraxia. Brothers at ages 31 and 33 years showing prominent forehead and large ears (A, B); enlarged lateral ventricles on cranial tomography of older brother (C).   Courtesy of Dr. Lisbeth Tranebjaerg, University Hospital, Tromsø, Norway.

DIFFERENTIAL MATRIX

Syndrome	Ataxia	Hypotonia	Tremors	Comments
XLID-Ataxia-Apraxia	+	+	+	Prominent forehead, large ears, uncoordinated movements, seizures
Pelizaeus-Merzbacher	+	+	+	Optic atrophy, nystagmus, spasticity, dystonia, CNS dysmyelination
Ataxia-Deafness-Dementia, X-linked	+	+	+	Optic atrophy, vision loss, hearing loss, spastic paraplegia, seizures, childhood death
Allan-Herndon-Dudley	+	+	0	Large ears with cupping or abnormal architecture, muscle hypoplasia, childhood hypotonia, contractures, dysarthria, athetosis, spastic paraplegia
Pettigrew	+	+	0	Dandy-Walker malformation, spasticity, microcephaly or hydrocephaly, long face with macrostomia, small testes, contractures, choreoathetosis, iron deposits in basal ganglia, seizures
XLID-Ataxia-Dementia	+	0	+	Spastic paraplegia, adult-onset dementia
XLID-Hypogonadism-Tremor	+	0	+	Short stature, prominent lower lip, muscle wasting of legs, abnormal gait, hypogonadism, obesity, seizures
Oral-Facial-Digital I	0	+	+	Sparse scalp hair, dystopia canthorum, flat midface, hypoplastic alae nasi, hypertrophic and aberrant oral frenuli, intra-oral clefts and pseudoclefts, lingual hamartomas, brachydactyly, syndactyly, clinodactyly, structural brain anomalies, polycystic kidneys

XLID-ATAXIA-DEMENTIA

(X-LINKED ATAXIA, SPINOCEREBELLAR ATAXIA, X-LINKED 4)

OMIM 301840

Definition. X-linked progressive ataxia, pyramidal signs, and adult-onset dementia. Close linkage has not been found, but most of Xp and distal Xq (Xq26-qter) have been excluded.

Somatic Features. Affected males have no distinctive facial features or growth aberrations. Motor and language milestones are moderately delayed, and clumsiness and tremors mark childhood. Incoordination of gait and intention tremor are demonstrable but mild during childhood. Ataxia and pyramidal tract signs progressively intensify during adult life and may lead to near total incapacitation in the fourth or fifth decades. Muscle weakness and extrapyramidal signs do not occur. Cognitive impairment is not apparent during childhood, although some affected persons have not completed secondary schooling. Dementia begins in early adulthood, heralded by forgetfulness, confusion, disorientation, and loss of cognitive skills. Mood swings with emotional lability accompany the dementia.

Growth and Development. No abnormalities of growth. Motor and language milestones are delayed, with walking and first words between ages 2 and 3 years.

Cognitive Function. No definite impairment during childhood, although testing not reported. Cognitive deterioration begins as early as the fourth decade and progresses.

Neurological Findings. Progressive neurological changes dominate the clinical picture. The clumsiness of childhood evolves by early adult life into frank incoordination, unsteady gait, intention tremors, increased tone and deep tendon reflexes, and Babinski signs. Lower limbs are affected to the greater degree.

Imaging. CT and MRI show cortical atrophy but no specific abnormality of cerebellum, olivary nuclei, or white matter.

Comment. The findings in X-linked ataxia-dementia have also been reported as cerebello-olivary degeneration. Patients with similar neurological course but without

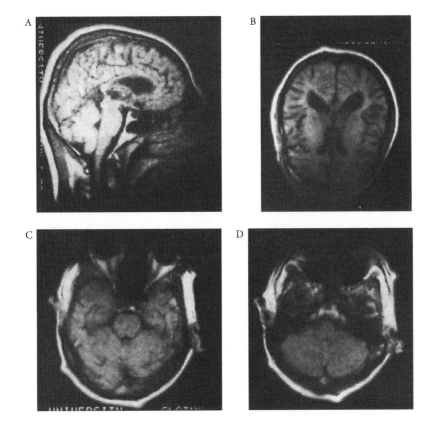

XLID-Ataxia-Dementia. Midsagittal **(A)** and axial **(B–D)** MRIs of brain of 55-year-old man showing generalized cortical atrophy, but normal pons and cerebellum.   Courtesy of Dr. Martin Farlow, Indiana University School of Medicine, Indianapolis.

dementia have been reported by Spira et al. (1979) and Shokier (1970). Malamud and Cohen (1958) reported more severe deterioration in a family with intellectual disability, ataxia, tremors, dysarthria, extrapyramidal signs, and death in childhood. Adult-onset dementia, ataxia, and pyramidal signs occur in Mohr-Tranebjaerg syndrome, but the optic atrophy, blindness, and mutation in the dystonia-deafness protein (*TIMM8A*) gene have not been found in the XLID-Ataxia-Dementia syndrome. Adrenoleukodystrophy may be excluded by normal long-chain fatty acids and the absence of leukodystrophy on brain imaging.

REFERENCES

Carter RH, Sukavanjana C: Familial cerebello-olivary degeneration with late development of rigidity and dementia. Neurology 6:876, 1956.

Farlow MR, DeMyer W, Dlouhy SR, et al.: X-linked recessive inheritance of ataxia and adult-onset dementia: Clinical features and preliminary linkage analysis. Neurology 37:602, 1987.

Malamud N, Cohen P: Unusual form of cerebellar ataxia with sex-linked inheritance. Neurology 8:261, 1958.

Shokeir MHK: X-linked cerebellar ataxia. Clin Genet 1:225, 1970.

Spira PJ, McLeod JG, Evans WA: A spinocerebellar degeneration with X-linked inheritance. Brain 102:27, 1979.

Tranebjaerg L, Lou H, Andreesen J: New X-linked syndrome with apraxia, ataxia, and mental deficiency: Clinical, cytogenetic and neuropsychological studies in two Danish families. Am J Med Genet 43:498, 1992.

DIFFERENTIAL MATRIX

Syndrome	Ataxia	Spasticity	Tremors or Rigidity	Comments
XLID-Ataxia-Dementia	+	+	+	Adult-onset dementia
Pelizaeus-Merzbacher	+	+	+	Optic atrophy, nystagmus, hypotonia, dystonia, CNS dysmyelination
Pettigrew	+	+	+	Dandy-Walker malformation, microcephaly or hydrocephaly, long face with macrostomia, small testes, contractures, choreoathetosis, iron deposits in basal ganglia, seizures
Adrenoleukodystrophy	+	+	0	Adrenal insufficiency, diffuse skin pigmentation, progressive neurological deterioration and dementia, elevated long-chain fatty acids in plasma
Allan-Herndon-Dudley	+	+	0	Large ears with cupping or abnormal architecture, muscle hypoplasia, childhood hypotonia, contractures, dysarthria, athetosis
Apak Ataxia-Spastic Diplegia	+	+	0	Short stature, clubfoot, muscle hypoplasia
Goldblatt Spastic Paraplegia	+	+	0	Optic atrophy, exotropia, nystagmus, dysarthria, muscle hypoplasia, contractures
Hydrocephaly-MASA Spectrum	+	+	0	Hydrocephaly, adducted thumbs, dysgenesis of corpus callosum
Mohr-Tranebjaerg	+	+	0	Hearing loss, vision loss, neurological deterioration with childhood onset, dystonia
Ataxia-Deafness-Dementia, X-linked	+	+	0	Optic atrophy, vision loss, hearing loss, hypotonia, seizures, childhood death
XLID-Ataxia-Apraxia	+	0	+	Prominent forehead, large ears, uncoordinated movements, hypotonia, seizures
XLID-Hypogonadism-Tremor	+	0	+	Short stature, prominent lower lip, muscle wasting of legs, abnormal gait, hypogonadism, obesity, seizures
Lesch-Nyhan	0	+	+	Choreoathetosis, self-mutilation, hyperuricemia
PPM-X	0	+	+	Macroorchidism, psychosis, Parkinsonian features
Waisman-Laxova	0	+	+	Macrocephaly, strabismus
XLID-Spastic Paraplegia-Athetosis	0	+	+	Nystagmus, weakness, dysarthria, muscle-wasting, contractures

XLID-BLINDNESS-SEIZURES-SPASTICITY

(HAMEL SYNDROME)

Xp11.3-q12

Definition. XLID with postnatal-onset microcephaly and poor growth, clubfoot, progressive loss of vision, spasticity, seizures, digital contractures, hypomyelination, and early childhood death. The gene has not been identified but is linked to markers DXS337 (Xp11.3) and PGK (Xq12).

Somatic Features. Major malformations and distinctive craniofacial changes do not occur. Apart from calcaneovalgus foot deformation, appearance at birth is normal. Neurological deterioration begins within a few months and is manifested as loss of vision, waning of interest in the environment, failure to achieve motor and language milestones, seizures, and spasticity. Global growth failure results in microcephaly and short stature. Pale optic discs, strabismus, and digital contractures are noted, and unexplained febrile episodes occur. Death occurs within a few years.

Growth and Development. Intrauterine growth appears normal, but slowing of all growth parameters occurs in infancy. Little developmental progress is made during infancy or the early childhood years.

Cognitive Function. Severe impairment.

Neurological Findings. The first neurological sign appears at about age 3 months, with progressive loss of vision, spasticity, and seizures. Hearing appears normal. Clubfoot is present at birth, and scoliosis and digital contractures develop secondary to the spasticity.

Heterozygote Expression. None

Imaging. Not available

Neuropathology. Brain examination has been possible in two cases. The brains were small and showed mild hypomyelination of the cerebrum and cerebellum.

Comment. Although a number of XLID syndromes are localized to the pericentromeric region, XLID-Blindness-Seizures-Spasticity is the only severe neurodegenerative disorder thus far linked to the region.

REFERENCE

Hamel BC, Wesseling P, Renier WO, et al.: A new X linked neurodegenerative syndrome with mental retardation, blindness, convulsions, spasticity, mild hypomyelination, and early death maps to the pericentromeric region. J Med Genet 36:140, 1999.

Syndrome	Optic Atrophy or Blindness	Spastic Paraplegia	Seizures	Comments
XLID-Blindness-Seizures-Spasticity	+	+	+	Poor growth, postnatal microcephaly, clubfoot, contractures, scoliosis, hypomyelination
Cerebro-Oculo-Genital	+	+	+	Microcephaly, hydrocephaly, short stature, agenesis of corpus callosum, microphthalmia, ptosis, hypospadias, cryptorchidism, clubfoot
Gustavson	+	+	+	Microcephaly, short stature, large ears, deafness, joint contractures, rockerbottom feet, brain undergrowth, hydrocephaly, cerebellar hypoplasia
Paine	+	+	+	Microcephaly, short stature, hearing loss
Pelizaeus-Merzbacher	+	+	+	Nystagmus, hypotonia, ataxia, dystonia, CNS dysmyelination
Proud	+	+	+	Microcephaly, hearing loss, agenesis of corpus callosum, cryptorchidism, inguinal hernias, ataxia
Schimke	+	+	+	Microcephaly, sunken eyes, downslanting palpebral fissures, narrow nose, wide spacing of teeth, cupped ears, hypotonia, abducens palsy, hearing loss, choreoathetosis, contractures
Ataxia-Deafness-Dementia, X-linked	+	+	+	Hearing loss, ataxia, hypotonia, childhood death
Adrenoleukodystrophy	+	+	0	Adrenal insufficiency, diffuse skin pigmentation, progressive neurological deterioration and dementia, elevated long-chain fatty acids in plasma
Goldblatt Spastic Paraplegia	+	+	0	Exotropia, nystagmus, ataxia, dysarthria, muscle hypoplasia, contractures
Mohr-Tranebjaerg	+	+	0	Hearing loss, neurological deterioration with childhood onset, dystonia
XLID-Spastic Paraplegia, type 7	+	+	0	Nystagmus, reduced vision, absent speech and ambulation, bowel and bladder dysfunction
Wittwer	+	0	+	Microcephaly, short stature, microphthalmia, hearing loss, hypertelorism, genitourinary anomalies, hypotonia

XLID-CHOREOATHETOSIS

(MRXS10)

OMIM 300220

Xp11.22

HSD17B10 (HADH2)

Definition. XLID with infantile onset choreoathetosis. The responsible gene encodes an hydroxyacyl-CoA-dehydrogenase.

Somatic Features. Malformations or craniofacial dysmorphism do not occur. One boy exhibited arachnodactyly, delayed development, dysarthric speech, spasticity, and irregular, purposeless, nonrhythmic, abrupt, and rapid involuntary movements. Once walking, the gait was widely based with lumbar lordosis. Bouts of aggressive behavior, agitation, and psychosis were described.

Growth and Development. Growth is not impaired. Development is moderately delayed.

Cognitive Function. Mild impairment

Heterozygote Expression. None

Comment. XLID-Choreoathetosis joins Lesch-Nyhan, Pelizaeus-Merzbacher and *AP1S2*-Associated XLID as X-linked conditions with choreoathetosis in which the molecular and biochemical bases are known. Other XLID syndromes with involuntary movements (Waisman-Laxova, Pettigrew, Gustavson, Schimke and XLID-Spastic Paraplegia-Athetosis) have yet to be tested for mutations in *HSD17B10*.

REFERENCES

Lenski C, Kooy RF, Reyniers E, et al.: The reduced expression of the HADH2 protein causes X-linked mental retardation, choreoathetosis, and abnormal behavior. Am J Hum Genet 80:372, 2007.

Reyniers E, Van Bogaert P, Peeters N, et al.: A new neurological syndrome with mental retardation, choreoathetosis, and abnormal behavior maps to chromosome Xp11. Am J Hum Genet 65:1406, 1999.

XLID-CHOROIDEREMIA-ECTODERMAL DYSPLASIA

(VAN DEN BOSCH SYNDROME)

OMIM 314500

Definition. XLID with ocular, ectodermal, and skeletal manifestations. The gene has not been localized.

Somatic Features. van den Bosch summarized the findings in two brothers as intellectual disability, choroideremia, horizontal nystagmus, myopia, abnormal retinogram, winged scapula, acrokeratosis verruciformis, heat intolerance, no sweat reaction to acetylcholine, and susceptibility to respiratory and cutaneous infections. Other males were affected in three generations.

Comment. A gene for choroideremia has been localized to Xq21.2, some 16 Mb distal to *EDA*, the gene for anhidrotic ectodermal dysplasia. The possibility that this condition is caused by a contiguous gene deletion or other rearrangement has not been investigated.

REFERENCES

Hodgson SV, Robertson ME, Fear CN, et al.: Prenatal diagnosis of X-linked choroideremia with mental retardation, associated with a cytologically detectable X-chromosome deletion. Hum Genet 75:286, 1987.

van den Bosch J: A new syndrome in three generations of a Dutch family. Ophthalmologica 137:422, 1959.

XLID-CLEFT LIP/CLEFT PALATE

(XLID-FACIAL CLEFTING, BRESLAU-SIDERIUS SYNDROME, SIDERIUS SYNDROME)

OMIM 300263

Xp11.2

PHF8

Definition. XLID with cleft lip and cleft palate, long face, broad nose, and large hands. The gene encodes a histone demethylase that acts as a transcriptional coactivator.

Somatic Features. The phenotype is based on a limited number of cases. Craniofacial manifestations include normal head circumference, long face, fullness of the nasal root, broad nasal tip, cleft lip, and cleft palate. Cupping of the ears was present in two cases, synophrys and low posterior hairline in one case, and thoracic scoliosis and postaxial polydactyly in one case. The testes were retractile in two cases and in one of these cases were small. Total hand length was near or above the 97th centile.

Growth and Development. Intrauterine and postnatal growth was normal. Although details are not available, developmental delay was noted from early childhood.

Cognitive Features. Mild to borderline impairment

Behavior. Behavior in two cases is described as unpredictable with aggressive outbursts and uncontrollable with short attention span.

Neurological Findings. None

Heterozygote Expression. None

Imaging. Normal

Comment. A number of X-linked intellectual disability syndromes (Aarskog, Aicardi, Lenz, Oral-Facial-Digital I, Simpson-Golabi-Behmel, and Telecanthus-Hypospadias syndromes) may have cleft lip and cleft palate, at least occasionally. Cleft palate alone has been reported in Alpha-Thalassemia Intellectual Disability, Otopalatodigital I, Otopalatodigital II, Snyder-Robinson and Vasquez syndromes. Isolated median cleft lip occurs in Pallister W syndrome.

REFERENCES

Abidi FE, Miano MG, Murray JC, et al.: A novel mutation in the PHF8 gene is associated with X-linked mental retardation with cleft lip/cleft palate. Clin Genet 72:19, 2007.

Fortschegger K, de Graaf P, Outchkourov NS, et al.: PHF8 targets histone methylation and RNA polymerase II to activate transcription. Mol Cell Biol 30:3286, 2010.

Laumonnier F, Holbert S, Ronce N, et al.: Mutations in PHF8 are associated with X linked mental retardation and cleft lip/cleft palate. J Med Genet 42:780, 2005.

Siderius LE, Hamel BCJ, van Bokhoven H, et al.: X-linked mental retardation associated with cleft lip/cleft palate maps to Xp11.3-q21.3. Am J Med Genet 85:216, 1999.

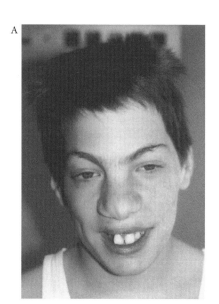
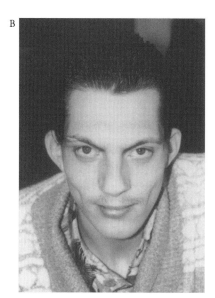
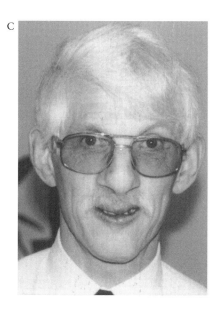

XLID-Cleft Lip/Cleft Palate. Teenager and adults with long face and broad nasal root and nasal tip (**A–C**). Teenager (**A**) has synophrys and repaired cleft lip and cleft palate. Adult (**C**) has repaired cleft lip and palate. Courtesy of Dr. Ben Hamel, University Hospital, Nijmegen, The Netherlands.

Syndrome	Orofacial Clefting	Hypertelorism or Broad Nose	Large Hands	Comments
XLID-Cleft Lip/ Cleft Palate	+	+	+	Long face, broad nasal tip, long hands
Oral-Facial-Digital I	+	+	0	Sparse scalp hair, dystopia canthorum, flat midface, hypoplastic alae nasi, hypertrophic and aberrant oral frenuli, lingual hamartomas, brachydactyly, syndactyly, clinodactyly, structural brain anomalies, polycystic kidneys
Otopalatodigital I	+	+	0	Short stature, conductive hearing impairment, prominent brow, apparent ocular hypertelorism, downslanting palpebral fissures, blunted distal phalanges, irregular curvature and spacing of digits, limitation of elbow movement
Otopalatodigital II	+	+	0	Short stature, hearing impairment, prominent forehead, downslanting palpebral fissures, flat midface, cleft palate, blunted flexed overlapping fingers, rockerbottom feet, hypoplastic fibulae, subluxed/dislocated joints
Simpson-Golabi-Behmel	+	+	0	Somatic overgrowth, supernumerary nipples, polydactyly
Telecanthus-Hypospadias	+	+	0	Dysplastic ears, abnormal cranial contour or symmetry

XLID-EPILEPSY (XIDE)

OMIM 300423

Xp11.4

ATP6AP2

Definition. XLID with infancy-onset epilepsy. The responsible gene encodes the renin receptor, *ATP6AP2*.

Somatic Features. Seizures and developmental delay dominate the clinical presentation. Growth and craniofacial features appear normal. Malformations do not occur. Motor and speech development is moderately delayed. Seizures begin between 4 and 14 months and include generalized tonic-clonic, brief atonic, and myoclonic attacks. Scoliosis and gait disturbance occur in a minority. Hyporeflexia has been noted in several males.

Growth and Development. Growth appears normal, but development lags after the onset of seizures.

Cognitive Function. IQ measurements in the 50–70 range.

Heterozygote Expression. None.

Comment. The major XLID syndromes in which seizures dominate the clinical picture have been resolved at the molecular level.

REFERENCES

Hedera P, Alvarado D, Beydoun A, et al.: Novel mental retardation-epilepsy syndrome linked to Xp21.1-p11.4. Ann Neurol 51:45, 2002.

Ramser J, Abidi FE, Burckle CA, et al.: A unique exonic splice enhancer mutation in a family with X-linked mental retardation and epilepsy points to a novel role of the renin receptor. Hum Mol Genet 14:1019, 2005.

DIFFERENTIAL MATRIX

Syndrome	Developmental Regression	Stereotypical Movements	Seizures	Comments
XLID-Epilepsy	+	+	+	Hyporeflexia
Rett	+	+	+	Acquired microcephaly, truncal ataxia, autistic features
Ornithine Transcarbamoylase Deficiency	+	0	+	Microcephaly, chronic or intermittent hyperammonemia, protein-induced vomiting and lethargy, ataxia
Pyruvate Dehydrogenase Deficiency	+	0	+	Microcephaly, ataxia, dysarthria, structural brain anomalies, hypotonia, lactic acidosis

XLID-HYDROCEPHALY-BASAL GANGLIA CALCIFICATIONS (*SEE ALSO AP1S2*-ASSOCIATED XLID)

(MRX59, FRIED SYNDROME, TURNER XLID)

OMIM 300630

Xp22.2

AP1S2

Definition. XLID with hydrocephaly, calcification of the basal ganglia, and spastic diplegia. Mutations in the sigma-2 subunit of the Adaptor Protein 1 Complex (*AP1S2*), which is involved in the assembly of endocytic vesicles, have been demonstrated. Hence, Fried syndrome is allelic to MRX59 and to the XLID-Hypotonia-Aggression syndrome reported by Turner et al. (2003).

Somatic Features. Except for macrocephaly, which is found only among those with hydrocephaly, the craniofacial manifestations are not distinctive. The ears may be prominent, with outfolding of the upper portion. In adult life, the face may appear elongated with some coarsening. From early childhood, the muscles appear hypoplastic or atrophic. The small muscles of the hands are especially affected. Kyphoscoliosis, genu valgum, and pes planus are also evident.

Growth and Development. On the basis of limited information, intrauterine growth appears to be normal. Adult stature is variable, with some measurements below the 3rd centile. Head circumference is normal, except in the presence of hydrocephaly. Developmental milestones lag from birth in most cases.

Cognitive Features. Severe impairment

Neurological Findings. Although the onset of spasticity has not been well-documented, increased muscle tone, weakness, hyperactive deep tendon reflexes, and clonus are apparent by early adult life. Sensory loss and impairment of coordination have also been documented.

Heterozygote Expression. None

Imaging. Cranial tomography shows enlarged ventricles and calcification of the basal ganglia.

Comment. Prior to localization of the gene in Xp22, this entity was considered to be the same as the MASA syndrome. There are thus at least two XLID syndromes with hydrocephaly and spastic paraplegia as predominant manifestations. Elevated CSF protein has been reported.

REFERENCES

Borck G, Mollà-Herman A, Boddaert N, et al.: Clinical, cellular, and neuropathological consequences of AP1S2 mutations: further delineation of a recognizable X-linked mental retardation syndrome. Hum Mutat 29:966, 2008.

Carpenter NJ, Brown WT, Qu Y, et al.: Regional localization of a nonspecific X-linked mental retardation gene (MRX59) to Xp21.2-p22.2. Am J Med Genet 85:266, 1999.

Fried K: X-linked mental retardation and/or hydrocephalus. J Med Genet 10:17, 1973.

Saillour Y, Zanni G, Des Portes V, et al.: Mutations in the AP1S2 gene encoding the sigma 2 subunit of the adaptor protein 1 complex are associated with syndromic X-linked mental retardation with hydrocephalus and calcifications in basal ganglia. J Med Genet 44:739, 2007.

Strain L, Wright AF, Bonthron DT: Fried syndrome is a distinct X linked mental retardation syndrome mapping to Xp22. J Med Genet 34:535, 1977.

Tarpey PS, Stevens C, Teague J, et al.: Mutations in the gene encoding the Sigma 2 subunit of the adaptor protein 1 complex, AP1S2, cause X-linked mental retardation. Am J Hum Genet 79:1119, 2006.

Turner G, Gedeon A, Kerr B, et al.: Syndromic form of X-linked mental retardation with marked hypotonia in early life, severe mental handicap, and difficult adult behavior maps to Xp22. Am J Med Genet A 117A:245, 2003.

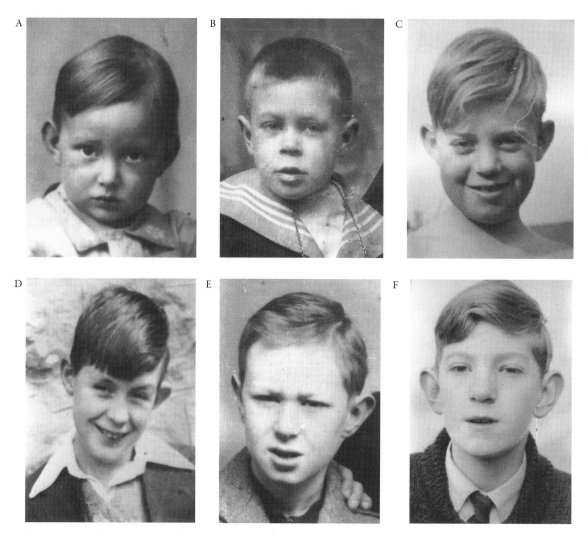

XLID-Hydrocephaly-Basal Ganglia Calcifications. Facial appearance in six affected males showing no consistent distinctive manifestations other than cupping of the ears.   Courtesy of Dr. Kalman Fried, ASAF Harofe Hospital, Zerifin, Israel.

DIFFERENTIAL MATRIX

Syndrome	Muscle Hypoplasia	Iron Deposits or Calcification of Basal Ganglia	Spastic Paraplegia	Comments
XLID-Hydrocephaly-Basal Ganglia Calcifications (*AP1S2*-Associated XLID)	+	+	+	Hydrocephaly, sensory impairment
Gustavson	+	+	+	Microcephaly, short stature, optic atrophy with blindness, large ears, deafness, joint contractures, rockerbottom feet, brain undergrowth, hydrocephaly, cerebellar hypoplasia, seizures
Pelizaeus-Merzbacher	+	+	+	Optic atrophy, hypotonia, dystonia, CNS dysmyelination, ataxia, nystagmus
Pettigrew	0	+	+	Dandy-Walker malformation, microcephaly or hydrocephaly, long face with macrostomia, small testes, contractures, choreoathetosis, cerebellar hypoplasia, seizures
Schimke	0	+	+	Microcephaly, sunken eyes, downslanting palpebral fissures, narrow nose, wide spacing of teeth, cupped ears, hypotonia, abducens palsy, hearing loss, vision loss, choreoathetosis, contractures

ATLAS OF X-LINKED INTELLECTUAL DISABILITY SYNDROMES

XLID-HYPOGAMMAGLOBULINEMIA

(CHUDLEY HYPOGAMMAGLOBULINEMIA SYNDROME, XLID-HYPOGAMMAGLOBULINEMIA-ATAXIA-SEIZURES)

Xq21.33-q23

Definition. XLID with prominent glabella, synophrys, prognathism, single palmar creases, hirsutism, progressive weakness, gait disturbance, seizures, and hypogammaglobulinemia.

Somatic Features. Major malformations do not occur. The craniofacies are characterized by normal head size, hypertelorism, prominent glabella, synophrys, and prognathism. Single palmar creases and generalized hirsutism may also be present. Small cerebellar size was present in one case. Another case had a bifid uvula, diastasis rectus, an undescended testis, mild scoliosis, and macrocephaly, the latter finding evident in his father as a benign trait.

Growth and Development. Intrauterine and postnatal growth appears normal. Developmental milestones lag from infancy, with speech delayed to a greater degree than motor skills.

Cognitive Function. Moderate impairment

Neurological Findings. Generalized tonic-clonic seizures date from childhood or early adolescence. Two older males had progressive weakness and ataxia with gait disturbance in their 40s, findings not present in a younger cousin at age 22 years. Tight heel cords and brisk deep tendon reflexes were demonstrated in one of the older males and abnormal peripheral nerve conduction by the other.

Heterozygote Expression. None

Imaging. Cranial tomography showed cerebellar atrophy in one case and normal anatomy in another. The latter was the youngest of the three cases reported and had not yet developed progressive weakness and ataxia.

A
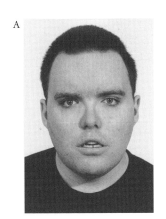
B
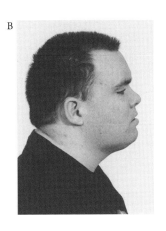
C
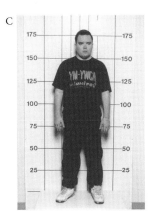
D
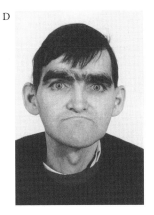

E
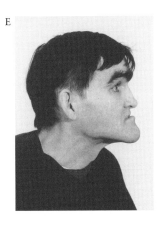
F
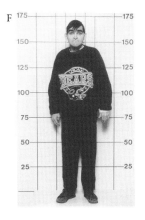

XLID-Hypogammaglobulinemia. Hyertelorism, mild synophrys, underbite, and prognathism at age 22 years (**A–C**); heavy eyebrows, synophrys, hypertelorism, short philtrum, and prognathism in a 43-year-old maternal uncle (**D–F**). Courtesy of Dr. Albert Chudley, Children's Hospital, Winnipeg, Manitoba, Canada.

Laboratory. Hypogammaglobulinemia with low IgG and absent secretory IgA was present in two of the three cases reported. The third case had low normal IgM, IgG, and IgA.

Comment. The gene for Bruton Type, X-Linked Agammaglobulinemia (*BTK*) is located within the mapping limits of Chudley Hypogammaglobulinemia syndrome. Because Bruton Agammaglobulinemia is not associated with intellectual disability, ataxia, and seizures, the possibility of a contiguous gene deletion syndrome was considered by Chudley et al. (1999). A search for a deletion involving the 5'-UTR and 3'-UTR of the *BTK* gene was negative.

REFERENCE

Chudley AE, Tackels DC, Lubs HA, et al.: X-linked mental retardation with dysmorphic features, seizures, hypogammaglobulinemia, and progressive gait disturbance is regionally mapped between Xq21.33 and Xq23. Am J Med Genet 85:255, 1999.

DIFFERENTIAL MATRIX

Syndrome	Ataxia	Seizures	Hypogamma-globulinema	Comments
XLID-Hypogamma-globulinemia	+	+	+	Prominent glabella, synophrys, prognathism, hirsutism, weakness, gait disturbance
Arts	+	+	0	Growth deficiency, poor muscle development, hypotonia, areflexia, deafness, vision loss, childhood death
Gustavson	+	+	0	Microcephaly, short stature, optic atrophy with blindness, large ears, deafness, joint contractures, rockerbottom feet, brain undergrowth, hydrocephaly, cerebellar hypoplasia, spasticity
Pelizaeus-Merzbacher	+	+	0	Optic atrophy, nystagmus, hypotonia, spasticity, dystonia, CNS dysmyelination
Proud (*ARX*-Associated XLID)	+	+	0	Microcephaly, hearing loss, vision loss, agenesis of corpus callosum, cryptorchidism, inguinal hernias, spasticity
Ataxia-Deafness-Dementia, X-linked	+	+	0	Optic atrophy, vision loss, hearing loss, spastic paraplegia, hypotonia, childhood death
XLID-Hypogonadism-Tremor	+	+	0	Short stature, prominent lower lip, muscle wasting of legs, abnormal gait, hypogonadism, obesity, tremor

XLID-HYPOGONADISM-TREMOR

(CABEZAS SYNDROME)

OMIM 300354

Xq24

CUL4B

Definition. XLID with short stature, prominent lower lip, muscle wasting of legs, abnormal gait, hypogonadism, obesity, seizures, and tremor. The responsible gene, *CUL4B*, encodes an E3 ubiquitin ligase.

Somatic Features. Craniofacial findings are not distinctive, but macrocephaly is common, as is prominence of the lower lip. Some males have kyphosis, hyperextensible joints, small feet, pes cavus, gap between toes 1 and 2, and wasting of the legs. The testes are small, and gynecomastia may be present. Central obesity and seizures are common. A fine tremor of the upper limbs, decreased motor coordination, wasting of the legs, and abnormal gait help to distinguish this condition from other X-linked hypogonadism syndromes.

Growth and Development. Intrauterine growth may be normal. Postnatal stature measures at or below the 10th centile, whereas head circumference is normal or increased. Central obesity is typical. Development is globally delayed.

Cognitive Function. Intelligence is usually severely impaired, but some males have had IQs above 50. Attention deficit and hyperactivity are common. Mood swings and bouts of aggressive behavior have been reported.

Heterozygote Expression. Some carriers have a mild tremor and learning disability.

Comment. A number of XLID-hypogonadism syndromes are recognized. Tremor and muscle wasting of the legs are helpful in distinguishing this entity from others.

Vitale et al. (2001) reported a family with quite similar findings that links to Xq24. Affected males had short stature, variable head circumference, widow's peak and low frontal hairline, synophrys, narrow and downslanting palpebral fissures, prominent nasal tip, hypoplastic earlobes, short philtrum, macrostomia, and misaligned teeth. Skeletal findings included short thick neck, sloping shoulders, scoliosis or kyphosis, small hands and feet with short digits, proximal placement of toes 3 or 4 and fifth-finger clinodactyly. The abdomen was prominent and the penis small. The males had aphasia or severely limited speech and severe intellectual disability. They were generally friendly, but some had poor adaptive skills and bouts of aggressiveness or impulsivity. One had seizures, another had tremors, and all were considered clumsy. Two female carriers had learning disabilities, minor craniofacial dysmorphology, and digital anomalies but normal speech and cognitive performance.

REFERENCES

Badura-Stronka M, Jamsheer A, Materna-Kiryluk A, et al.: A novel nonsense mutation in CUL4B gene in three brothers with X-linked mental retardation syndrome. Clin Genet 77:141, 2010.

Cabezas DA, Slaugh R, Abidi F, et al.: A new X linked mental retardation (XLMR) syndrome with short stature, small testes, muscle wasting, and tremor localizes to Xq24-q25. J Med Genet 37:663, 2000.

Tarpey PS, Raymond FL, O'Meara S, et al.: Mutations in *CUL4B*, which encodes a ubiquitin E3 ligase subunit, cause an X-linked mental retardation syndrome associated with aggressive outbursts, seizures, relative macrocephaly, central obesity, hypogonadism, pes cavus, and tremor. Am J Hum Genet 80:345, 2007.

Vitale E, Specchia C, Devoto M, et al.: Novel X-linked mental retardation syndrome with short stature maps to Xq24. Am J Med Genet 103:1, 2001.

Zou Y, Liu Q, Chen B, et al.: Mutation in CUL4B, which encodes a member of cullin-RING ubiquitin ligase complex, causes X-linked mental retardation. Am J Hum Genet 80:561, 2007.

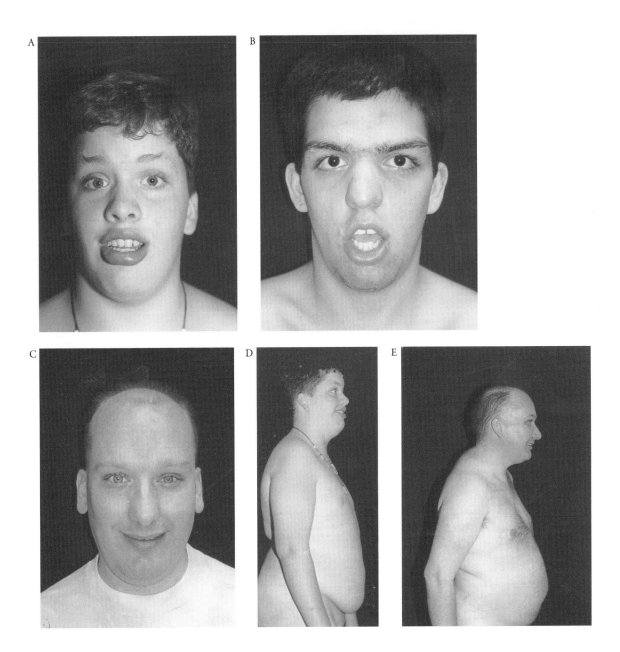

XLID-Hypogonadism-Tremor. Nineteen-year-old with prominent lips (A); 21-year-old cousin with synophrys, broad nasal bridge, bulbous nose, open mouth and prominent lower lip (B); 40-year-old cousin with balding, overhanging columella and prominent lower lip (C). Lateral views of 19-year-old and 40-year-old showing truncal obesity (D,E).

Syndrome	Short Stature	Hypogonadism	Tremor	Comments
XLID-Hypogonadism-Tremor	+	+	+	Prominent lower lip, muscle wasting of legs, abnormal gait, obesity, seizures
ATRX-Associated XLID	+	+	0	Microcephaly, telecanthus/hypertelorism, small triangular nose, tented upper lip, open mouth, wide spacing of teeth, abnormal genitalia, minor musculoskeletal anomalies, hypotonia, erythrocyte HbH inclusions in some
Börjeson-Forssman-Lehmann	+	+	0	Microcephaly, coarse face, large ears, gynecomastia, narrow sloped shoulders, visual impairment, tapered digits, hypotonia, obesity
MEHMO	+	+	0	Microcephaly, edematous hands and feet, equinovarus deformity, seizures, early childhood death, obesity, hypotonia
Urban	+	+	0	Small hands and feet, digital contractures, osteoporosis, obesity
Vasquez	+	+	0	Microcephaly, gynecomastia, obesity, hypotonia
XLID-Microcephaly-Testicular Failure	+	+	0	Microcephaly, prominent supraorbital ridges, high nasal bridge, prominent nose, macrostomia
XLID-Panhypopituitarism	+	+	0	Small sella turcica, deficiency of pituitary, thyroid, adrenal, and gonadal hormones, hypogenitalism, obesity
Young-Hughes	+	+	0	Small palpebral fissures, cupped ears, ichthyosiform scaling, obesity, hypogenitalism

XLID-HYPOSPADIAS

Definition. XLID with microcephaly, trigonocephaly, and hypospadias. The gene has not been identified or localized.

Goldblatt et al. (1987) reported three brothers with normal stature, microcephaly, trigonocephaly, synophrys, midface hypoplasia, beaked nose, posteriorly rotated ears with folded helix, and arched palate. Hypotonia and joint hypermobility were present. There was fifth-finger clinodactyly and the nail "beaking." Two of the brothers had glandular hypospadias, and the third had a hooded prepuce.

Mild-to-moderate developmental impairment was present. Other cases have not been reported. Craniofacial features are different from the telecanthus-hypospadias syndrome (Opitz G/BBB, C syndrome), which maps to Xp22.2.

REFERENCE

Goldblatt J, Wallis C, Viljoen D: A new hypospadias - mental retardation syndrome in three brothers. Am J Dis Child 141:1168, 1987.

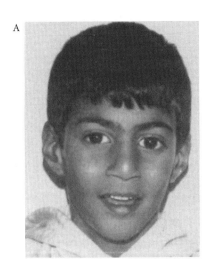 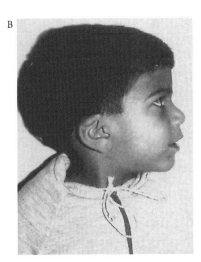 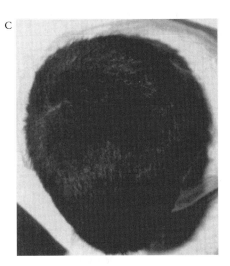

XLID-Hypospadias. Six-year-old male with microcephaly, synophrys, maxillary hypoplasia **(A)**; 4-year-old brother with microcephaly, trigonocephaly, posteriorly-rotated ear with flattened upper helix and depressed nasal tip **(B, C)**.   Courtesy of Dr. Dennis Viljoen, University of the Witwatersrand, Johannesburg, South Africa.

XLID-HYPOTONIA-RECURRENT INFECTIONS

(LUBS-ARENA SYNDROME)

OMIM 300260

Xq28

dup MECP2

Definition. XLID with hypotonic facies, hypertelorism, downslanting palpebral fissures, gastroesophageal reflux, recurrent respiratory infections, and seizures. Duplication of several genes in Xq28, including *MECP2*, has been found in the original family and in a number of other families.

Somatic Features. Major malformations do not occur. Hypotonic facies with hypertelorism, downslanting palpebral fissures, posteriorly rotated or abnormally sculpted ears, short nose with a flat nasal bridge, and large open mouth are the major somatic findings. Cardiomegaly was present at post mortem examination in two cases. Cerebral atrophy is the only abnormality present on cranial imaging. Swallowing problems and gastroesophageal reflux appear to be caused by cerebral dysfunction rather than structural anomalies of the gastrointestinal tract. Similarly, recurrent infections appear to be caused by aspiration rather than a defect in the immune system. A relentless deterioration of nervous system function leads to death by age 10 years.

Growth and Development. Although birth weight is impaired, the velocity of all growth parameters appears normal postnatally. Developmental milestones are delayed from infancy and developmental regression begins prior to age 5 years.

Cognitive Function. Severe impairment

Neurological Findings. Hypotonia exists from infancy and rapid neurological deterioration manifested by loss of motor and language skills, seizures, loss of vision and hearing, spasticity, and unresponsiveness usually begins before age 5 years. The neurological deterioration likely underlies a course complicated with swallowing difficulty, gastroesophageal reflux, and recurrent respiratory infections.

Heterozygote Expression. Carrier females may have mild cognitive impairment but do not experience neurological abnormalities or recurrent infections. Language function was affected to the greatest degree and emotional lability was evident. Carriers have highly skewed X-inactivation which can be utilized as a marker for this syndrome.

Neuropathology. Three postmortem examinations have yielded inconsistent findings. No gross or microscopic changes other than ischemia and vascular congestion were present in two cases, both of whom died at age 8 years. Normal cerebral cortex, small hippocampi, loss of Purkinje cells, meningitis and encephalitis, and changes of anoxia were present in a third case wherein the patient died at age 5 years.

Imaging. Cerebral atrophy

Laboratory. Immunoglobulins, acylcarnitine profile, and lysosomal enzymes are normal. In one case, skeletal muscle obtained at post mortem showed variability in size of muscle fiber with centralization of nuclei. In two other cases, there was cardiomegaly with biventricular hypertrophy.

Comment. Although several genes in Xq28 are usually duplicated, it appears that duplication of *MECP2* is the essential phenotype-inducing abnormality. Pai et al. (1997) reported a family with hypertelorism, seizures, recurrent infections, and childhood death that mapped to the Xq28. The clinical manifestations were sufficiently inconsistent, however, to prompt the authors to consider the phenotype nonsyndromal (MRX64). This notwithstanding, demonstration of an Xq28 duplication in the family confirmed that the two conditions are allelic.

REFERENCES

Friez MJ, Jones JR, Clarkson K, et al.: Recurrent infections, hypotonia, and mental retardation caused by duplication of MECP2 and adjacent region in Xq28. Pediatrics 118:e1687, 2006.

Lubs H, Abidi F, Blaymore J, et al.: An XLMR syndrome characterized by multiple respiratory infections, hypertelorism, severe CNS deterioration and early death localizes to distal Xq28. Am J Med Genet 85:243, 1999.

Lugtenberg D, Kleefstra T, Oudakker AR, et al.: Structural variation in Xq28: MECP2 duplications in 1% of patients with unexplained XLMR and in 2% of male patients with severe encephalopathy. Eur J Hum Genet 17:444, 2009.

Pai GS, Häne B, Joseph M, et al.: A new X-linked recessive syndrome of mental retardation and mild dysmorphism maps to Xq28. Am J Med Genet 34:529, 1997.

Van Esch H, Bauters M, Ignatius J, et al.: Duplication of the MECP2 region is a frequent cause of severe mental retardation and progressive neurological symptoms in males. Am J Hum Genet 77:442, 2005.

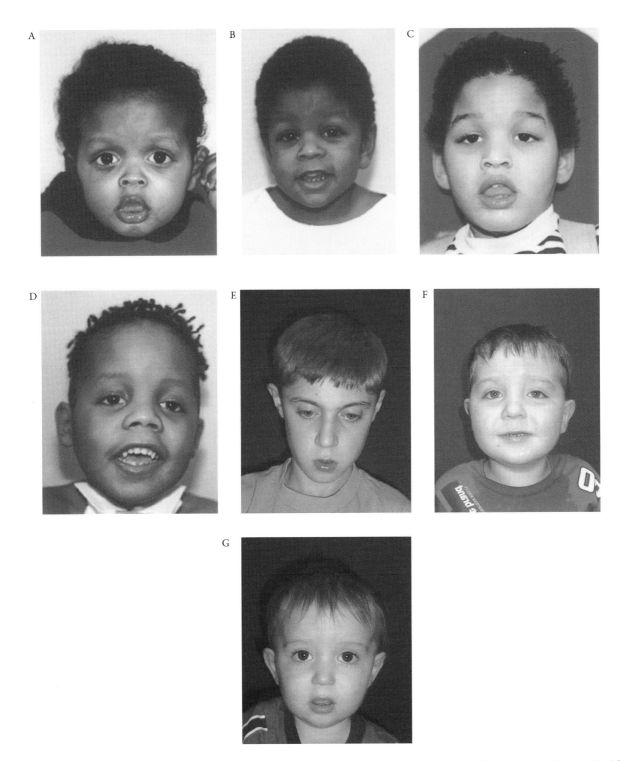

XLID-Hypotonia-Recurrent Infections. Affected males at ages 2, 3, 5, and 7 years (**A–D**) showing hypertelorism, downslanted palpebral fissures, short nose with anteverted nostrils, and tenting of the upper lip. Brothers ages 11.5 years (**E**), 4 years (**F**), and 1.5 years (**G**). Note hypotonic face and small mouth in **E** and **G** but absence of those features in **F**.

Syndrome	Hypotonic Facies	Developmental Regression	Seizures	Comments
XLID-Hypotonia-Recurrent Infections	+	+	+	Hypertelorism, downslanting palpebral fissures, gastroesophageal reflux, recurrent infections, childhood death
Proud (*ARX*-Associated XLID)	+	0	+	Microcephaly, hearing loss, vision loss, agenesis of corpus callosum, cryptorchidism, inguinal hernias, ataxia, spasticity
Smith-Fineman-Myers	+	0	+	Microcephaly, ptosis, flat philtrum, scoliosis, midfoot varus, narrow feet, hypotonia
XLID-Psoriasis	+	0	+	Hypertelorism, open mouth, large ears, hypotonia, psoriasis
Rett	0	+	+	Acquired microcephaly, truncal ataxia, repetitive hand movements, autistic features
XLID-Epilepsy	0	+	+	Repetitive stereotypical hand movements, hyporeflexia

XLID-ICHTHYOSIS-HYPOGONADISM
(RUD SYNDROME)

OMIM 308200

Definition. XLID with ichthyosis, hypogonadism, anosmia and seizures. This combination of manifestations probably results from deletions of variable magnitude in Xp22.3 rather than from mutations in a single gene. The entry is included for historical reasons.

Somatic Features. Craniofacial features appear normal, although alopecia including absent eyebrows and eyelashes has been reported. Ichthyosis is present from birth or very soon thereafter. It may begin as a general erythema and progress to thick scales that darken with age. The trunk and extensor surfaces are most extensively affected; the palms, soles and flexion creases are spared. Most patients have underdevelopment of the genitalia and hypogonadism. The penis is small and testes small or undescended. Uncommonly, hypospadias is present. Sexual hair does not develop and gynecomastia occurs in a minority. Generalized or psychomotor seizures occur in most patients, with usual onset at the end of the first decade. Nystagmus and anosmia have been noted in some cases.

Growth and Development. Short stature occurs in most cases.

Cognitive Function. Variable impairment has been described with IQs ranging from low normal range to severe impairment.

Neurological Findings. Seizures occur in most cases. Nystagmus, strabismus and anosmia are less consistently present.

Heterozygote Expression. Carriers have normal cognitive function and no somatic manifestations.

Laboratory. Deletions of Xp22 may result in reduced levels of steroid sulfatase, testosterone, and gonadotropins. Normal steroid sulfatase and hypergonadotrophic hypogonadism are likely caused by nondeletion genocopies.

Comment. Traupe (1989) has pointed out that the two patients, a male and an unrelated female, described by Rud (1927, 1929) had dissimilar disorders and neither had intellectual disability. Thus, the diagnosis of Rud syndrome to describe ichthyosis, hypogonadism, intellectual disability, and seizures is inappropriate. Further, it appears probable that this constellation of findings cannot be attributed to a single gene mutation, but rather to a contiguous gene deletion. The clinical heterogeneity is based in large measure on the extent of the deletion. Ichthyosis is associated with deletion of the steroid sulfatase (aryl sulfatase C) gene, hypogonadotrophic hypogonadism and anosmia with deletion of the Kallman syndrome gene and, presumably, intellectual disability and seizures with a different gene in the Xq22 region.

REFERENCES

Münke M, Kruse K, Goos M, et al.: Genetic heterogeneity of the ichthyosis, hypogonadism, mental retardation, and epilepsy syndrome. Eur J Pediatr 141:8, 1983.

Perrin JCS, Idemoto JY, Sotos JF, et al.: X-linked syndrome of congenital ichthyosis, hypogonadism, mental retardation and anosmia. Birth Defects: Orig Art Ser XII(5):267, 1976.

Rud E: Et Tilfaelde af Hypogenitalisme (Eunuchoidismus feminus) med partiel Gigantisme og Ichthyosis. Hospitalstidende 72:426, 1929.

Rud E: Et Tilfaelde af Infantilisme med Tetani, Epilepsi, Polyneuritis, Ichthyosis og Anaemi of Pernicios Type. Hospitalstidende 70:525, 1927.

Traupe H: The Ichthyoses. A Guide to Clinical Diagnosis, Genetic Counseling, and Therapy. Springer-Verlag, Berlin, 1989.

XLID-INFANTILE SPASMS (*SEE ALSO ARX*-ASSOCIATED XLID)

(WEST SYNDROME)

OMIM 308350

Xp21.3

ARX

Definition. XLID with infantile spasms and hypsarrhythmia. Mutations in *ARX* have also been found in a spectrum of XLID entities, including X-Linked Lissencephaly with Abnormal Genitalia, Partington syndrome and Nonsyndromal XLID.

Somatic Features. Malformations or distinctive craniofacial manifestations do not occur.

Growth and Development. Intrauterine and postnatal growth is normal. Developmental milestones slow after the onset of infantile spasms, usually within the first 6 months of life.

Cognitive Function. Severe impairment

Neurological Findings. Prior to the onset of seizures, affected males appear normal and experience normal growth and development. Seizures, usually in the form of infantile spasms, begin between 2 and 8 months. Typically, infantile spasms follow a brief period of atonia and consist of clusters of flexion and extension movements of the limbs, neck, and trunk. Early childhood death is not uncommon.

Heterozygote Expression. None

Laboratory. Metabolic studies are normal. A hypsarrhythmia pattern – multifocal spikes and high-voltage slow waves throughout the cortex – is usually found on electroencephalography.

Imaging. Cranial imaging is usually normal, with the exception of mild dilation of the cerebral ventricles.

Comment. A period of normal infantile development followed by stagnation of developmental progress and loss of skills is seen in few XLID syndromes. This phenomenon appears related to the seizures in XLID-Infantile Spasms and in XLID-Epilepsy. In other cases, the regression appears secondary to episodic or persistent metabolic abnormalities. XLID-Infantile Spasms (West syndrome) is allelic to Partington syndrome and X-linked Lissencephaly with Abnormal Genitalia. Mutations in *ARX* have been found in a number of families with Nonsyndromal XLID.

REFERENCES

Claes S. Devriendt K, Lagae L, et al.: The X-linked infantile spasms syndrome (MIM 308350) maps to Xp11.4-Xpter in two pedigrees. Ann Neurol 42:360, 1997.

Feinberg AP, Leahy WR: Infantile spasms: case report of sex-linked inheritance. Dev Med Child Neurol 19:524, 1977.

Kitamura K, Yanazawa M, Sugiyama N, et al.: Mutation of ARX causes abnormal development of forebrain and testes in mice and X-linked lissencephaly with abnormal genitalia in humans. Nat Genet 32:359, 2002.

Nawara M, Szczaluba K, Poirier K, et al.: The ARX mutations: a frequent cause of X-linked mental retardation. Am J Med Genet A 140:727, 2006.

Rugtveit J: X-linked mental retardation and infantile spasms in two brothers. Dev Med Child Neurol 28:544, 1986.

Strømme P, Mangelsdorf ME, Shaw MA, et al.: Mutations in the human ortholog of Aristaless cause X-linked mental retardation and epilepsy. Nat Genet 30:441, 2002.

Turner G, Partington M, Kerr B, et al.: Variable expression of mental retardation, autism, seizures, and dystonic hand movements in two families with an identical ARX gene mutation. Am J Med Genet 112:405, 2002.

DIFFERENTIAL MATRIX

Syndrome	Developmental Regression	Seizures	Hypsarrhythmia	Comments
XLID-Infantile Spasms	+	+	+	Early childhood death
Bertini	+	+	0	Macular degeneration, hypotonia, ataxia, childhood death, hypoplasia of cerebellar vermis and corpus callosum, postnatal growth impairment
Menkes	+	+	0	Growth deficiency, sparse kinky hair, hypothermia, pallor, limited movement, hypertonicity, metaphyseal widening and spurs, arterial tortuosity, childhood death
Ornithine Transcarbamoylase Deficiency	+	+	0	Chronic or intermittent hyperammonemia, microcephaly, protein-induced vomiting and lethargy, ataxia
Pelizaeus-Merzbacher	+	+	0	Optic atrophy, nystagmus, hypotonia, spasticity, ataxia, dystonia, CNS dysmyelination
Pyruvate Dehydrogenase Deficiency	+	+	0	Microcephaly, ataxia, dysarthria, structural brain anomalies, hypotonia, lactic acidosis
Rett	+	+	0	Acquired microcephaly, truncal ataxia, repetitive hand movements, autistic features
XLID-Epilepsy	+	+	0	Repetitive stereotypical hand movements, hyporeflexia

XLID-ISOLATED GROWTH HORMONE DEFICIENCY

OMIM 300123

Xq27.1

SOX3

Definition. XLID with short stature, gynecomastia, isolated growth hormone deficiency, and infantile behavior. *SOX3* mutations have been found in XLID-Isolated Growth Hormone Deficiency and XLID-Panhypopituitarism.

Somatic Features. Short stature is obvious from childhood, and gynecomastia occurs after puberty.

Growth and Development. Intrauterine growth may be normal, but height lags from birth. Ultimate height reaches 135 to 159 centimeters. Bone age lags significantly behind, and statural growth may continue into the mid-20s. The age of puberty has not been documented, but genitalia appear normal in adults, although secondary sexual characteristics may be incompletely virilized.

Neurological Findings. None

Heterozygote Expression. None

Imaging. Radiographs show a small sella turcica.

Laboratory. Isolated growth hormone deficiency with normal thyroid, adrenal, and gonadal hormones.

Comment. XLID-Isolated Growth Hormone Deficiency is allelic with XLID-Panhypopituitarism. Duplications resulting in increased *SOX3* dosage as well as mutations that reduce dosage have been described.

REFERENCES

Hamel BCJ, Smits APT, Otten BJ, et al.: Familial X-linked mental retardation and isolated growth hormone deficiency. Am J Med Genet 64:35, 1996.

Laumonnier F, Ronce N, Hamel BC, et al.: Transcription factor SOX3 is involved in X-linked mental retardation with growth hormone deficiency. Am J Hum Genet 71:1450, 2002.

Solomon NM, Ross SA, Morgan T, et al.: Array comparative genomic hybridisation analysis of boys with X linked hypopituitarism identifies a 3.9 Mb duplicated critical region at Xq27 containing SOX3. J Med Genet 41:669, 2004.

Woods KS, Cundall M, Turton J, et al.: Over- and underdosage of SOX3 is associated with infundibular hypoplasia and hypopituitarism. Am J Hum Genet 76:833, 2005.

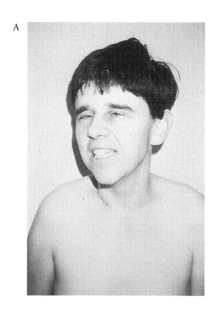
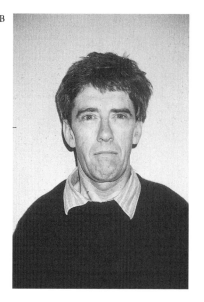
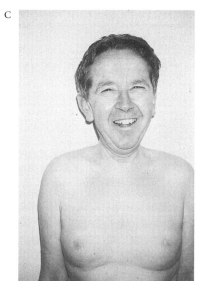
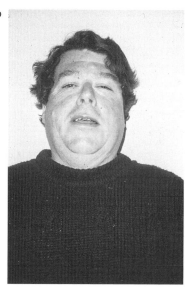

XLID-Isolated Growth Hormone Deficiency. Narrow palpebral fissures but otherwise variable facial appearance in brothers at ages 39, 45, and 50 years (A-C) and a maternal cousin at age 45 years (D).   Courtesy of Dr. Ben Hamel, University Hospital, Nijmegen, The Netherlands.

DIFFERENTIAL MATRIX

Syndrome	Short Stature	Gynecomastia	Growth Hormone Deficiency	Comments
XLID-Isolated Growth Hormone Deficiency	+	+	+	–
Börjeson-Forssman-Lehmann	+	+	0	Obesity, hypotonia, hypogonadism, microcephaly, coarse facies, large ears, narrow sloped shoulders, visual impairment, tapered digits
Chudley-Lowry (*ATRX*-Associated XLID)	+	+	0	Bitemporal narrowing, almond-shaped eyes, depressed nasal bridge, tented upper lip, open mouth, hypogonadism, hypotonia, obesity
Vasquez	+	+	0	Microcephaly, obesity, hypotonia, hypogonadism
XLID-Panhypopituitarism	+	0	+	Hypogenitalism, small sella turcica, deficiency of pituitary, thyroid, adrenal, and gonadal hormones

XLID-MACROCEPHALY

OMIM 300706

Xp11.22

HUWE1

Definition. XLID with macrocephaly in affected males and carrier females. The *HUWE1* gene is involved in ubiquitination of histones.

Somatic Features. Macrocephaly occurs in males and carrier females but not in nonaffected siblings. Apart from macrocephaly, downslanting palpebral fissures, obesity, and elbow limitation, the phenotype is not notable. Testicular volume is normal. Tapered fingers with short terminal phalanges and nails were present in one case.

Growth and Development. Details of childhood growth are not available. Although all developmental milestones are delayed, speech lags to a greater degree than motor skills.

Cognitive Features. Mild-to-moderate impairment

Neurological Findings. None

Heterozygote Expression. Carrier females have macrocephaly, obesity, and mild intellectual disability. Seizures have occurred in one carrier.

Imaging. Cranial tomography in one male was normal at age 1 year.

Comment. Macrocephaly of all causes occurs twice as frequently among individuals with intellectual disability as in the general population. Commonly, the macrocephaly results from hydrocephaly. Macrocephaly caused by a large brain without hydrocephaly occurs in a number of XLID syndromes, including Atkin-Flaitz, Clark-Baraitser, Fragile X, Mucopolysaccharidosis IIA, PPM-X, Waisman-Laxova, XLID-Macrocephaly and XLID-Macrocephaly-Macroorchidism syndromes.

REFERENCES

Turner G, Gedeon A, Mulley J: X-linked mental retardation with heterozygous expression and macrocephaly: Pericentromeric gene localization. Am J Med Genet 51:575, 1994.

Froyen G, Corbett M, Vandewalle J, et al.: Submicroscopic duplications of the hydroxysteroid dehydrogenase HSD17B10 and the E3 ubiquitin ligase HUWE1 are associated with mental retardation. Am J Hum Genet 82:432, 2008.

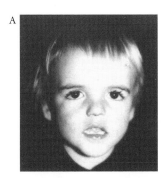
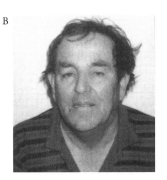
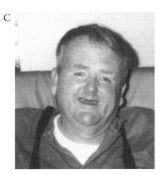
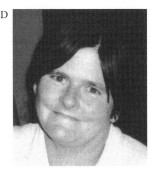
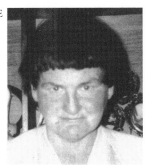

XLID-Macrocephaly. Macrocephaly and downslanting palpebral fissures in a boy age 2 years (**A**); macrocephaly and downslanting palpebral fissures and prominence of the tip of the chin in adult cousins (**B, C**); macrocephaly and prominence of the tip of the chin in adult carrier females (**D, E**). Courtesy of Dr. Gillian Turner, Prince of Wales Children's Hospital, Randwick, New South Wales, Australia.

DIFFERENTIAL MATRIX

Syndrome	Macrocephaly	Obesity	Carrier Female Manifestations	Comments
XLID-Macrocephaly	+	+	+	Downslanting palpebral fissures, elbow limitation
Atkin-Flaitz	+	+	+	Short stature, hypertelorism, downslanting palpebral fissures, broad nasal tip, thick lower lip, brachydactyly, seizures
Clark-Baraitser	+	+	+	Large stature, dental abnormalities, broad nasal tip, thick lower lip, macroorchidism
Fragile X	+	0	+	Normal or excessive growth, prominent forehead, long face, midface hypoplasia, large ears, prominent mandible, macro-orchidism
Lujan	+	0	+	Marfanoid habitus, asthenic build, long face, prominent forehead, high palate, micrognathia, long digits, pectus excavatum, joint hyperextensibility, seizures, hyperactivity
Waisman-Laxova	+	0	+	Spasticity, strabismus
XLID-Macrocephaly-Macroorchidism	+	0	+	Elongated face, prominent mandible, macroorchidism, clumsiness, repetitive movements

XLID-MACROCEPHALY-MACROORCHIDISM

(XLID-MACROORCHIDISM)

OMIM 309530

Xp11-q21

Definition. XLID with normal stature, variable macrocephaly and macroorchidism, and normal FMR1 analysis. Although multiple causes may produce this phenotype, one gene has been mapped to the pericentromeric region between DXS991 (Xp11) and DXS1002 (Xq21).

Somatic Features. Macrocephaly contributes to the triangular facial shape and downslanting palpebral fissures. Prominence of the mandible has been noted in some cases. Macroorchidism becomes obvious after puberty.

Growth and Development. Details of childhood growth and development are not available. In adulthood, stature is normal and head circumference large. Speech appears impaired to a greater degree than motor skills.

Cognitive Function. Moderate impairment is usual with IQ measurements between 35 and 50.

Heterozygote Expression. Mild cognitive impairment may occur in carrier females.

Comment. Once the phenotype of the Fragile X syndrome was delineated, individuals with similar phenotypes but negative Fragile X testing were identified. Prominent among these individuals were those with intellectual disability and macroorchidism with or without macrocephaly or other craniofacial manifestations of the Fragile X syndrome. Proops et al. (1983), Tariverdian et al. (1991), and Johnson et al. (1998) have reported affected brothers or families that appear to follow a pattern of X-linked transmission. Proops (1983) described three adult brothers who were small with relatively large heads, square facial shape, prominent ears, high-arched palate, stubby hands and feet, macroorchidism, limited language, and pleasant quiet demeanors. Three nephews also had intellectual disability and short stature but showed a less consistent phenotype. Carrier females appeared to have mild intellectual disability. This family, designated MRX2, shows linkage to DXS989 in Xp22 (Hu et al., 1994).

Tariverdian et al. (1991) reported two half-brothers with elongated face, dense eyebrows, long nose, prominent jaw, and macroorchidism. Growth was normal. Severe intellectual disability, aggressive behaviors, clumsy "unskilled movement" and gait, repetitive hand movements, dysarthria, and echolalia were present. The mother had a prominent chin and mild mental impairment. Cranial tomography in the younger brother showed slight enlargement of the third ventricle, a subarachnoid cyst in the left temporal region, and an area of density in the pons.

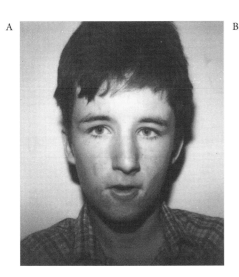
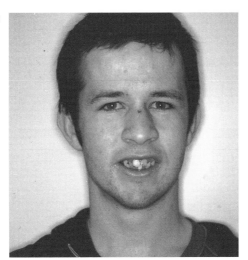
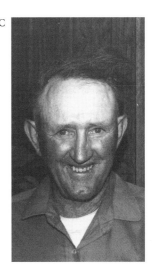

XLID-Macrocephaly-Macroorchidism. Brothers at ages 17 and 22 years showing macrocephaly and downslanting palpebral fissures (**A, B**); maternal uncle at age 56 years with macrocephaly and prominence of the mandible (**C**).   Courtesy of Dr. John Johnson, Shodair Hospital, Helena, Montana.

Johnson et al. (1998) studied a family with 10 males with moderate intellectual disability, macrocephaly, and macroorchidism. However, not all affected males had macrocephaly and macroorchidism, whereas some of the non-affected brothers did. Several carrier females had mild intellectual disability. The responsible gene was mapped to the pericentromeric region between Xp11 and Xq12.

Fryns et al. (1986) and Chiurazzi et al. (1994) have reported similar sporadic or familial cases. Macroorchidism has also been reported in Atkin-Flaitz, Clark-Baraitser, Lujan, and PPM-X syndromes.

REFERENCES

Chiurazzi P, de Graaff E, Ng J, et al.: No apparent involvement of the FMR1 gene in five patients with phenotypic manifestations of the fragile X syndrome. Am J Med Genet 51:309, 1994.

Froyen G, Corbett M, Vandewalle J, et al.: Submicroscopic duplications of the hydroxysteroid dehydrogenase HSD17B10 and the E3 ubiquitin ligase HUWE1 are associated with mental retardation. Am J Hum Genet 82:432, 2008.

Fryns JP, Dereymaeker A, Hoefnagels M, et al.: Partial fragile(X) phenotype with megalotestes in fragile(X)-negative patients with acquired lesions of the central nervous system. Am J Med Genet 23:213, 1986.

Hu L-J, Blumenfeld-Heyberger S, Hanauer A, et al.: Non-specific X-linked mental retardation: Linkage analysis in MRX2 and MRX4 families revisited. Am J Med Genet 51:569, 1994.

Johnson JP, Nelson R, Schwartz CE: A family with mental retardation, variable macrocephaly and macroorchidism, and linkage to Xq12-q21. J Med Genet 35:1026, 1998.

Proops R, Mayer M, Jacobs PA: A study of mental retardation in children in the Island of Hawaii. Clin Genet 23:81, 1983.

Tariverdian G, Froster-Iskenius U, Deuschl G, et al.: Mental retardation, acromegalic face, and megalotestes in two half-brothers: A specific form of X-linked mental retardation without fra(X) (q)? Am J Med Genet 38:208, 1991.

DIFFERENTIAL MATRIX

Syndrome	Macrocephaly	Macroorchidism	Carrier Female Manifestations	Comments
XLID-Macrocephaly-Macroorchidism	+	+	+	Elongated face, prominent mandible, clumsiness, repetitive movements
XLID-Macrocephaly	+	+	+	Downslanting palpebral fissures, obesity, elbow limitation
Atkin-Flaitz	+	+	+	Short stature, hypertelorism, downslanting palpebral fissures, broad nasal tip, thick lower lip, brachydactyly, seizures
Clark-Baraitser	+	+	+	Large stature, obesity, dental abnormalities, broad nasal tip, thick lower lip
Fragile X	+	+	+	Normal or excessive growth, prominent forehead, long face, midface hypoplasia, large ears, prominent mandible
Waisman-Laxova	+	0	+	Spasticity, strabismus
PPM-X	0	+	+	Spastic paraplegia, psychosis, Parkinsonian features

XLID-MICROCEPHALY-TESTICULAR FAILURE

Xq25-q26

Definition. Mild intellectual disability with microcephaly, short stature, and hypogonadism. The gene has not been identified.

Somatic Features. The craniofacies are characterized by microcephaly, prominent supraorbital ridges, high nasal bridge, prominent nose, and macrostomia. The hands are small, with fifth-finger clinodactyly and small nails. The testes are small, hypospadias occurred in one male, and undescended testes were present in two males.

Growth and Development. Intrauterine growth is normal, but short stature and microcephaly become apparent in infancy or shortly thereafter.

Cognitive Function. Learning difficulty becomes apparent in the school years and is mild.

Comment. This XLID-Hypogonadism syndrome maps to the same region as Börjeson-Forssman-Lehmann and XLID-Hypogonadism-Tremor syndromes.

REFERENCE

Cilliers DD, Parveen R, Clayton P, et al.: A new X-linked mental retardation (XLMR) syndrome with late-onset primary testicular failure, short stature and microcephaly maps to Xq25-q26. Eur J Med Genet 50:216, 2007.

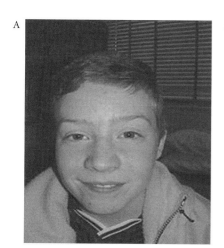
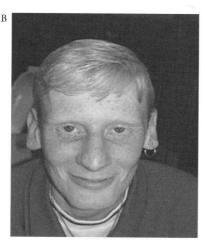
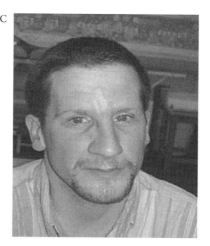

XLID-Microcephaly-Testicular Failure. Thirteen-year-old male with prominent forehead and supraorbital ridges and wide nose and mouth **(A)**. 28-year-old uncle with deep-set eyes, prominent supraorbital ridges, and high nasal bridge **(B)**. Similar facial findings in 34-year-old uncle **(C)**.
Courtesy of Dr. Jill Clayton-Smith, St. Mary's Hospital, Manchester, UK.

DIFFERENTIAL MATRIX

Syndrome	Microcephaly	Short Stature	Hypogonadism	Comments
XLID-Microcephaly-Testicular Failure	+	+	+	Prominent supraorbital ridges, high nasal bridge, prominent nose, macrostomia
ATRX-Associated XLID	+	+	+	Telecanthus/hypertelorism, small triangular nose, tented upper lip, open mouth, wide spacing of teeth, abnormal genitalia, minor musculoskeletal anomalies, hypotonia, erythrocyte HbH inclusions in some
Börjeson-Forssman-Lehmann	+	+	+	Coarse face, large ears, gynecomastia, narrow sloped shoulders, visual impairment, tapered digits, hypotonia, obesity
MEHMO	+	+	+	Coarse face, large ears, gynecomastia, narrow sloped shoulders, visual impairment, tapered digits, obesity, hypotonia
Vasquez	+	+	+	Gynecomastia, obesity, hypotonia
Renpenning	+	+	0	Upslanting palpebral fissures, small testes
Ahmad	0	+	+	Obesity, tapered fingers
Urban	0	+	+	Small hands and feet, digital contractures, osteoporosis, hypotonia, obesity
XLID-Hypogonadism-Tremor	0	+	+	Prominent lower lip, muscle wasting of legs, abnormal gait, obesity, seizures, tremor
XLID-Panhypopituitarism	0	+	+	Small sella turcica; deficiency of pituitary, thyroid, adrenal, and gonadal hormones; hypogenitalism; obesity
Young-Hughes	0	+	+	Small palpebral fissures, cupped ears, ichthyosiform scaling, obesity, hypogenitalism

XLID-NAIL DYSTROPHY-SEIZURES

MIM

Xq24-q25

UBE2A

Definition. XLID with distinctive face, generalized hirsutism, small penis, dry skin and nail dystrophy, and seizures. Mutations and deletions of *UBE2A*, a member of the ubiquitin proteasome pathway, have been described in several families.

Somatic Features. The head circumference is normal or large; the face is characterized by its wide appearance, upslanted palpebral fissures, synophrys, midface hypoplasia with low nasal bridge, large mouth, and thin lips. The neck is broad and short with a low pattern hairline. Nipples are widely spaced. The penis is small. The feet are small, with swelling of the dorsum. The skin is dry, and there is marked generalized hirsutism and nail dystrophy.

Growth and Development. Intrauterine growth is not impaired, but the height eventually settles in the lower centiles; the head circumference and weight are in the higher centiles.

Cognitive Function. Measurements are not available, but speech is severely impaired or absent.

Heterozygote Expression. None

Comment. The distinctive face, generalized hirsutism, and nail dystrophy should be helpful in clinical diagnosis of suspected cases.

REFERENCES

Budny B, Badura-Stronka M, Materna-Kiryluk A, et al.: Novel missense mutations in the ubiquitination-related gene UBE2A cause a recognizable X-linked mental retardation syndrome. Clin Genet 77:541, 2010.

de Leeuw N, Bulk S, Green A, et al.: UBE2A deficiency syndrome: Mild to severe intellectual disability accompanied by seizures, absent speech, urogenital, and skin anomalies in male patients. Am J Med Genet 152A:3084, 2010.

Honda S, Orii KO, Kobayashi J, et al.: Novel deletion in Xq24 including the UBE2A gene in a patient with X-linked mental retardation. J Hum Genet 55:244, 2010.

Nascimento RMP, Otto PA, de Brouwer APM, et al.: UBE2A, which encodes a ubiquitin-conjugating enzyme, is mutated in a novel X-linked mental retardation syndrome. Am J Hum Genet 79:549, 2006.

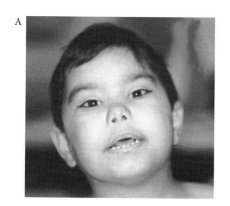
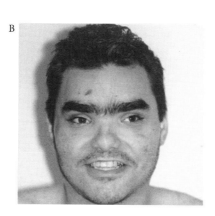
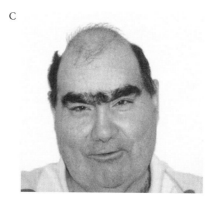

XLID-Nail Dystrophy-Seizures. Five-year-old male with wide face, upslanted palpebral fissures, hypertelorism, low nasal bridge, large mouth, thin lips, and short broad neck **(A)**. Maternal cousin at age 20 years with similar facial findings and dense eyebrows and synophrys **(B)**. Maternal uncle at age 46 years with thick bushy eyebrows and synophrys, upslanted palpebral fissures and thin lips. Courtesy of the *American Journal of Human Genetics*. Copyright 2006, American Society of Human Genetics.

DIFFERENTIAL MATRIX

Syndrome	Distinctive Face	Hair/Cutaneous Abnormalities	Seizures	Comments
XLID-Nail Dystrophy-Seizures	+	+	+	Small penis, dry skin, nail dystrophy
Young-Hughes	+	+	+	Small palpebral fissures, cupped ears, ichthyosiform scaling, short stature, obesity, hypogenitalism
Goltz	+	+	0	Linear areas of dermal aplasia, dystrophic nails, abnormal teeth and hair, vertebral anomalies, limb reduction defects, ocular abnormality, urogenital anomalies
MIDAS	+	+	0	Microphthalmia, ocular dysgenesis, corneal opacification, dermal aplasia, dysgenesis of corpus callosum, cardiac defects, cardiomyopathy, ectodermal dysplasia, ocular anomaly, CNS anomaly
Hereditary Bullous Dystrophy, X-linked	+	+	0	Short stature, microcephaly, cardiac defects, upslanting palpebral fissures, protruding ears, short and tapered digits, bullous dystrophy, small testes, early death from pulmonary infection
Cantu	0	+	+	Microcephaly, short stature, cortical atrophy, follicular keratosis, alopecia
Incontinentia Pigmenti	0	+	+	Cutaneous vesicles, verrucous lesions, and irregular hyperpigmentation, microcephaly, ocular anomalies, oligodontia, abnormally shaped teeth, spasticity, ocular anomalies, dental anomalies

XLID-NYSTAGMUS-SEIZURES

(XLID-MICROCEPHALY WITH PONTINE AND CEREBELLAR HYPOPLASIA)

OMIM 300749

Xp11.4

CASK

Definition. XLID of variable severity associated with nystagmus, abnormal growth, and seizures.

Somatic Features. No consistent craniofacial abnormalities have been noted. Several individuals have had microcephaly or macrocephaly, but the head size is usually within the normal range. Synophrys, upslanting palpebral fissures, and wide mouth have been reported.

Growth and Development. Measures of prenatal growth have not been reported. In adulthood, short stature occurs in less than half of patients.

Cognitive Function. Mild intellectual disability is the rule, although more severe impairment has been noted, particularly in those patients with microcephaly.

Neurological Findings. Ocular manifestations in the form of nystagmus, strabismus, and reduced visual acuity are present in about half of patients. Unsteady gait, tremor, and seizures occur less frequently.

Heterozygote Expression. It is not uncommon for carrier females to be affected with mild intellectual disability, nystagmus, and tremor.

Imaging. Cerebellar and midbrain hypoplasia, dysgenesis of the corpus callosum, and pachygyria have been described in several individuals.

Comment. There appears to be no mandatory or consistently occurring manifestations other than intellectual disability. Yet, the abnormalities in growth parameters and neurological function preclude designation as Nonsyndromal XLID. Although nystagmus occurs in several XLID syndromes with impaired vision, it may be a helpful finding, present in about half of cases.

REFERENCES

Hackett A, Tarpey PS, Licata A, et al.: CASK mutations are frequent in males and cause X-linked nystagmus and variable XLMR phenotypes. Eur J Hum Genet 18:544, 2010.

Hayashi S, Mizuno S, Migita O, et al.: The CASK gene harbored in a deletion detected by array-CGH as a potential candidate for a gene causative of X-linked dominant mental retardation. Am J Med Genet A 146A:2145, 2008.

Najm J, Horn D, Wimplinger I, et al.: Mutations of CASK cause an X-linked brain malformation phenotype with microcephaly and hypoplasia of the brainstem and cerebellum. Nat Genet 40:1065, 2008.

Takanashi J, Arai H, Nabatame S, et al.: Neuroradiologic features of CASK mutations. AJNR Am J Neuroradiol 31:1619, 2010.

Syndrome	Nystagmus	Cerebellar and Midbrain Hypoplasia	Seizures	Comments
XLID-Nystagmus-Seizures	+	+	+	Variable head circumference, vision loss, dysgenesis of corpus callosum, neuronal migration disturbance, ataxia
Pelizaeus-Merzbacher	+	+	+	Ataxia, spastic paraplegia, optic atrophy, hypotonia, dystonia, CNS dysmyelination
Pettigrew	+	O	+	Dandy-Walker malformation, microcephaly or hydrocephaly, long face with macrostomia, small testes, contractures, choreoathetosis, cerebellar hypoplasia, spastic paraplegia, iron deposits or calcification of basal ganglia
Cerebro-Oculo-Genital	+	O	+	Microcephaly, hydrocephaly, short stature, agenesis of corpus callosum, microphthalmia, ptosis, hypospadias, cryptorchidism, clubfoot, spasticity, ocular anomaly, genitourinary anomaly
Proud (*ARX*-Associated XLID)	+	O	+	Microcephaly, cryptorchidism, inguinal hernias, ataxia, dysgenesis of corpus callosum, impaired vision and/or hearing, spasticity
Paine	+	O	+	Microcephaly, short stature, optic atrophy, blindness and/or deafness, spasticity

XLID-PANHYPOPITUITARISM

OMIM 312000

Xq27.1

SOX3

Definition. XLID with short stature and hypogenitalism associated with panhypopituitarism. Mutations in *SOX3* have been demonstrated in XLID-Panhypopituitarism and XLID-Isolated Growth Hormone Deficiency.

Somatic Features. Major malformations or craniofacial abnormalities do not occur. The sella turcica is small. Short stature becomes apparent in infancy and, untreated, persists into adult life. Hypogenitalism may be obvious before puberty and thereafter is associated with variable degrees of hypogonadism, including decreased sexual hair and truncal obesity. Some affected males have died during the newborn period, with hypoplasia of the adrenal glands documented at autopsy.

Growth and Development. Intrauterine growth is usually normal, but slowing of bone growth occurs during the first year. Puberty is delayed and virilization is incomplete. Language skills lag behind motor skills.

Cognitive Function. Lower cognitive function than in nonaffected siblings can be expected, but with intellectual disability of mild degree present in a minority.

Heterozygote Expression. None

Laboratory. Growth hormone deficiency consistently occurs. Other endocrine abnormalities are more variable but may include low levels of other pituitary hormones, thyroxine, cortisol, and sex hormones.

Comment. The location of XLID-Panhypopituitarism overlaps the mapping limits of XLID-Isolated Growth Hormone Deficiency, suggesting the possibility that these two XLID syndromes are allelic. This has now been confirmed. Secondary hypothyroidism may contribute, at least in part, to the intellectual disability in XLMR-Panhypopituitarism.

REFERENCES

Hamel BC, Smits AP, Otten BJ, et al.: Familial X-linked mental retardation and isolated growth hormone deficiency: clinical and molecular findings. Am J Med Genet 64:35, 1996.

Lagerström-Fermér M, Sundvall M, Johnsen E, et al.: X-linked recessive panhypopituitarism associated with a regional duplication in Xq25-q26. Am J Hum Genet 60:910, 1997.

Laumonnier F, Ronce N, Hamel BC, et al.: Transcription factor SOX3 is involved in X-linked mental retardation with growth hormone deficiency. Am J Hum Genet 71:1450, 2002.

Phelan PD, Connelly J, Martin FIR, et al.: X-linked recessive hypopituitarism. Birth Defects: Orig Art Ser VII(6):24, 1971.

Woods KS, Cundall M, Turton J, et al.: Over- and underdosage of SOX3 is associated with infundibular hypoplasia and hypopituitarism. Am J Hum Genet 76:833, 2005.

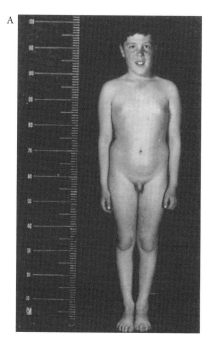
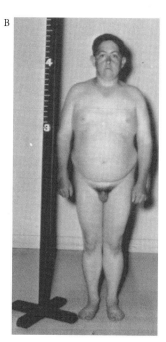

XLID-Panhypopituitarism. Eleven-year-old male with short stature (A); 30-year-old uncle with short stature, obesity, and diminished virilization as manifestation of panhypopituitarism (B). Courtesy of *Birth Defects Original Article Series*. Copyright 1971, March of Dimes National Foundation.

DIFFERENTIAL MATRIX

Syndrome	Short Stature	Hypogenitalism	Obesity	Comments
XLID-Panhypopituitarism	+	+	+	Small sella turcica, deficiency of pituitary, thyroid, adrenal, and gonadal hormones
Börjeson-Forssman-Lehmann	+	+	+	Hypotonia, microcephaly, coarse facies, large ears, gynecomastia, narrow sloped shoulders, visual impairment, tapered digits
Chudley-Lowry	+	+	+	Bitemporal narrowing, almond-shaped eyes, depressed nasal bridge, tented upper lip, open mouth, hypotonia
Urban	+	+	+	Small hands and feet, digital contractures, osteoporosis
Young-Hughes	+	+	+	Small palpebral fissures, cupped ears, ichthyosiform scaling
Vasquez	+	+	+	Microcephaly, gynecomastia, hypotonia
XLID-Hypogonadism-Tremor	+	+	+	Prominent lower lip, muscle wasting of legs, abnormal gait, seizures, tremor
Abidi	+	+	0	Microcephaly, sloping forehead, cupped ears
ATRX-Associated XLID	+	+	0	Microcephaly, telecanthus/hypertelorism, small triangular nose, tented upper lip, open mouth, wide spacing of teeth, minor musculoskeletal anomalies, hypotonia, erythrocyte HbH inclusions in some
Cerebro-Oculo-Genital	+	+	0	Microcephaly, hydrocephaly, agenesis of corpus callosum, microphthalmia, ptosis, hypospadias, cryptorchidism, clubfoot, spasticity
Hereditary Bullous Dystrophy, X-linked	+	+	0	Microcephaly, upslanting palpebral fissures, protruding ears, short and tapered digits, cardiac defects, bullous dystrophy, early death from pulmonary infection
Renpenning	+	+	0	Microcephaly, upslanting palpebral fissures
XLID-Microcephaly-Testicular Failure	+	+	0	Microcephaly, prominent supraorbital ridges, high nasal bridge, prominent nose, macrostomia, hypogonadism
Wilson-Turner	0	+	+	Normal growth, small hands and feet, tapered digits, gynecomastia, hypotonia, emotional lability

XLID-PRECOCIOUS PUBERTY

Hockey (1986) described a normally developing boy with precocious penile and testicular enlargement at age 3 years. The bone age was advanced and testosterone, LH, and FSH rose in response to gonadotropin stimulation. One maternal uncle experienced precocious puberty at age 4 years, showed advanced bone age, and deteriorated in school performance with measured IQs (Binet LM) decreasing from 96 at age 4 years to 59 at age 9.5 years. A second maternal uncle at age 14 years had penile enlargement, Tanner 2 scrotum, and a few pubic hairs. His IQ was 41. It is uncertain when penile enlargement began.

The mother of the first boy was subsequently found to have Prader-Willi syndrome with a deletion of 15p11-q13. The lack of details and molecular studies precludes certainty is assigning this condition XLID status.

REFERENCE

Hockey A: X-linked intellectual handicap and precocious puberty with obesity in carrier females. Am J Med Genet 23:127, 1986.

XLID-PSORIASIS
(TRANEBJAERG SYNDROME I)

OMIM 309480

Definition. XLID with hypertelorism, large ears, macrostomia with arched upper lip, prominent lips, hypotonia, childhood-onset psoriasis, and seizures. The gene has not been mapped.

Somatic Features. Patients have hypotonic facies with hypertelorism, large open mouth and prominent lips, thickening of the alae nasi, and large ears. The nares may be anteverted and the palate high. Skeletal features include horizontal palmar creases, proximally placed thumbs, hyperextensible joints, and fifth-finger clinodactyly. Cryptorchidism may occur. Psoriasis occurs during childhood, affecting the scalp, trunk, elbows, knees, palms, soles, genital area, and popliteal fossas. The cutaneous changes begin as nonspecific and generalized erythroderma or dry scaling skin and progress to typical localized psoriatic plaques.

Growth and Development. Intrauterine and postnatal growth progresses at a normal rate. Marked delay of developmental milestones is evident from infancy.

Cognitive Function. Severe impairment

Neurological Findings. Seizures with onset in early childhood are described.

Heterozygote Expression. None

Laboratory. Skin biopsy shows changes of psoriasis. Normal steroid sulfatase activity has been demonstrated in fibroblasts.

Comment. With the exception of the normal cranial circumference, the craniofacial manifestations resemble those of Alpha-Thalassemia Intellectual Disability. Psoriasis has not been described in any other XLID syndrome.

REFERENCE

Tranebjaerg L, Svejgaard A, Lykkesfeldt G: X-linked mental retardation associated with psoriasis: A new syndrome? Am J Med Genet 30:263, 1988.

A 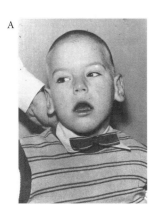 B 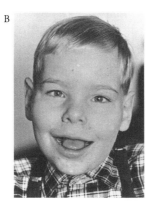 C 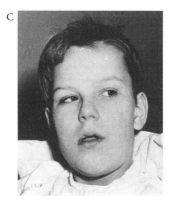 D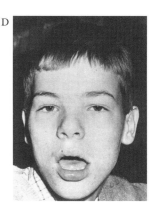

XLID-Psoriasis. Short nose, tented upper lip, prominent ears, and everted lower lip in four affected members of the same family at ages 6, 8, 10, and 14 years. Courtesy of Dr. Lisbeth Tranebjaerg, University Hospital, Tromsø, Norway, and the *American Journal of Medical Genetics*, Copyright 1988, Wiley-Liss, Inc.

Syndrome	Hypotonic Facies	Hypogenitalism	Ectodermal Changes	Comments
XLID-Psoriasis	+	+	+	Hypertelorism, open mouth, large ears, hypotonia, seizures, psoriasis
ATRX-Associated XLID	+	+	0	Microcephaly, short stature, telecanthus/hypertelorism, small triangular nose, tented upper lip, open mouth, wide spacing of teeth, abnormal genitalia, minor musculoskeletal anomalies, hypotonia, erythrocyte HbH inclusions in some
Wittwer	+	+	0	Microcephaly, short stature, microphthalmia, hearing loss, vision loss, hypertelorism, genitourinary anomalies, hypotonia, seizures
Hereditary Bullous Dystrophy, X-linked	0	+	+	Microcephaly, short stature, upslanting palpebral fissures, protruding ears, short and tapered digits, cardiac defects, bullous dystrophy, early death from pulmonary infection

XLID-RETINITIS PIGMENTOSA

(XLID-MICROCEPHALY-RETINITIS PIGMENTOSA SYNDROME)

Definition. XLID with microcephaly and retinitis pigmentosa. The gene has not been localized, although preliminary evidence suggests a location between Xp21 and Xq21.

Somatic Features. Microcephaly, possibly of postnatal onset, occurs as the only consistent nonocular manifestation. Myopia, pigmentary retinopathy, narrowing of the retinal arterioles, choroidal degeneration, and pallid optic discs may be noted in the first two years of life. Nystagmus may be present from infancy. Constricted visual fields, night blindness, and poor vision result from the retinitis pigmentosa. Cataracts may develop in adulthood.

Growth and Development. Growth impairment appears to be a variable component of this syndrome. Low birth weight has been recorded in one case and adult short stature in another.

Cognitive Function. Mild impairment

Neurological Findings. Seizures have occurred in one case. Although poor vision may be apparent from infancy or early childhood, blindness may be delayed until late childhood or early adult life. Nystagmus has occurred in infancy in one case and in later childhood in another.

Heterozygote Expression. Cognitive function is normal, but in early adult life myopia, constricted visual fields, choroidal degeneration, and night blindness may develop.

Laboratory. Electroretinogram and vision-evoked responses are abnormal.

Comment. Two X-linked genes for retinitis pigmentosa have been mapped, *RP2* (OMIM 312600) at Xp11.23 and *RP3* (OMIM 300029) at Xp11.4. The possibility that XLID-Microcephaly-Retinitis Pigmentosa is caused by a deletion of contiguous genes cannot be excluded at present.

REFERENCES

Aldred MA, Dry KL, Knight-Jones EB, et al.: Genetic analysis of a kindred with X-linked mental handicap and retinitis pigmentosa. Am J Hum Genet 55:916, 1994.

Pelletier V, Jambou M, Delphin N, et al.: Comprehensive survey of mutations in RP2 and RPGR in patients affected with distinct retinal dystrophies: genotype-phenotype correlations and impact on genetic counseling. Hum Mutat 28:81, 2007.

Schwahn U, Lenzner S, Dong J, et al.: Positional cloning of the gene for X-linked retinitis pigmentosa 2. Nat Genet 19:327, 1998.

DIFFERENTIAL MATRIX

Syndrome	Microcephaly	Vision Loss	Nystagmus	Comments
XLID-Retinitis Pigmentosa	+	+	+	Bone-spicule-type retinitis pigmentosa
Cerebro-Oculo-Genital	+	+	+	Hydrocephaly, short stature, agenesis of corpus callosum, microphthalmia, ptosis, hypospadias, cryptorchidism, clubfoot, spasticity
Paine	+	+	+	Short stature, optic atrophy, hearing loss, spasticity, seizures
Proud (*ARX*-Associated XLID)	+	+	+	Hearing loss, agenesis of corpus callosum, cryptorchidism, inguinal hernias, ataxia, spasticity, seizures
Gustavson	+	+	0	Short stature, large ears, deafness, joint contractures, rockerbottom feet, brain undergrowth, hydrocephaly, cerebellar hypoplasia, spasticity, seizures
Lenz Microphthalmia	+	+	0	Microphthalmia, ocular dysgenesis, malformed ears, cleft lip/palate, cardiac and genitourinary anomalies, thumb duplication or hypoplasia, narrow shoulders
Schimke	+	+	0	Sunken eyes, downslanting palpebral fissures, narrow nose, wide spacing of teeth, cupped ears, hypotonia, abducens palsy, hearing loss, spasticity, choreoathetosis, contractures
Wittwer	+	+	0	Short stature, microphthalmia, hearing loss, hypertelorism, genitourinary anomalies, hypotonia, seizures
Goldblatt Spastic Paraplegia	0	+	+	Optic atrophy, exotropia, ataxia, spastic paraplegia, dysarthria, muscle hypoplasia, contractures
Lowe	0	+	+	Short stature, cataracts, hypotonia, aminoaciduria, progressive renal failure

XLID-ROLANDIC SEIZURES

OMIM 300643

Xq22.1

SRPX2

Definition. XLID with Rolandic seizures and speech dyspraxia. The gene, *SRPX2*, encodes a sushi-repeat containing protein.

Somatic Features. Craniofacial dysmorphism and malformations do not occur. The presentation is developmental and neurological in nature. Speech development is primarily affected, with males and females showing overall speech delay, oro-facial dyspraxia, impaired comprehension, and inattention. Seizures originate adjacent to the Rolandic or Sylvian fissures and are characterized electroencephalographically by clusters of centrotemporal spikes that are activated during sleep.

Growth and Development. Prenatal and postnatal growth is normal.

Cognitive Function. Cognitive function is variably impaired generally in the mild-to-moderate range.

Heterozygote Expression. Females appear to be affected with equal severity as males.

Comment. XLID-Rolandic Seizures is one of numerous X-linked seizure disorders. Some may be distinguished by somatic manifestations: for example, Armfield, Oral-Facial-Digitial I, Pallister W, Cerebro-Oculo-Genital, Incontinentia Pigmenti, Lowe, Wittwer, Brooks, Gustavson, Cantu, Schimke, Bertini, Christianson, and other syndromes. Others, like XLID-Rolandic Seizures, lack somatic findings that help in clinical diagnosis: Rett, XLID-Epilepsy, West, XIDE, Pyruvate Dehydrogenase Deficiency, and others. The type of seizures may be most helpful in distinguishing those in this latter category.

REFERENCE

Roll P, Rudolf G, Pereira S, et al.: SRPX2 mutations in disorders of language cortex and cognition. Hum Mol Genet 15:1195, 2006.

XLID-SPASTIC PARAPLEGIA, TYPE 7

(X-LINKED SPASTIC PARAPLEGIA)

Xq11.2-q23

Definition. XLID with nystagmus, reduced vision, absent speech and ambulation, bowel and bladder dysfunction, and spastic quadriplegia. The gene has not been identified but is located between markers AR (Xq11.2-q12) and DXS458 (Xq23).

Somatic Features. Malformations or distinctive craniofacial features have not been described.

Growth and Development. Head circumference is normal; details of statural growth are not available. Language and motor milestones are severely delayed from infancy, with failure of speech and independent ambulation.

Cognitive Function. Severe impairment

Neurological Findings. Nystagmus is present for a time but disappears before adolescence. Spasticity, evident during the second 6 months of life, appears first in the lower limbs and progresses to affect all limbs.

Heterozygote Expression. None

Imaging. Not available

Comment. Spastic Paraplegia Type 7 is the most recently described X-linked type. The proteolipid protein gene responsible for the Pelizaeus-Merzbacher type of spastic paraplegia (SPG2) is located within the mapping limits. Extensive search for a mutation in the *PLP1* gene has been negative.

REFERENCES

Saugier-Veber P, Munnich A, Bonneau D, et al.: X-linked spastic paraplegia and Pelizaeus-Merzbacher disease are allelic disorders at the proteolipid protein locus. Nat Genet 6:257, 1994.

Steinmüller R, Lantigua-Cruz A, Garcia-Garcia R, et al.: Evidence of a third locus in X-linked recessive spastic paraplegia. Hum Genet 100:287, 1997.

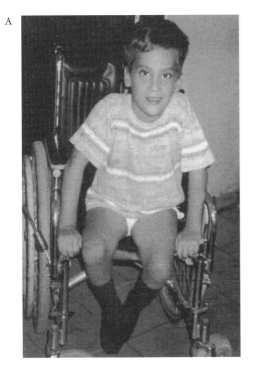
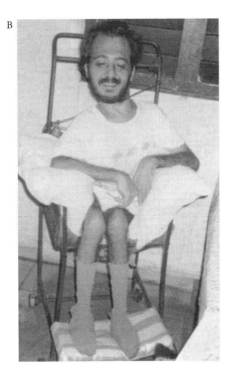

XLID-Spastic Paraplegia, Type 7. Affected males in childhood and adult life showing progressive muscle wasting and spasticity.   Courtesy of Dr. Ulrich Müller, Universität Giessen, Giessen, Germany.

Syndrome	Spasticity	Impaired Vision	Absent Ambulation	Comments
XLID-Spastic Paraplegia, type 7	+	+	+	Nystagmus, absent speech, bowel and bladder dysfunction
Cerebro-Oculo-Genital	+	+	+	Microcephaly, hydrocephaly, short stature, agenesis of corpus callosum, microphthalmia, ptosis, hypospadias, cryptorchidism, clubfoot
Goldblatt Spastic Paraplegia	+	+	+	Optic atrophy, exotropia, nystagmus, ataxia, dysarthria, muscle hypoplasia, contractures
Gustavson	+	+	+	Microcephaly, short stature, optic atrophy with blindness, large ears, deafness, joint contractures, rockerbottom feet, brain undergrowth, hydrocephaly, cerebellar hypoplasia, seizures
Paine	+	+	+	Microcephaly, short stature, optic atrophy, hearing loss, seizures
Ataxia-Deafness-Dementia, X-linked	+	+	+	Optic atrophy, ataxia, hypotonia, seizures, childhood death
XLID-Blindness-Seizures-Spasticity	+	+	+	Poor growth, postnatal microcephaly, clubfoot, seizures, contractures, scoliosis, hypomyelination
Pelizaeus-Merzbacher	+	+	0	Optic atrophy, nystagmus, hypotonia, ataxia, dystonia, CNS dysmyelination
Apak Ataxia-Spastic Diplegia	+	0	+	Short stature, clubfoot, muscle hypoplasia, ataxia

XLID-SPASTIC PARAPLEGIA-ATHETOSIS
(BAAR-GABRIEL SYNDROME)

OMIM 312890

Definition. XLID with spastic paraplegia, weakness, dysarthria, and nystagmus. A gene locus has not been mapped.

Somatic Features. No distinctive facial features or major malformations occur. Facial muscles show very little movement. Positional abnormalities of the limbs may be present at birth. Wasting, contractures and kyphoscoliosis accompany the neurological abnormalities.

Growth and Development. Prenatal growth is normal or nearly so. Speech development may appear at the normal time but is slurred. Weakness, wasting, and contractures prevent normal ambulation.

Cognitive Function. Considerable variability of cognitive function, both intra- and interfamilial, has been observed. Severe impairment, however, is the rule.

Neurological Findings. Neurological signs dominate the clinical picture from early in childhood. Spastic tetraparesis with greater involvement of the lower limbs is typical. Muscle tone and deep tendon reflexes are increased and Babinski signs present. Secondary muscle wasting, weakness, and kyphoscoliosis may occur. Cerebellar signs include nystagmus, unsteadiness, and dysmetria of the upper limbs. Athetoid movements of the upper limbs occur as well. Speech is dysarthric, gag reflex is exaggerated, and tongue movements spastic. Even among infants whose limbs appear spared at birth, nystagmus or unsteadiness of gaze indicates involvement.

Heterozygote Expression. None

Imaging. Not available

Comment. The X-linked spastic paraplegias with intellectual disability are a large and heterogeneous group. Two major types – Complicated Spastic Paraplegia 1 and Complicated Spastic Paraplegia 2 – have been mapped and the genes, L1 cell adhesion molecule (*L1CAM*) and proteolipid protein (*PLP1*), cloned. SPG1 is allelic to X-Linked Hydrocephaly-MASA Spectrum and SPG2 to Pelizaeus-Merzbacher Syndrome. XLID-Spastic Paraplegia-Athetosis may, in fact, be allelic to one of these syndromes. The numerous additional XLID syndromes with spastic paraplegia as a prominent finding include Allan-Herndon-Dudley, Apak, Lesch-Nyhan, Mohr-Tranebjaerg, Pettigrew, and many others. X-linked spastic paraplegias without intellectual disability may represent separate or allelic disorders (e.g., the condition reported by Johnston and McKusick [1962] and updated by Thurmon et al. [1971] and Zatz et al. [1976] is caused by a mutation in *PLP1*).

REFERENCES

Baar HS, Gabriel AM: Sex-linked spastic paraplegia. Am J Ment Defic 71:13 1966.

Bundy S, Griffiths MT: Recurrence risks in families of children with symmetrical spasticity. Dev Med Child Neurol 19:179, 1977.

Haldane JBS: The partial sex-linkage of recessive spastic paraplegia. J Genet 41:141, 1941.

Johnston AW, McKusick VA: A sex-linked recessive form of spastic paraplegia. Am J Human Genet 14:83, 1962.

Paskind HA, Stone TT: Familial spastic paralysis. Arch Neuro Psychia 30:481, 1933.

Thurmon TF, Walker BA, Scott CI, et al.: Two kindreds with a sex-linked recessive form of spastic paraplegia. Birth Defects: Orig Art Ser VII(1):219, 1971.

Zatz M, Penha-Serrano C, Otto PA: X-linked recessive type of pure spastic paraplegia in a large pedigree: absence of detectable linkage with Xq. J Med Genet 13:217, 1976.

DIFFERENTIAL MATRIX

Syndrome	Spasticity	Cerebellar Signs	Seizures	Comments
XLID-Spastic Paraplegia-Athetosis	+	+	+	Nystagmus, weakness, dysarthria, spastic paraplegia, muscle wasting, contractures
Christianson	+	+	+	Short stature, microcephaly, general asthenia, contractures, ophthalmoplegia
Goldblatt Spastic Paraplegia	+	+	+	Optic atrophy, exotropia, nystagmus, ataxia, spastic paraplegia, dysarthria, muscle hypoplasia, contractures
Gustavson	+	+	+	Microcephaly, short stature, optic atrophy with blindness, large ears, deafness, joint contractures, rockerbottom feet, brain undergrowth, hydrocephaly, cerebellar hypoplasia
Paine	+	+	+	Microcephaly, short stature, optic atrophy, vision and hearing loss
Pelizaeus-Merzbacher	+	+	+	Optic atrophy, nystagmus, hypotonia, ataxia, dystonia, CNS dysmyelination
Pettigrew	+	+	+	Dandy-Walker malformation, microcephaly or hydrocephaly, long face with macrostomia and prognathism, small testes, contractures, choreoathetosis, iron deposits in basal ganglia
Ataxia-Deafness-Dementia, X-linked	+	+	+	Optic atrophy, vision loss, hearing loss, ataxia, hypotonia, childhood death
Apak Ataxia-Spastic Diplegia	+	+	0	Short stature, clubfoot, muscle hypoplasia, ataxia
Cerebro-Oculo-Genital	+	+	0	Microcephaly, hydrocephaly, short stature, agenesis of corpus callosum, microphthalmia, ptosis, hypospadias, cryptorchidism, clubfoot
Mohr-Tranebjaerg	+	+	0	Hearing loss, vision loss, neurological deterioration with childhood onset, dystonia
Schimke	+	+	0	Microcephaly, sunken eyes, downslanting palpebral fissures, narrow nose, wide spacing of teeth, cupped ears, hypotonia, choreo-athetosis, contractures
Bertini	0	+	+	Macular degeneration, hypotonia, ataxia, childhood death, hypoplasia of cerebellar vermis and corpus callosum, developmental delays and regression, postnatal growth impairment
Cerebro-Cerebello-Coloboma	0	+	+	Hydrocephaly, cerebellar vermis hypoplasia, retinal coloboma, hypotonia, abnormal respiratory pattern

XLID-SPONDYLOEPIMETAPHYSEAL DYSPLASIA

OMIM 300232

Bieganski and associates (1999) reported three males with a diffuse spondyloepimetaphyseal dysplasia and progressive intellectual disability making its appearance in the second half of infancy. After normal pregnancy, delivery, and initial months of development, these boys developed facial coarsening, chest deformation, slowing of developmental progress, and progressive skeletal deformation. Radiographs showed widespread dysplasia of the spine, epiphyses, and metaphyses. Both the skeletal dysplasia and

mental deterioration appeared relentless. No molecular studies were performed. Cranial imaging demonstrated a small corpus callosum, delayed myelination, and cerebral atrophy.

REFERENCE

Bieganski T, Dawydzik B, Kozlowski K: Spondylo-epimetaphyseal dysplasia: a new X-linked variant with mental retardation. Eur J Pediatr 158:809, 1999.

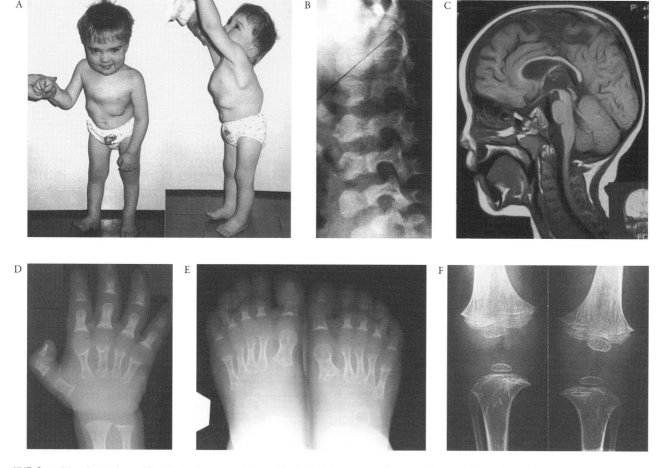

XLID-Spondyloepimetaphyseal Dysplasia. Four-year-old boy with short stature, square face, prominent eyebrows, hypertelorism, depressed nasal bridge, broad nose, short trunk, deformed chest, and short broad hands and feet (**A**). Lumbar spine at age 18 months showing hexagonal vertebral bodies (**B**). MRI at age 5 years showing increased subarachnoid space, thin corpus callosum, and delayed myelination (**C**). Hand at age 18 months showing short metacarpals and phalanges with cupped metaphyses and thin cortices and delayed bone age (**D**), and similar findings in bones of feet (**E**). Knees at age 30 months showing widened femoral metaphyses, small epiphyses, and asymmetric widening of tibial metaphyses (**F**). Courtesy of Dr. Tadeusz Bieganski, Polish Mother's Memorial Hospital, Research Institute, Lodz.

DIFFERENTIAL MATRIX

Syndrome	Coarse Facies	Chest Deformation	Skeletal Dysplasia	Comments
XLID-Spondyloepi-metaphyseal Dysplasia	+	+	+	Small corpus callosum, cerebral atrophy
Mucopolysaccharidosis IIA	+	0	+	Short stature, hepatosplenomegaly, hernias, joint stiffness, thick skin, hirsutism, macrocephaly, behavioral aberrations

XLID-THYROID APLASIA-CUTIS VERTICIS GYRATA

(ÅKESSON SYNDROME)

OMIM 304200

Åkesson (1965) reported a single case with short stature, cutis gyrata over the vertex of the scalp, signs of myxedema, diastasis rectus, ulnar deviation of the hands, and severe intellectual disability with aphasia. The head circumference was normal. Autopsy showed thyroid aplasia and no gross brain abnormalities. Four other males in two generations were intellectually disabled by history, but it is not known whether they had cretinism or cutis gyrata of the scalp.

REFERENCE

Åkesson HO: Cutis verticis gyrata thyroaplasia and mental deficiency. Acta Genet Med Gem 14:200, 1965.

XLID WITH THYROXINE-BINDING GLOBULIN DEFICIENCY
(TBG DEFICIENCY-INTELLECTUAL DISABILITY)

OMIM 314200

Xq22.3

Definition. XLID with thyroxine-binding globulin deficiency.

Somatic Features. No consistent somatic manifestations have been reported among males with TBG deficiency and intellectual disability. Individual cases have had short stature, muscular build, hypertelorism, high palate, seizures, conductive hearing loss, and ataxic gait.

Growth and Development. If prenatal growth impairment occurs, it is mild. In some cases, postnatal stature has been normal; in others, it has been significantly shortened. Developmental milestones lag from the outset, with speech delay being more severe than motor delay.

Cognitive Function. Moderate impairment

Heterozygote Expression. Carrier females may have low thyroxine-binding capacity but have normal growth and cognitive function.

Laboratory. Growth hormone, adrenal steroids, and glucose metabolism are normal. Serum thyroxine is low, and TBG is low or absent. Delayed bone age may be found in patients with short stature.

Comment. Thyroxine-binding globulin is the major serum binding protein for triiodothyronine (T_3) and thyroxine (T_4). When absent or deficient, serum total T_3 and T_4 may be low, whereas free T_3 and T_4 may be elevated. Patients with TBG deficiency are generally euthyroid and do not have intellectual or neurological impairments. For this reason, it might be suspected that XLID associated with TBG deficiency is caused by a contiguous gene deletion rather than by a mutation of the *TBG* gene.

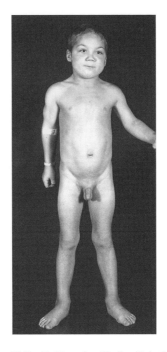

XLID with Thyroxine-Binding Globulin Deficiency. Short stature, hypertelorism, and muscular build in a 7-year-old male with TBG deficiency.   Courtesy of Dr. Theodore AvRuskin, Brookdale Hospital Medical Center, Brooklyn, New York.

REFERENCE

AvRuskin TW, Braverman LE, Crigler JF: Thyroxine-binding globulin deficiency and associated neurological deficit. Pediatrics 50:638, 1972.

YOUNG-HUGHES SYNDROME

Definition. XLID with short stature, obesity, hypergonadotropic hypogonadism, chronic dermatitis, strabismus, and seizures. The gene has not been localized.

Somatic Features. The facies show short palpebral fissures, strabismus, and low-set and cupped ears. Optic nerve hypoplasia, nystagmus, and myopia may be present. Short stature, obesity, underdevelopment of the genitalia, and scant sexual hair dominate the phenotype. The skin is chronically and variably affected with dryness, atopia, ichthyosiform scaling, and excoriation. Generalized seizures appear common. The voice is high-pitched.

Growth and Development. Low birth weight is followed by short stature and obesity during childhood and beyond. Developmental milestones are globally delayed. Speech development appears more delayed than motor development.

Cognitive Features. Severe cognitive impairment with IQ measurements below 30.

Behavior. All affected males have been good-natured, gentle, and affectionate.

Neurological Findings. No neurologic manifestations except seizures have been noted.

Heterozygote Expression. Carrier females have normal intelligence and normal stature and exhibit none of the somatic features seen in affected males.

Laboratory. Low testosterone, elevated gonadotropins, and normal steroid sulfatase.

Comment. Short stature and obesity commonly accompany XLID syndromes with hypogonadism. The type of hypogonadism, severity of cognitive impairment, and association with other somatic or neurological manifestations are useful in discriminating these syndromes. The underlying gene has been identified in Börjeson-Forssman-Lehmann and MEHMO syndromes, but not so for Urban and Vasquez syndromes.

REFERENCE

Young ID, Hughes HE: Sex-linked mental retardation, short stature, obesity and hypogonadism: report of a family. J Ment Defic Res 26:153, 1982.

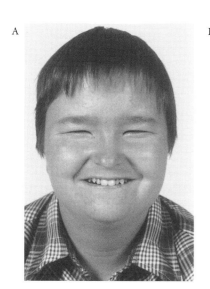 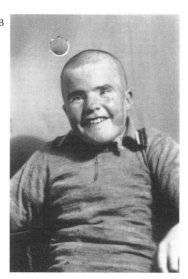 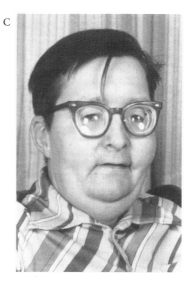

Young-Hughes Syndrome. Short stature, obesity, and narrow palpebral fissures in an adolescent at age 16 years (A); narrow palpebral fissures and strabismus in a 25-year-old maternal great-uncle (B); rounded face with obesity in a 45-year-old maternal cousin (C).   Courtesy of Dr. Ian Young, Centre for Medical Genetics, Nottingham, United Kingdom, and Dr. Helen Hughes, University Hospital of Wales, Cardiff.

DIFFERENTIAL MATRIX

Syndrome	Short Stature	Obesity	Hypogenitalism	Comments
Young-Hughes	+	+	+	Small palpebral fissures, cupped ears, ichthyosiform scaling
Börjeson-Forssman-Lehmann	+	+	+	Hypotonia, hypogonadism, microcephaly, coarse facies, large ears, gynecomastia, narrow sloped shoulders, visual impairment, tapered digits
MEHMO	+	+	+	Hypotonia, microcephaly, edematous hands and feet, equinovarus deformity, seizures, early childhood death
Urban	+	+	+	Small hands and feet, digital contractures, osteoporosis
Vasquez	+	+	+	Microcephaly, gynecomastia, hypotonia
ATRX-Associated XLID	+	0	+	Microcephaly, telecanthus/hypertelorism, small triangular nose, tented upper lip, open mouth, wide spacing of teeth, abnormal genitalia, minor musculoskeletal anomalies, hypotonia, erythrocyte HbH inclusions in some
Cerebro-Oculo-Genital	+	0	+	Microcephaly, hydrocephaly, agenesis of corpus callosum, microphthalmia, ptosis, hypospadias, cryptorchidism, clubfoot, spasticity
Hereditary Bullous Dystrophy, X-linked	+	0	+	Microcephaly, upslanting palpebral fissures, protruding ears, short and tapered digits, cardiac defects, bullous dystrophy, early death from pulmonary infection
Renpenning	+	0	+	Microcephaly, upslanting palpebral fissures
Wilson-Turner	0	+	+	Normal growth, small hands and feet, tapered digits, gynecomastia, hypotonia, emotional lability

APPENDIX I

GENES INVOLVED IN X-LINKED INTELLECTUAL DISABILITY (BY ORDER OF DISCOVERY)

Year	Gene Name	Gene Symbol	XLID Entity	Function	How Found
1983	Hypoxanthine guanine phosphoribosyl transferase	HPRT	Lesch-Nyhan	Enzyme	Met-Fu
1983	Phosphoglycerokinase 1	PGK1	Phosphoglycerokinase Deficiency	Enzyme	Met-Fu
1985	Proteolipid protein	PLP1	PMP, SPG1	Myelination	Mol-Fu
1986	Ornithine transcarbamoylase	OTC	Ornithine Transcarbamoylase Deficiency	Enzyme	Met-Fu
1987	Dystrophin	DMD	Duchenne Muscular Dystrophy	Structure of skeletal muscle membrane	Chr-rea
1989	Pyruvate dehydrogenase	PDHA1	Pyruvate Dehydrogenase Deficiency	Enzyme	Met-Fu
1990	Iduronate sulfatase	IDS	Hunter	Lysosomal enzyme	Met-Fu
1991	Fragile X mental retardation 1	FMR1	Fragile X	RNA-binding protein, gene regulation	Chr-rea L-can
1992	Cell adhesion molecule, L1	L1CAM	Hydrocephaly-MASA, SPG2, XL-ACC	Neuronal migration, cell adhesion	L-can
1992	Norrie	NDP	Norrie	Neuroectodermal cell interaction	Chr-rea
1992	Oculorenal	OCRL1	Lowe	Enzyme	Chr-rea
1993	Adrenoleukodystrophy protein	ABCD1 (ALDP)	Adrenoleukodystrophy	Peroxisomal transport protein	L-can
1993	Copper transporting ATPase 7A	ATP7A	Menkes, Occipital Horn	Copper transport	Chr-rea
1993	Monoamine oxidase A	MAOA	Monoamine Oxidase A Deficiency	Enzyme	L-can
1995	X-linked nuclear protein, X-linked helicase 2	ATRX (XNP, XH2)	Alpha-Thalassemia Intellectual Disability, Carpenter-Waziri, Chudley-Lowry, Holmes-Gang, XLID-Hypotonic Facies, XLID-Spastic Paraplegia, XLID-Arch Fingerprints-Hypotonia	Transcription factor, helicase activities	L-can
1996	Dystonia-deafness peptide	TIMM8A (DDP)	Mohr-Tranebjaerg, Jensen	Transcription factor	L-can
1996	Faciogenital dysplasia	FGD1 (FGDY)	Aarskog-Scott	Guanine nucleotide exchange factor	Chr-rea

(continued)

Year	Gene Name	Gene Symbol	XLID Entity	Function	How Found
1996	Fragile X mental retardation 2	AFF2 (FMR2)	Fragile XE	Unknown	Chr-rea
1996	Glycerol kinase deficiency	GKD	Glycerol Kinase Deficiency	Metabolism, glycerol uptake	Met-Fu
1996	Glypican 3	GPC3	Simpson-Golabi-Behmel	Cell adhesion, motility	L-can
1996	Myotubularin	MTM1	Myotubular Myopathy	Tyrosine phosphatase	L-can
1997	Midline 1	MID1	Telecanthus-Hypospadias, Opitz G/BBB	Zinc finger gene	L-can, Chr-rea
1997	Rab GDP-dissociation inhibitor 1	GDI1	MRX41, 48	Stabilizes GDP bound conformations	L-can
1997	Threonine-serine kinase 2	RPS6KA3 (RSK2)	Coffin-Lowry, MRX19	Kinase signaling pathway	L-can
1998	Doublecortin	DCX	Lissencephaly, X-linked	Neuronal migration	Chr-rea (del)
1998	Dyskerin	DKC1	Dyskeratosis Congenita	Cell cycle and nucleolar functions	L-can
1998	Filamin 1	FLNA (FLN1)	Periventricular Heterotopias, OPD I, OPD II	Actin-binding protein	L-can
1998	Oligophrenin 1	OPHN1	MRX60	GTPase activating protein	L-can
1998	P21-activated kinase	PAK3	MRX30, 47	Rac/Cdc 42 effector	Chr-rea
1999	IL-1 receptor accessory protein-like	IL1RAPL	MRX21	Unknown	Chr-rea
2000	Lysosomal-associated membrane protein 2	LAMP2	Danon Cardiomyopathy	Membrane, lysosome	L-can
2000	NF-$_\kappa$B essential modulator	NEMO (IKB6KG)	Incontinentia Pigmenti	Activates the transcription factor NF-$_\kappa$B	L-can
2000	Rho guanine nucleotide exchange factor 6	ARHGEF6 (α-PIX)	MRX46	Effector of the rho GTPases	Chr-rea
2000	Transmembrane 4 superfamily member 2	TM4SF2	MRX58	Interacts with integrins	Chr-rea
2001	Creatine transporter	SLC6A8	XLID with Seizures	Creatine transporter	Met-Fu
2001	Methyl-CpG binding protein 2	MECP2	Rett, MRX16, 79	Binds methylated CpGs	L-can
2001	Oral-facial-digital syndrome 1	OFD1	Oral-Facial-Digital I	Unknown	L-can
2002	Angiotensin-II receptor type 2	AGTR2	Optic Atrophy, X-linked, MRX	Angiotensin II receptor	Chr-rea
2002	Aristaless-related X chromosome gene	ARX	Hydranencephaly, Partington, Proud, West, Lissencephaly and Abnormal Genitalia, X-linked, MRX29, 32, 33, 36, 43, 54, 76	Neuronal migration	Chr-rea (del)
2002	Fatty acid acyl CoA synthetase type 4	ACSL4 (FACL4)	MRX63, 68	Fatty acid CoA ligase 4	Chr-rea (del)
2002	Kruppel-like factor 8	KLF8 (ZNF741)	MRX		Chr-rea

(*continued*)

Year	Gene Name	Gene Symbol	XLID Entity	Function	How Found
2002	PHD-like zinc finger gene 6	PHF6	Börjeson-Forssman-Lehmann	Unknown	L-can
2002	Serine-threonine kinase 9	CDKL5 (STK9)	Rett-Like Seizures-Hypotonia	Unknown	Chr-rea
2002	SRY-box 3	SOX3	XLID-Growth Hormone Deficiency	Pituitary function, transcription factor	Chr-rea, L-can
2003	Immunoglobulin-binding protein 1	IGBP1	Graham Coloboma		L-can
2003	Nance-Horan syndrome gene	NHS	Nance-Horan	-	L-can
2003	Neuroligin 3	NLGN3	Autism	Cell adhesion	L-can
2003	Neuroligin 4	NLGN4	Autism	Cell adhesion	L-can
2003	Polyglutamine tract binding protein 1	PQBP1	Renpenning, Sutherland-Haan, Hamel Cerebro-Palato-Cardiac, Golabi-Ito-Hall, Porteous, MRX55	Polyglutamine binding, regulates transcription	L-can
2003	Spermine synthase	SMS	Snyder-Robinson	Synthesis of spermine	L-can
2003	Zinc finger 41	ZNF41	MRX	Zinger finger	Chr-rea
2003	Zinc finger 81	ZNF81	MRX45	Zinc finger	Chr-rea
2004	BCL6 corepressor	BCOR	Lenz Microphthalmia (1 type)	Histone/protein deacetylation	L-can
2004	Jumonji, AT-rich interactive domain 1C	KDM5C (JARID1C, SMX)	MRX	Regulates transcription, chromatin remodelling	L-can
2004	K1AA1202 protein	SHROOM4 (KIAA1202)	Stoccos dos Santos	Roles in cellular architecture, neurulation, and ion channel function	Chr-rea
2004	KIAA2022 protein	KIAA2022	Cantagrel Spastic Paraplegia	DNA synthesis, DNA polymerase activity	Chr-rea
2004	Methyl transferase	FTSJ1	MRX9	Methylase	L-can
2004	Neuroendocrine DLG	DLG3	MRX	NMDA-receptor, mediated signaling, synaptic plasticity	X seq
2004	PFD finger protein 8	PHF8	XLID-Cleft Lip-Cleft Palate	Regulates transcription, binds DNA	L-can
2004	Renin receptor	ATP6AP2 (ATP6A8–9)	XLID-Infantile Epilepsy	Renin receptor	L-can
2004	Rho guanine nucleotide exchange factor 9	ARHGEF9	XLID-Hypotonia-Seizures	Regulation of Rho protein signal transduction	Chr-rea
2004	Synapsin 1	SYN1	Epilepsy-Macrocephaly	Synaptic vesicle protein	L-can
2004	T3 transporter	SLC16A2 (MCT8)	Allan-Herndon-Dudley	T3 receptor	L-can
2005	Zinc finger DHHC domain-containing protein 15	ZDHHC15	MRX91		Chr-rea

(continued)

Year	Gene Name	Gene Symbol	XLID Entity	Function	How Found
2006	Fanconi anemia complementation group B protein	FANCB	VACTERL-Hydrocephaly	DNA repair	Mol-Fu
2006	Holocytochrome C synthase	HCCS	MIDAS	Energy production, cytochrome homolyase	Chr-rea (del)
2006	Sigma 2 subunit of adaptor protein/complex	AP1S2	Turner XLID, Hydrocephaly-Basal Ganglia Calcification	Assembly of endocytic vesicles	X-seq
2006	SMC1 structural maintenance of chromosomes 1-like	SMC1A/ SMC1L1	Cornelia de Lange, X-linked	Cell cycle, mitotic spindle organization and biogenesis, chromosome segregation	Mol-Fu
2006	Sushi repeat containing protein, X-linked	SRPX2	XLID-Rolandic Seizures	Signal transduction, growth factor 2	Mol-Fu
2006	Ubiquitin-conjugating enzyme E2A	UBE2A	XLID-Nail Dystrophy-Seizures	Ubiquitin cycle, ubiquitin-protein ligase	L-can
2006	Zinc finger protein 674*	ZNF674	XLID-Retinal Dystrophy-Short Stature and MRX92	Transcription regulation	Chr-rea (del)
2007	Bromodomain and WD repeat domain-containing protein 3	BRWD3	XLID-Macrocephaly-Large Ears	Transcription factor	X-seq
2007	Cullin 4B	CUL4B	XLID-Hypogonadism-Tremor	Cell cycle, ubiquitin cycle, E3 ubiquitin ligase	X-seq
2007	Drosophila porcupine homolog	PORCN	Goltz	Wnt receptor signaling pathway, acyltransferase activity, integral to membrane of endoplasmic reticulum	Chr-rea (del)
2007	Glutamate receptor ionotropic AMPA 3	GRIA3	Chiyonobu XLID	Signal transduction, ion transport, glutamate signaling pathway	Chr-rea, Exp-Arr, X seq
2007	Hydroxyacyl-coenzyme A dehydrogenase, type III	HSD17B10 (HADH2)	XLID-Choreoathetosis	Lipid metabolism	L-can
2007	Mediator of RNA polymerase II transcription, subunit 12	MED12 (HOPA)	Opitz FG, Lujan	Transcription regulation, RNA polymerase II transcription mediator activity, ligand-dependent nuclear receptor transcription coactivator activity, vitamin D receptor and thyroid hormone receptor binding	L-can
2007	NADH dehydrogenase (ubiquinone) 1 alpha subcomplex	NDUFA1	Mitochondrial Complex 1 Deficiency	Energy production, oxidoreductase activity	Mol-Fu
2007	Nuclear RNA export factor 5	NXF5	XLID-Short Stature-Muscle Wasting	mRNA processing, mRNA export from nucleus	Chr-rea

(continued)

Year	Gene Name	Gene Symbol	XLID Entity	Function	How Found
2007	Phosphoribosyl pyrophosphate synthetase 1	PRPS1	Arts, PRPS1 Superactivity	Ribonucleotide monophosphate biosynthesis	L-can
2007	Ribosomal protein L10	RPL10	Autism	Protein synthesis, ribosomal protein	X seq
2007	UPF3 regulator of nonsense transcript homolog B	UPF3B	MRX, Lujan/FG Phenotype	mRNA catabolism, nonsense-mediated decay	X-seq
2007	Zinc finger, DHHC-domain containing protein 9	ZDHHC9	XLID-Macrocephaly-Marfanoid Habitus	?	X-seq
2008	E3 ubiquitin-protein ligase	HUWE1	MRX, XLID-Macrocephaly, Juberg-Marsidi-Brooks	Ubiquitin-protein ligase, mRNA transport	M-CGH
2008	Protocadherin 19	PCDH19	Epilepsy-Intellectual Disability Limited to Females		L-can
2008	Sodium-hydrogen exchanger NHE6	SLC9A6	Christianson, X-linked Angelman-like	Sodium-hydrogen antiporter activity, lysosome organization and biogenesis, regulation of endosome volume	L-can
2009	Magnesium transporter 1	MAGT1			
2009	Intramembrane zinc metalloprotease	MBTPS2	Ichthyosis Follicularis, Atrichia, Photophobia (IFAP)	Protease activity, activates signaling proteins	L-can
2009	NAD(P)H steroid dehydrogenase-like	NSDHL	CK (microcephaly, pachygyria, facial dysmorphism, seizures), also in CHILD syndrome	Sterol metabolism	L-can
2010	Small GTPase gene	RAB39B	MRX72 and a syndrome with macrocephaly, seizures, and autism	Formation and maintenance of synapse	L-can
2010	Guanine nucleotide exchange factor	IQSEC2	MRX1, MRX18, and other Nonsyndromal XLID	Regulation of vesicular transport and organelle structure	X-seq
2010	Patched domain-containing 1	PTCHD1	Autism-XLID	Transmembrane protein related to hedgehog receptors	Array CGH
2011	Ras-associated protein RAB40A-like	RAB40AL	Martin-Probst	Ras-like GTPase protein	X-seq
2011	RNA-binding motif protein	RBM10	TARP	RNA-binding	X-seq
2011	N-acetyltransferase subunit 10	NAA10	N-Alpha-Acetyltransferase Deficiency	N-terminal acetylation	X-seq
2011	Las1-like protein	LAS1L	Wilson-Turner	Nucleolar protein, cell proliferation and ribosome biogenesis	X-seq
2011	Eukaryotic translation initiation factor 2	EIF2S3	MEHMO	Initiates translation	X-seq

(continued)

Year	Gene Name	Gene Symbol	XLID Entity	Function	How Found
2011	Host cell factor C1	*HCFC1*	MRX3	Cell proliferation	X-seq
2011	THO complex, subunit 2	*THOC2*	MRX12	mRNA transcription or export	X-seq
2011	Chloride channel voltage-gated 4	*CLCN4*	MRX49	Chloride transport	X-seq
2011	Histone deacetylase 8	*HDAC8*	Cornelia de Lange, X-linked	Chromatin cohesion	Mol-Fu

* Association of ZNF674 and XLID considered uncertain.

Chr-rea = chromosome rearrangement

Exp-Arr = expression array

L-can = linkage and candidate gene testing

M-CGH = array-comparative genomic hybridization

Met-Fu = exploitation of metabolic alteration

Mol-Fu = exploitation of molecular finding

X-seq = brute force sequencing

APPENDIX II

XLID SYNDROMES WITH MICROCEPHALY

MICROCEPHALY USUALLY PRESENT

ATRX-Associated XLID [301040, 309580, *ATRX*]

Börjeson-Forssman-Lehmann [301900, *PHF6*]

Branchial Arch, X-linked [301950]

Cantu [308830]

Cerebro-Oculo-Genital

Christianson [300243, *SLC9A6*]

CK [300831, *NSDHL*]

Coffin-Lowry [303600, *RPS6KA3*]

Cornelia de Lange, X-linked [300590, 300269, *SMC1A, HDAC8*]

Craniofacioskeletal [300712]

Giuffrè-Tsukahara [603438]

Goltz [305600, *PORCN*]

Gustavson [309555]

Hereditary Bullous Dystrophy, X-linked [302000]

Juberg-Marsidi-Brooks [300612, *HUWE1*]

Kang

Lenz Microphthalmia [309800]

Lissencephaly, X-linked [300067, *DCX*]

Martin-Probst [300519, *RAB40AL*]

MEHMO [300148, *EIF2S3*]

Menkes [309400, *ATP7A*]

Miles-Carpenter [309605]

Paine [311400]

Pettigrew [304340]

Pyruvate Dehydrogenase Deficiency [312170, *PDHA1*]

Renpenning [309500, *PQBP1*]

Rett [312750, *MECP2*]

Roifman [300258]

Say-Meyer [314320]

Schimke [312840]

Shrimpton [300709]

Smith-Fineman-Myers

Turner XLID (Fried, *AP1S2*-Associated XLID) [300630, *AP1S2*]

Vasquez

Warkany

Wittwer [300421]

XLID-Blindness-Seizures-Spasticity

XLID-Hypospadias

XLID-Microcephaly-Testicular Failure

XLID-Retinitis Pigmentosa

MICROCEPHALY UNCOMMONLY PRESENT

Abidi [300262]

ARX-Associated XLID (*ARX* spectrum) [309510, *ARX*]

Hyde-Forster [300064]

MIDAS [309801, *HCCS*]

Ornithine Transcarbamoylase Deficiency [311250, *OTC*]

Telecanthus-Hypospadias [300000, *MID1*]

APPENDIX III

XLID SYNDROMES WITH MACROCEPHALY

MACROCEPHALY USUALLY PRESENT

Atkin-Flaitz [300431]

Clark-Baraitser [300602]

Fragile X [309550, *FMR1*]

Hydrocephaly-MASA Spectrum (H) [303350, 304100, 307000, *L1CAM*]

Lujan [309520, *MED12*]

Mucopolysaccharidosis IIA [309900, IDS]

Opitz FG [305450, *MED12*]

VACTERL-Hydrocephalus (H) [314390, *FANCB*]

Waisman-Laxova [311510]

XLID-Macrocephaly [300706, *HUWE1*]

XLID-Macrocephaly-Macroorchidism [309530]

MACROCEPHALY UNCOMMONLY PRESENT

AP1S2-Associated XLID (H) [300630, *AP1S2*]

ARX-Associated XLID (H) [309510, *ARX*]

Pettigrew (H) [304340]

Simpson-Golabi-Behmel [312870, *GPC3*]

Snyder-Robinson [309583, *SMS*]

H = hydrocephaly

APPENDIX IV

XLID SYNDROMES WITH OCULAR ANOMALIES AND/OR VISUAL IMPAIRMENT

ABNORMALITIES OF THE LIDS AND OCULAR ADNEXAE

Cantu [308830]

Cerebro-Oculo-Genital

CK [300831, *NSDHL*]

Cornelia de Lange, X-linked [300590, 300269, *SMC1A, HDAC8*]

Dyskeratosis Congenita [305000, *DKC1*]

Graham Anophthalmia [301590]

Hall Orofacial

Hereditary Bullous Dystrophy, X-linked [302000]

Juberg-Marsidi-Brooks [300612, *HUWE1*]

Lenz [309800]

Norrie [310600, *NDP*]

Shashi [300238]

Wieacker-Wolff [314580]

XLID-Nail Dystrophy-Seizures [312180, *UBE2A*]

ORBITAL CYSTS

MIDAS [309801, *HCCS*]

ANOPHTHALMIA/MICROPHTHALMIA

Aicardi [304050]

Ataxia-Deafness-Dementia, X-linked [301790]

Cerebro-Oculo-Genital

Chassaing-Lacombe Chondrodysplasia

Goltz [305600, *PORCN*]

Graham Anophthalmia [301590]

Incontinentia Pigmenti [308310, *IKBKG*]

Lenz [309800]

MIDAS [309801, *HCCS*]

Nance-Horan (O) [302350, *NHS*]

VACTERL-Hydrocephalus [314390, *FANCB*]

COLOBOMAS/RETINAL LACUNAE

Aicardi [304050]

Cerebro-Cerebello-Coloboma

Goltz [305600, *PORCN*]

Graham Coloboma

Lenz [309800]

MIDAS [309801, *HCCS*]

Renpenning (O) [309500, *PQBP1*]

CATARACTS

Armfield [300261]

Cerebro-Oculo-Genital

Goltz [305600, *PORCN*]

Hereditary Bullous Dystrophy, X-linked [302000]

Hypoparathyroidism, X-linked [307700]

Incontinentia Pigmenti [308310, *IKBKG*]

Lenz [309800]

Lowe [309000, *OCRL1*]

MIDAS [309801, *HCCS*]

Nance-Horan [302350, *NHS*]

(*continued*)

Norrie [310600, *NDP*]

Shashi [300238]

OPTIC ATROPHY

Aicardi [304050]

Arts [301835, *PRPS1*]

Ataxia-Deafness-Dementia, X-linked [301790]

Cerebro-Oculo-Genital

Goldblatt [312920]

Goltz [305600, *PORCN*]

Gustavson [309555]

Incontinentia Pigmenti [308310, *IKBKG*]

Mohr-Tranebjaerg [304700, *TIMM8A*]

Optic Atrophy, X-linked [311050]

Paine [311400]

Pelizaeus-Merzbacher [312080, *PLP1*]

Prieto [309610]

TARP [311900, *RBM10*]

Wittwer (O) [300421]

RETINOPATHY

Cerebro-Oculo-Genital

MIDAS [309801, *HCCS*]

Mohr-Tranebjaerg [304700, *TIMM8A*]

Norrie [310600, *NDP*]

Roifman [300258]

XLID-Choroideremia-Ectodermal Dysplasia [314500]

XLID-Retinitis Pigmentosa

MACULAR DEGENERATION

Bertini

Hereditary Bullous Dystrophy, X-linked [309100]

RETINAL DETACHMENT

Aicardi [304050]

Lenz [309800]

MIDAS [309801, *HCCS*]

OCULAR PALSY

Aicardi [304050]

Ataxia-Deafness-Dementia, X-linked [301790]

Christian [309620]

Christianson [300243, *SLC9A6*]

CK [300831, *NSDHL*]

Schimke [312840]

Wieacker-Wolff [314580]

XLID-Blindness-Seizures-Spasticity

NYSTAGMUS

Aicardi [304050]

Allan-Herndon-Dudley [300523, *SLC16A2*]

Apak

Arts [301835, *PRPS1*]

Cerebro-Oculo-Genital

Goldblatt Spastic Paraplegia [312920]

Incontinentia Pigmenti [308310, *IKBKG*]

Nance-Horan [302350, *NHS*]

Pelizaeus-Merzbacher [312080, *PLP1*]

Proud [300004, *ARX*]

XLID-Choroideremia-Ectodermal-Dysplasia [314500]

XLID-Nystagmus-Seizures [300749, *CASK*]

XLID-Retinitis Pigmentosa

XLID-Spastic Paraplegia, type 7

XLID-Spastic Paraplegia-Athetosis [312890]

(continued)

CORNEAL CLOUDING

Cerebro-Oculo-Genital

MIDAS [309801, *HCCS*]

Wittwer [300421]

DISLOCATED LENS

Lenz [309800]

O – occasionally present

GLAUCOMA

Armfield [300261]

Lowe [309000, *OCRL1*]

MIDAS [309801, *HCCS*]

Nance-Horan (O) [302350, *NHS*]

APPENDIX V

XLID SYNDROMES WITH HEARING LOSS

HEARING LOSS OFTEN PRESENT

Adrenoleukodystrophy [300100, *ABCD1*]

Arts [301835, *PRPS1*]

Ataxia-Deafness-Dementia, X-linked [301790]

Branchial Arch, X-linked [301950]

Charcot-Marie-Tooth, Cowchock Variant [310490]

FLNA-Associated XLID [300077, *FLNA*]

Gustavson [309555]

Juberg-Marsidi-Brooks [300612, *HUWE1*]

Martin-Probst [300519, *RAB40AL*]

Mohr-Tranebjaerg [304700, *TIMM8A*]

Norrie [310600, *NDP*]

Paine [311400]

Schimke [312840]

Wittwer [300421]

HEARING LOSS IN SOME INDIVIDUALS

ARX-Associated XLID [309510, *ARX*]

Coffin-Lowry [303600, *RPS6KA3*]

TARP [311900, *RBM10*]

APPENDIX VI

XLID SYNDROMES WITH FACIAL CLEFTING

FACIAL CLEFTING OFTEN PRESENT

FLNA-Associated XLID (P) [300077, *FLNA*]

TARP (P) [311900, *RBM10*]

Telecanthus-Hypospadias (CL/P) [300000, *MID1*]

FACIAL CLEFTING IN MINORITY OF PATIENTS

Aicardi (CL/P) [304050]

Armfield (P) [300261]

ATRX-Associated XLID (P) [301040, 309580, *ATRX*]

Cerebro-Palato-Cardiac (P) [309500, *PQBP1*]

Cornelia de Lange, X-linked (P) [300590, 300269, *SMC1A, HDAC8*]

Craniofacioskeletal (P) [300712]

Goltz (CL/P) [305600, *PORCN*]

Hall Orofacial (CL/P)

Lenz (CL/P) [309800]

Oral-Facial-Digital I (P) [311200, *CXORF5*]

Pallister W (CL/P) [311450]

Simpson-Golabi-Behmel (P) [312870, *GPC3*]

Snyder-Robinson (P) [309583, *SMS*]

VACTERL-Hydrocephalus (P) [314390, *FANCB*]

XLID-Cleft Lip/Cleft Palate (CL/P) [300263, *PHF8*]

CL = cleft lip; P = palate

APPENDIX VII

XLID SYNDROMES WITH CARDIAC MALFORMATIONS OR OTHER CARDIOVASCULAR ABNORMALITIES

CARDIAC MALFORMATION OFTEN PRESENT

Bergia Cardiomyopathy (CM)

Cerebro-Palato-Cardiac [309500, *PQBP1*]

Craniofacioskeletal (in males) [300712]

MIDAS [309801, *HCCS*]

Myotubular Myopathy (CM) [310400, *MTM1*]

TARP [311900, *RBM10*]

CARDIAC MALFORMATION OR OTHER CARDIOVASCULAR ABNORMALITIES PRESENT IN SOME PATIENTS

ATRX-Associated XLID [301040, 309580, *ATRX*]

Creatine Transporter Deficiency (CM) [300036, *SLC6A8*]

Duchenne Muscular Dystrophy (CM) [310200, *DMD*]

Hereditary Bullous Dystrophy, X-linked [302000]

Lenz Microphthalmia [309800]

Lujan [309520, *MED12*]

Opitz FG [305450, *MED12*]

Renpenning [309500, *PQBP1*]

Simpson-Golabi-Behmel [312870, *GPC3*]

Telecanthus-Hypospadias [300000, *MID1*]

CM = cardiomyopathy

APPENDIX VIII

XLID SYNDROMES WITH UROGENITAL ANOMALIES

Aarskog [305400, *FGD1*]

Abidi [300262]

Ahmad

Armfield [300261]

ARX-Associated XLID [309510, *ARX*]

Atkin-Flaitz [300431]

ATRX-Associated XLID [301040, 309580, *ATRX*]

Börjeson-Forssman-Lehmann [301900, *PHF6*]

Branchial Arch, X-linked [301950]

Cerebro-Oculo-Genital

Clark-Baraitser [300602]

Craniofacioskeletal (in males) [300712]

Dyskeratosis Congenita [305000, *DKC1*]

Fragile X [309550, *FMR1*]

Goltz [305600, *PORCN*]

Hall Orofacial

Hereditary Bullous Dystrophy, X-linked [302000]

Lenz Microphthalmia [309800]

Lissencephaly and Abnormal Genitalia, X-linked [300215, *ARX*]

Lissencephaly, X-linked [300067, *DCX*]

Lujan [309520, *MED12*]

Martin-Probst [300519, *RAB40AL*]

MEHMO [300148, *EIF2S3*]

Myotubular Myopathy [310400, *MTM1*]

Oral-Facial-Digital I [311200, *CXORF5*]

PPM-X [300055, *MECP2*]

Prieto [309610]

Renpenning [309500, *PQBP1*]

Shashi [300238]

Simpson-Golabi-Behmel [312870, *GPC3*]

Telecanthus-Hypospadias [300000, *MID1*]

Urban

VACTERL-Hydrocephalus [314390, *FANCB*]

Vasquez

Wilson-Turner [309585, *LAS1L*]

Wittwer [300421]

XLID-Hypogonadism-Tremor [300354, *CUL4B*]

XLID-Hypospadias

XLID-Macrocephaly-Macroorchidism [309530]

XLID-Microcephaly-Testicular Failure

XLID-Panhypopituitarism [312000]

XLID-Precocious Puberty

Young-Hughes

APPENDIX IX

XLID SYNDROMES WITH NEURONAL MIGRATION DISTURBANCE

Aicardi [304050]

ARX-Associated XLID [309510, *ARX*]

CK [300831, *NSDHL*]

FLNA-Associated XLID [300077, *FLNA*]

Kang

Lissencephaly and Abnormal Genitalia, X-linked [300215, *ARX*]

Lissencephaly, X-linked [300067, *DCX*]

APPENDIX X

XLID SYNDROMES WITH SPASTIC PARAPLEGIA

Adrenoleukodystrophy [300100, *ABCD1*]

Allan-Herndon-Dudley [300523, *SLC16A2*]

AP1S2-Associated XLID [300630, *AP1S2*]

Apak

ARX-Associated XLID [309510, *ARX*]

Ataxia-Deafness-Dementia, X-linked [301790]

ATRX-Associated XLID [301040, 309580, *ATRX*]

Cerebro-Oculo-Genital

Christianson [300243, *SLC9A6*]

Fitzsimmons [309560]

Goldblatt Spastic Paraplegia [312920]

Gustavson [309555]

Hydrocephaly-MASA Spectrum [303350, 304100, 307000, *L1CAM*]

Incontinentia Pigmenti [308310, *IKBKG* (*NEMO*)]

Juberg-Marsidi-Brooks (O) [300612, *HUWE1*]

Kang

Lesch-Nyhan [300322, *HPRT*]

Lissencephaly, X-linked [300067, *DCX*]

Menkes [309400, *ATP7A*]

Miles-Carpenter [309605]

Mohr-Tranebjaerg [304700, *TIMM8A*]

Optic Atrophy, X-linked [311050]

Paine [311400]

Pallister W [311450]

Pelizaeus-Merzbacher [312080, *PLP1*]

Pettigrew [304340]

PPM-X [300055, *MECP2*]

Pyruvate Dehydrogenase Deficiency [312170, *PDHA1*]

Rett [312750, *MECP2*]

Rett-Like Seizures-Hypotonia [300672, *CDKL5*]

Schimke [312840]

Shrimpton (O) [300709]

Smith-Fineman-Myers

Snyder-Robinson (O) [309583, *SMS*]

Sutherland-Haan [309470, *PQBP1*]

Waisman-Laxova [311510]

XLID-Ataxia-Dementia [301840]

XLID-Blindness-Seizures-Spasticity

XLID-Epilepsy (O) [300423, *ATP6AP2*]

XLID-Hydrocephaly-Basal Ganglia Calcifications [300630, *AP1S2*]

XLID-Hypotonia-Recurrent Infections [300260, *dup MECP2*]

XLID-Spastic Paraplegia, Type 7 [312890]

XLID-Spastic Paraplegia-Athetosis [312890]

O = occasional

APPENDIX XI

XLID SYNDROMES WITH SEIZURES

SEIZURES USUALLY PRESENT

Aicardi [304050]

Armfield [300261]

Arts [301835, *PRPS1*]

ARX-Associated XLID [309510, *ARX*]

Ataxia-Deafness-Dementia, X-linked [301790]

Bertini

Börjeson-Forssman-Lehmann [301900, *PHF6*]

Cantu [308830]

Cerebro-Cerebello-Coloboma

Christianson [300243, *SLC9A6*]

CK [300831, *NSDHL*]

Creatine Transporter Deficiency [300036, *SLC6A8*]

Epilepsy-Intellectual Disability in Females [300088, *PCDH19*]

FLNA-Associated XLID [300077, *FLNA*]

Fragile X [309550, *FMR1*]

Gustavson [309555]

Homfray Seizures-Contractures

Hydrocephaly-Cerebellar Agenesis [307010]

Juberg-Marsidi-Brooks [300612, *HUWE1*]

Lissencephaly and Abnormal Genitalia, X-linked [300215, *ARX*]

Lissencephaly, X-linked [300215, *DCX*]

MEHMO [300148, *EIF2S3*]

Menkes [309400, *ATP7A*]

Ornithine Transcarbamoylase Deficiency [311250, *OTC*]

Paine [311400]

Pallister W [311450]

Pettigrew [304340]

Phosphoglycerokinase Deficiency [311800, *PGK1*]

PPM-X [300055, *MECP2*]

Pyruvate Dehydrogenase Deficiency [312170, *PDHA1*]

Rett [312750, *MECP2*]

Rett-Like Seizures-Hypotonia [300672, *CDKL5*]

Say-Meyer [314320]

Shashi [300238]

Smith-Fineman-Myers

Wittwer [300421]

XLID-Blindness-Seizures-Spasticity

XLID-Epilepsy [300423, *ATP6AP2*]

XLID-Hypogonadism-Tremors [300354, *CUL4B*]

XLID-Hypotonia-Recurrent Infections [300260, *dup MECP2*]

XLID-Ichthyosis-Hypogonadism [308200]

XLID-Infantile Spasms [308350, *ARX*]

XLID-Nail Dystrophy-Seizures [312180, *UBE2A*]

XLID-Nystagmus-Seizures [300749, *CASK*]

XLID-Psoriasis [309480]

XLID-Rolandic Seizures [300643, *SRPX2*]

Young-Hughes

SEIZURES IN LESS THAN HALF OF PATIENTS

Allan-Herndon-Dudley [300253, *SLC16A2*]

Atkin-Flaitz [300431]

ATRX-Associated XLID [301040, 309580, *ATRX*]

(continued)

Coffin-Lowry [303600, *RPS6KA3*]

Cornelia de Lange, X-linked [300590, 300269, *SMC1A, HDAC8*]

Hyde-Forster [300064]

Hydrocephaly-MASA Spectrum [303350, 304100, 307000, *L1CAM*]

Incontinentia Pigmenti [308310, *IKBKG*]

Lesch-Nyhan [300322, *HPRT*]

Lujan [309520, *MED12*]

MIDAS [309801, *HCCS*]

Mucopolysaccaridosis IIA [309900, *IDS*]

Opitz FG [305450, *MED12*]

Oral-Facial-Digital I [311200, *CXORF5*]

Pelizaeus-Merzbacher [312080, *PLP1*]

Prieto [309610]

Renpenning [309500, *PQBP1*]

Simpson-Golabi-Behmel [312870, *GPC3*]

Snyder-Robinson [309583, *SMS*]

Vasquez

Waisman-Laxova [311510]

XLID-Ataxia-Apraxia

XLID-Retinitis Pigmentosa

XLID-Thyroxine-Binding Globulin Deficiency [314200]

APPENDIX XII

XLID SYNDROMES WITH HYPOTONIA

Allan-Herndon-Dudley [300523, *SLC16A2 (MCT8)*]

AP1S2-Associated XLID [300630, *AP1S2*]

Arts [310835, *PRPS1*]

Ataxia-Deafness-Dementia, X-linked [301790]

ATRX-Associated XLID [301040, 309580, *ATRX*]

Bertini

Borjeson-Forssman-Lehmann [301900, *PHF6*]

Cerebro-Cerebello-Coloboma [309500, *PQBP1*]

CK [300831, *NSDHL*]

Coffin-Lowry [303600, *RPS6KA3*]

Fragile X [309550, *FMR1*]

Hydrocephaly-Cerebellar Agenesis [307010]

Juberg-Marsidi-Brooks [300612, *HUWE1*]

Lissencephaly and Abnormal Genitalia, X-linked [300315, *ARX*]

Lissencephaly, X-linked [300067, *DCX*]

Lowe [309000, *OCRL1*]

Martin-Probst [300519, *RAB40AL*]

MEHMO [300148, *EIF2S3*]

Myotubular Myopathy [310400, *MTM1*]

N-Alpha Acetyltransferase Deficiency [300013, *NAA10*]

Opitz FG [305450, *MED12*]

Pallister W [311450]

Pelizaeus-Merzbacher [3120800, *PLP1*]

Pettigrew [304340]

Prieto [309610]

Pyruvate Dehydrogenase Deficiency [312170, *PDHA1*]

Rett [312750, *MECP2*]

Rett-Like Seizures-Hypotonia [300672, *CDKL5 (STK9)*]

Roifman [300258]

Schimke [312840]

Simpson-Golabi-Behmel [312870, *GPC3*]

Smith-Fineman-Myers

Snyder-Robinson [309583, *SMS*]

Stoll

TARP [311900, *RBM10*]

Vasquez

Wilson-Turner [309585, *LASIL*]

Wittwer Syndrome [300421]

XLID-Ataxia-Apraxia

XLID-Hypospadias

XLID-Hypotonia-Recurrent Infections [300260, *dup MECP2*]

XLID-Psoriasis [309480]

APPENDIX XIII

XLID SYNDROMES PREDOMINANTLY AFFECTING FEMALES

Aicardi [304050]

Craniofacioskeletal [300712]

Epilepsy-Intellectual Disability in Females [300088, *PCDH19*]

Goltz [305600, *PORCN*]

Incontinentia Pigmenti [308310, *IKBKG*]

MIDAS [309801, *HCCS*]

Oral-Facial-Digital I [311200, *CXORF5*]

Periventricular Nodular Heterotopia [300049, *FLNA*]

Rett [312750, *MECP2*]

Rett-Like Seizures-Hypotonia [300672, *CDKL5*]

APPENDIX XIV

DUPLICATION OF XLID GENES AND REGIONS OF THE X-CHROMOSOME GENOME

Segmental duplications involving one or more genes on the X-chromosome have been associated with intellectual disability. In some instances, it is unclear whether the whole gene duplication, partial duplication of adjacent gene(s), or other position effect is most important in the causation of ID. In many cases of clinically important segmental duplications of the X-chromosome, marked skewing of X-inactivation has been documented in carrier females.

- **Xp22.31**. Wagenstaller et al. (Am J Hum Genet 81:738, 2007) reported a 1.4-Mb duplication in a boy with severe language delay and acquired microcephaly. The duplicated genes were *VCX3A, HDHD1A, STS, VCX, PNPLA4,* and *VCX2*. The healthy mother carried the duplication. Horn et al. (Mediz Genetik 19:62, 2007) reported similar duplications in two unrelated males with ID: one with ID and "autistic aggressive" behavior, the other with ID, hypotonia, overgrowth, hypertelorism, bifid nasal tip, long philtrum, and aggressive behavior.

- **Xp22.2-p21.3**. Two families with 69-kb duplications including *REPS2, NHS,* and *ILRAPL1* were reported by Honda et al. (J Hum Genet 55:590, 2010). The clinical findings appeared different in the two families. In the first family, a male had severe ID, infantile spasms, absent speech, and atrophy of the hippocampus. In the other family, twin boys had moderate ID, speech delay, and autistic features.

- **Xp22.13-p22.11**. A 12.5-Mb duplication of Xp22.11-p22.13 that included *AP1S2, CDKL5, SCML1, PDAA1, RPS6KA3, SMX,* and *ARX* was found in two brothers with moderate ID, hypotonia, seizures, submucus cleft palate, long face with flat midface, asthenic habitus, scoliosis, and long digits (Gijsbers et al., Clin Genet 79:71, 2011). A 3.8-Mb duplication that includes *RPS6KA3, MBTDS2,* and *SMS* in one family with Nonsyndromal XLID was reported by Whibley et al. (Am J Hum Genet 87:173, 2010).

- **Xp21.3**. A 41-kb duplication that includes *ARX* and *POLA1* (partial) has been found in one family with Nonsyndromal XLID (Whibley et al., Am J Hum Genet 87:173, 2010).

- **Xp11.3**. A 0.5-Mb duplication that includes *MAOA, MAOB,* and *NDP* was reported by Klitten et al. (Eur J Hum Genet 19:1, 2011) in a male with severe intellectual disability, intractable seizures, osteoporosis, scoliosis, friendliness, and high-pitched voice. Tzschach et al. (Am J Med Genet 146A:197, 2008) reported an inherited 9.3-Mb duplication of this area in a male with intellectual disability and seizures.

- **Xp11.3-p11.23**. A number of duplications, varying in size from 0.8 to 9.2 Mb, have been reported in this region (Froyen et al., Hum Mut 28:1034, 2007; Bonnet et al., J Hum Genet 51:815, 2006; Marshall et al., Am J Hum Genet 82:427, 2008; Giorda et al., Am J Hum Genet 85:394, 2009; El-Hattab et al., Clin Genet 79:531, 2011). Clinical findings in the 11 families and 4 males with these duplications have shown the severity of intellectual disability has varied widely as have stature, head circumference, and facial dysmorphism. A minority have had deformation of the lower limbs, hypotonia, seizures, and autistic features.

- **Xp11.22**. Froyen et al. (Am J Hum Genet 82:432, 2008) reported variable length duplications in Xp11.22 in six families with Nonsyndromal XLID, including MRX17 and MRX31. The duplications ranged in size from about 300 kb to about 800 kb. Three genes were included in the common region of duplication: *RIBC1, HSD17B10,* and *HUWE1*. Duplication of *RIBC1* was excluded as a cause of ID because it is not brain-expressed. Missense mutations in *HUWE1* were also found in three additional families with XLID. Four additional families with Nonsyndromal XLID with 400- to 1000-kb duplications of this region were reported by Whibley et al. (Am J Hum Genet 87:373, 2010). Honda et al. (J Hum Genet 55:590, 2010) reported a 1.37-Mb duplication that included *FTSJ1, PQBP1,* and *SYP* in a male with speech delay and moderate ID. His sister was said to be affected, but details were not provided. Other large duplications of this region (5.0 Mb and 4.7 Mb) have been reported by Bonnet et al. (J Hum Genet 51:815, 2006) and Flynn et al. (Am J Med Genet 155A:141, 2010).

- **Xq12-q13.1.** An 800-kb duplication that includes *OPHN1* was found in a 20-year-old male with prenatal and postnatal undergrowth, global developmental delay, hypertelorism, deep-set eyes, downslanting palpebrae, narrow nasal bridge, broad nasal tip, long philtrum, thin upper lip, thick lower lip, cupped left ear, joint laxity, truncal hypotonia, leg length asymmetry, muscular underdevelopment, and hyperreflexia. MRI showed normal posterior fossa but abnormalities of corpus callosum, cerebral white matter, internal capsules, and pontine tegmentum (Bedeschi et al., Am J Med Genet 146A:1718, 2008).

- **Xq13.2-q21.1.** A 7-Mb duplication in Xq13.2-q21.1 was found in a male with severe ID, growth retardation, and facial dysmorphism by Koolen et al. (Hum Mutat 30:283, 2009). The duplication was de novo, but no other details were provided. An 11.5-Mb duplication of Xq13.1-q21.1 that included *MED12, NLGN3, SLC16A2, KIAA2022, ATRX,* and *BRWD3* was reported in one family with unspecified syndromal manifestations (Whibley et al. Am J Hum Genet 87:173, 2010).

- **Xq21-q22.** The most common segmented duplication on the X-chromosome involves the *PLP1* gene at Xq22 and is responsible for the majority of cases of Pelizaeus-Merzbacher disease (Mimault et al., Am J Hum Genet 65:360, 1999). The duplications range in size from less than 200 kb to 1650 kb and affect adjacent genes because the *PLP1* gene spans only 17 kb (Woodward et al., Am J Hum Genet 63:207, 1998). The size of the duplication has not been correlated with clinical severity of the disease (Regis et al., Clin Genet 72:279, 2008).

- **Xq22.3.** Jehee et al. (Am J Med Genet 139A:221, 2005) described a 4-Mb duplication in Xq22.3 in a male with cognitive disability, hypotonia, trigonocephaly (premature metopic closure), upslanted palpebrae, short nose, long philtrum, hypospadias, recurrent hyperthermia, and constipation. They considered the child to have FG syndrome and designated the Xq22.3 as FGS locus 5. We consider this diagnosis to be incorrect (Schwartz and Stevenson: David W. Smith Workshop on Malformations and Morphogenesis, Mont Tremblant, Ontario, August 2008).

- **Xq24.** A 190-Mb duplication in Xq24 was reported in a male with moderate ID, macrocephaly, facial dysmorphism, hypotonia, and pectus excavatum and his normal mother by Koolen et al. (Hum Mutat 30:283, 2009). The significance was unclear.

- **Xq25.** A de novo 255-kb duplication encompassing four known genes (*BCORL1, ELF4, PDCD8,* and *RAB33A*) was identified in a female with clinical features suggestive of Rett syndrome. The patient had skewed X-inactivation with the abnormal X being preferentially active based on expression studies of the genes involved. Further studies have suggested that overexpression of *PDCD8* and *RAB33A* are most likely involved in the etiology of the clinical features in this patient (D. Cohn, personal communication).

- **Xq25-q26.3.** A 4.7-Mb duplication was found in a male with moderate ID, growth retardation, microcephaly, cleft palate, hypospadias, and cryptorchidism and his normal mother by Koolen et al. (Hum Mutat 30:283, 2009). The significance was unclear.

- **Xq27.2-q27.3.** Several families in which males have had ID and panhypopituitarism have been found to have duplications in Xq27 (Lagerström-Fermér et al., Am J Hum Genet 60:910, 1997; Hol et al., Genomics 69:174, 2000; Laumonnier et al., Am J Hum Genet 71:1450, 2002; Solomon et al., J Med Genet 41:669, 2004). The duplication critical region appears to span a 3.9-Mb interval in Xq27.2-q27.3. The duplicated region contains *SOX3*, the transcription factor known to be associated with XLID-Panhypopituitarism.

- **Xq27.3-q28.** A small duplication of about 5 Mb was identified in a family in which affected males had short stature, hypogonadism, and some facial dysmorphism (deep-set eyes, bulbous nasal tip, and thin lips) (Rio et al., Eur J Hum Genet 18:285, 2010). Some genes encompassed within the duplication are *FMR1, AFF2, IDS,* and *MTM.*

- **Xq28.** Van Esch et al. (Am J Hum Genet 77:442, 2005), Friez et al. (Pediatrics 118:e1687, 2006), Lugtenberg et al. (Eur J Hum Genet 17:444, 2009), and others have reported a number of males with ID and duplications of variable size, including and adjacent to *MECP2*. The phenotype includes severe cognitive disability (sometimes with autism or autistic manifestations), hypotonia, absent/limited speech, absent/limited ambulation, spasticity, seizures, and recurrent respiratory infections. Two previously described XLID entities, XLID-Hypotonia-Recurrent infections (Lubs et al., Am J Hum Genet 85:243, 1999) and MRX64 (Pai et al., J Med Genet 34:529, 1997), are caused by these duplications. The duplications range in size from 0.3 Mb to 2.3 Mb (Bauters et al., Genome Res 18:847, 2008). The phenotype appears related primarily to duplications of MECP2 (Van Esch et al., Am J Hum Genet 77:442, 2005; Meins et al., J Med Genet 42:e12, 2005; Kirk et al., Clin Genet 75:301, 2009; Velinou et al., Clin Dysmorphol 18:9, 2008; Smyk et al., Am J Med Genet B 147B:799, 2008).

Clayton-Smith et al. (Eur J Hum Genet 17:434, 2009) described several families in which the duplication included *SLC6A8* and *FLNA*. Affected males had intestinal pseudo-obstruction or bladder distension as additional findings.

Rosenberg et al. (J Med Genet 43:180, 2006) reported a 1.3-Mb duplication in Xq28 in a male with ID, large ears, high palate, hypoplasia of cerebellar vermis, Dandy-Walker anomaly, abdominal obesity, and flat feet. An affected maternal cousin also had the duplication.

Whibley et al. (Am J Hum Genet 87:173, 2010) have reported a 210-kb duplication that includes part of AFF2 in one family with Nonsyndromal XLID.

APPENDIX XV

X-INACTIVATION

X-chromosome inactivation (XCI) is the process by which females achieve dosage compensation with males and was originally hypothesized by Mary Lyon in 1961. Thus, females are mosaic for X-linked gene expression, with cells expressing genes from either the maternally or paternally derived X-chromosome. The inactivation of the maternal or paternal X-chromosome in an individual cell occurs at the blastocyst stage in the inner cell mass and is known as the primary choice. This process typically occurs randomly leading to a roughly 50:50 X-inactivation pattern.

XCI is initiated at the X-chromosome inactivation center and transcriptional silencing spreads because of upregulation of the *Xist* gene, which leads to the coating of the inactive X-chromosome (Xi) with the *Xist* RNA. Concomitantly, the gene *Tsix* (antisense to *Xist*) is upregulated on the active X-chromosome (Xa) and represses Xist expression on the active X. Hypoacetylated histones and hypermethylated CpG islands silence gene expression and maintain the Xi choice throughout the cell lineage. However, approximately 15% to 25% (roughly 250 to 400 genes on the Xi) may escape inactivation. The genes escaping inactivation are spread along the length of the X-chromosome, but the majority is located on the distal short arm, a region known as pseudo-autosomal region 1.

The XCI pattern is determined by evaluation of the methylation differences on the active and inactive X-chromosome. The androgen receptor (*AR*) gene contains a highly polymorphic trinucleotide (CAG) repeat for which the different repeat sizes can be easily separated and quantitated, thus making the *AR* gene ideal to determine the XCI pattern.

Skewed or nonrandom XCI is thought to occur as a secondary event caused by postinactivation cell selection, which typically confers a significant survival disadvantage to the cells containing the mutant allele. X-inactivation skewing (XIS) is defined as moderate (≥80:20) or marked (≥90:10). XIS has been described in many X-linked diseases, including X-linked dominant male-lethal disorders and some X-linked intellectual disability disorders. Although XIS has also been detected in the general female population, highly skewed XI occurs at a significantly higher frequency in carriers of XLID disorders. Plenge et al. (2002) reported that 9% of 205 control females demonstrated XIS of 80:20 and only 3% were highly skewed at 90:10, whereas 48% of carriers of an XLID condition had XIS >80:20 and 30% were highly skewed at >90:10. The frequency of XIS may vary because of tissue sampled but is substantially correlated in an individual. XIS also varies with age, and several studies have documented an increasing frequency with increasing age.

Several X-linked intellectual disability (XLID) syndromes have been associated with an increased frequency of skewing in carrier females (Tables 1 and 2 and Figure 1 of this Appendix). Conversely, there are many X-linked genes, including most of those that cause Nonsyndromal XLID, that are not associated with skewing.

Unfavorable skewing may be defined as the occurrence of preferential inactivation of the X-chromosome on which the wildtype gene is located. Unfavorable skewing may underlie the occurrence of an X-linked syndrome (Mucopolysaccharidosis II, Duchenne Muscular Dystrophy) in a heterozygous female, which is usually expressed only in males. Because these affected females are mosaic, they will typically present with a milder phenotype.

Skewed X-inactivation also occurs in carrier females of phenotypically important microduplications (e.g., dup *MECP2*) and in females that carry X-autosome translocations. In the latter, the X-chromosome involved in the translocation typically remains active to prevent inactivation of the autosome.

Although skewed X-inactivation in females represents a nonspecific finding, it may be viewed as a generally protective phenomenon. Its presence in mothers of males with intellectual disability of unknown cause strongly supports molecular investigation for an X-linked disorder.

REFERENCES

Amos-Landgraf JM, Cottle A, Plenge RM, et al.: X-chromosome inactivation patterns of 1,005 phenotypically unaffected females. Am J Hum Genet 79:493, 2006.

Brown CJ, Robinson WP: The causes and consequences of random and non-random X chromosome inactivation in humans. Clin Genet 58:353, 2000.

Lyon MF: Gene action in the X-chromosome of the mouse (Mus musculus). Nature 190:372, 1961.

Morleo M, Franco B: Dosage compensation of the mammalian X chromosome influences the phenotypic variability of X-linked dominant male-lethal disorders. J Med Genet 45:401, 2008.

Orstavik KH: X chromosome inactivation in clinical practice. Hum Genet 126:363, 2009.

Plenge RM, Stevenson RA, Lubs HA, et al.: Skewed X-chromosome inactivation is a common feature of X-linked mental retardation disorders. Am J Hum Genet 71:168, 2002.

Van den Veyver IB: Skewed X inactivation in X-Linked Disorders. Semin Reprod Med 19:183, 2001.

Figure. Location of XLID genes with skewing of X-inactivation in female carriers (left) and selected genes that typically are not skewed in female carriers (right).

TABLE 1 (APPENDIX XV). Comparison of Skewing (≥80%) of X-Inactivation in Carriers and Non-carriers of Mutations Associated with XLID

Gene	Locus	Carrier		Non-carrier		P-value**
		Skewed	Non skewed	Skewed	Non skewed	
*ACSL4 (FACL4)	Xq22.3	24	0	1	7	< 0.0001
*ATRX (XNP)	Xq21.1	23	0	2	8	< 0.0001
*CUL4B	Xq24	8	1	0	3	0.0182
*HUWE1	Xp11.22	17	11	4	4	0.0319
MED12 (R961W)	Xq13.1	9	4	2	8	0.0361
*MECP2 dup	Xq28	44	3	3	15	<0.0001
*MECP2 mut	Xq28	26	46	1	16	0.0147
*PQBP1	Xp11.23	8	3	1	11	0.0028
RPS6KA3 (RSK2)	Xp22.12	20	11	4	20	0.0004
*TIMMA8 (DDP1)	Xq22.1	10	1	5	7	0.0272
*UPF3B	Xq24	13	0	1	3	0.0059

* Indicates that marked skewing (≥90%) was noted in female carriers
** P-value is a two tailed value calculated from Fisher's exact test

TABLE 2 (APPENDIX XV). Clinical Diagnostic Matrix for Genes Associated with Skewing of X-Inactivation in Carrier Females.

Gene	Dysmorphic Facies	Abnormal Head Size	Abnormal Stature	Hypogonadism, Genital Abnormal-ities	Abnormal Tone or Movement	Seizures	Progressive Neurological Degeneration	Other
ACSL4	-	-	-	-	-	-	-	Nonsyndromal
ATRX	+	Micro	Short	+	+	+	-	-
CUL4B	-	Macro	Short	+	+	-	-	Tremor, ataxia
HUWE1	+	Micro or Macro	Short	-	+	+	-	Blepharophimosis, deafness
MED12 (R961W)	+	Macro	-	-	+	-	-	Agenesis of corpus callosum, anal anomalies, broad thumbs
MECP2 dup	-	-	-	-	+	+	+	Spasticity, recurrent infections
MECP2 mut	-	Micro (acquired)	-	-	+	+	+	Females, hand stereotypies
PQBP1	+	Micro	Short	-	+	-	-	Occasional structural anomalies
RPS6KA3	+	Micro	Short	-	+	+	-	Coarse facies, tapered fingers
TIMM8A	-	-	-	-	+	-	+	Deafness, dystonia
UPF3B	+	Macro	Tall	-	-	-	-	Marfanoid, hypernasality

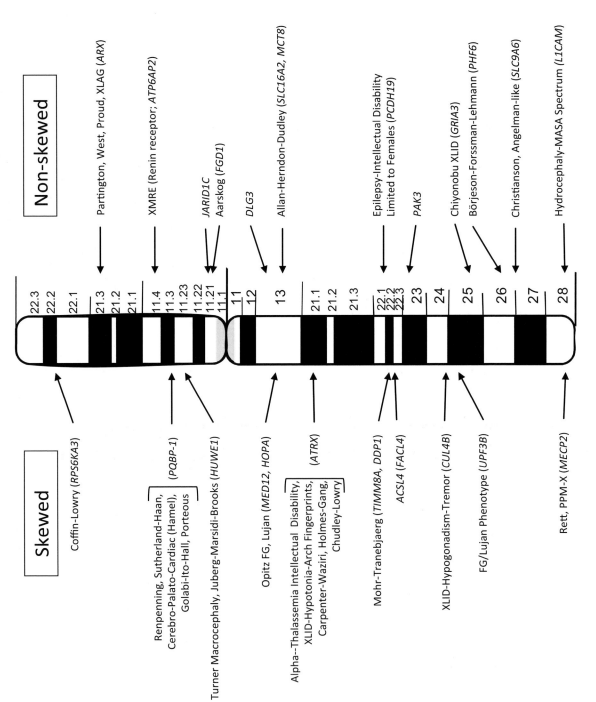

Appendix XV. Distribution of genes associated with XLID and skewed X-inactivation in carrier females is shown on the left. Selected genes associated with XLID that do not show skewed X-inactivation in carrier females are shown on the right.

APPENDIX XVI

SYNDROMAL XLID GENES

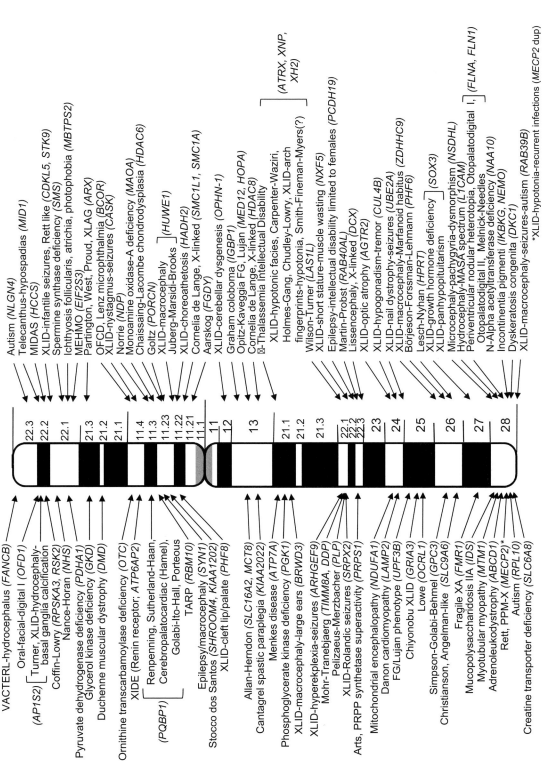

Appendix XVI Location of Genes Associated with XLID Syndromes

APPENDIX XVII

SYNDROMAL XLID (LINKAGE LIMITS)

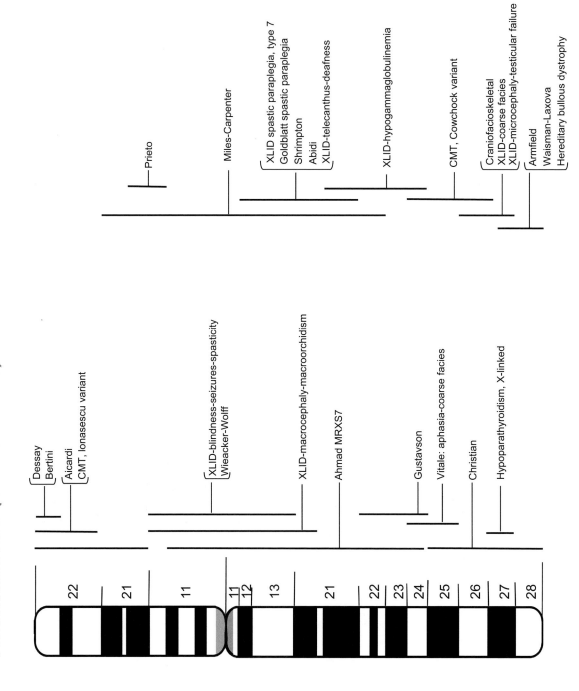

Appendix XVII. Linkage limits for loci in which the specific genes associated with XLID syndromes have not been identified.

APPENDIX XVIII

NONSYNDROMAL XLID FAMILIES

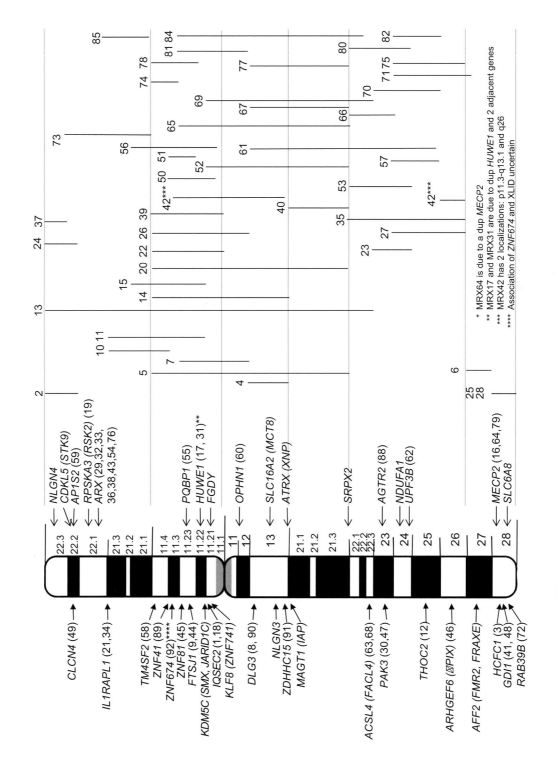

Appendix XVIII. Nonsyndromal XLID. Genes shown on the left of the X chromosome have been associated with nonsyndromal XLID; those shown on the right of the X chromosome have been associated with XLID syndromes and nonsyndromal XLID. Linkage limits shown at far right are for nonsyndromal XLID families assigned specific MRX numbers. See also (Appendix XIX)

* MRX64 is due to a dup *MECP2*
** MRX17 and MRX31 are due to dup *HUWE1* and 2 adjacent genes
*** MRX42 has 2 localizations: p11.3-q13.1 and q26
**** Association of *ZNF674* and XLID uncertain

APPENDIX XIX

NONSYNDROMAL XLID FAMILIES

Designation	Gene	Locus	Original Report	Gene Identification
MRX1	IQSEC2	Xp11.22	Suthers et al., Am J Med Genet 30:485, 1988	Shoubridge et al., Nat Genet 42:486, 2010
MRX2		Xp22.3	Proops et al., Clin Genet 23:81, 1983; Arveiler et al., Am J Med Genet 30:473, 1988; Hu et al., Am J Genet 51:569, 1994	
MRX3	HCFC1	Xq28	Gedeon et al., J Med Genet 28:372, 1991	Gecz et al. 15th International Workshop on Fragile X and Other Early-Onset Cognitive Disorders, Berlin, Sept. 4–7, 2011
MRX4		Xp11.22-Xq21.31	Arveiler et al., Am J Med Genet 30:473, 1988; Hu et al., Am J Genet 51:569, 1994	
MRX5		Xp21.1-Xq21.3	Samanns et al., Am J Med Genet 38:224, 1991	
MRX6		Xq27	Kondo et al., Cytogenet Cell Genet 58:2071, 1991	
MRX7		Xp11.23-Xq12	Jedele et al., Am J Med Genet 43:436, 1992	
MRX8	DLG3	Xq13.1	Schwartz et al., Am J Med Genet 43:467, 1992	Schwartz et al. (unpublished)
MRX9	FTSJ1	Xp11.23	Willems et al., Genomics 18:290, 1993	Ramser et al., J Med Genet 41:679, 2004
MRX10		Xp11.4-Xp21.3	Kerr et al., Am J Med Genet 43:392, 1992	
MRX11		Xp11.22-Xp21.3	Kerr et al., Am J Med Genet 43:392, 1992	
MRX12	THOC2	Xq25	Kerr et al., Am J Med Genet 43:392, 1992	Gecz, personal communication, October 2011
MRX13		Xp22.3-Xq22	Kerr et al., Am J Med Genet 43:392, 1992	
MRX14		Xp11.22-Xq12	Gendrot et al., Clin Genet 45:145, 1994	
MRX15		Xp22.1-Xq12	Moraine et al., Fifth International Workshop on Fragile X and X-Linked Mental Retardation. Strasbourg, 1991	
MRX16	MECP2	Xq28	Moraine et al., Fifth International Workshop on Fragile X and X-Linked Mental Retardation. Strasbourg, 1991	Couvert et al., Hum Mol Genet 15:941, 2002
MRX17	dup RIBC1, HSD17B10, HUWE1	Xp11.2	Gedeon et al., Am J Med Genet 51: 553, 1994	Froyen et al., Am J Hum Genet 82:432, 2008

Designation	Gene	Locus	Original Report	Gene Identification
MRX18	IQSEC2	Xp11.22	Suthers et al., Am J Med Genet 30:485, 1988	Shoubridge et al., Nat Genet 42:486, 2010
MRX19	RPS6KA3 (RSK2)	Xp22.12	Donnelly et al., Am J Med Genet 51:581, 1994	Merienne et al., Nat Genet 22:13, 1999
MRX20		Xp21.1-Xq23	Lazzarini et al., Am J Med Genet 57:552, 1995	
MRX21	IL1RAPL1	Xp22.1-Xp21.3	Kozak et al., J Med Genet 30:866, 1993	Tabolacci et al., Am J Med Genet 140A:482, 2006
MRX22		Xp11-cent	Passos-Bueno et al., Am J Med Genet 46:172, 1993	
MRX23		Xq23-Xq24	Gregg et al., Hum Mol Genet 5:411, 1996	
MRX24		Xp22.2-Xp22.3	Martinez et al., Am J Med Genet 55:387, 1995	
MRX25		Xq27.3	Nordstrom et al., Hum Genet 90:263, 1992	
MRX26		Xp11.4-Xq23	Robledo et al., Am J Med Genet 64:107, 1996	
MRX27		Xq24-Xq27.1	Glass et al., Am J Med Genet 38:240, 1991; Gedeon et al., Am J Med Genet 64:121, 1996	
MRX28		Xq27.3-qter	Holinski-Feder et al., Am J Med Genet 64:125, 1996	
MRX29	ARX	Xp21.3	Häne et al., Clin Genet 50:176, 1996	Stepp et al., BMC Med Genet 6:16, 2005
MRX30	PAK3	Xq21.3-Xq24	Donnelly et al., Am J Med Genet 64:113, 1996; Allen et al., Nat Genet 20:25, 1998	Allen et al., Nat Genet 20:25, 1998
MRX31	dup RIBC1, HSD17B10, HUWE1	Xp11.2	Donnelly et al., Am J Med Genet 64:113, 1996	Froyen et al., Am J Hum Genet 82:432, 2008
MRX32	ARX	Xp21.3	Howard-Peebles et al., Am J Hum Genet 31:214, 1979; Häne et al., Am J Med Genet 85:271, 1999	Stepp et al., BMC Med Genet 6:16, 2005
MRX33	ARX	Xp21.3	Holinski-Feder et al., Am J Med Genet 64:125, 1996	Stepp et al., BMC Med Genet 6:16, 2005
MRX34	IL1RAPL1	Xp21.3	Kozak et al., J Med Genet 30:866, 1993	Raeymaekers et al., Am J Med Genet 64:16, 1996
MRX35		Xq21.3-Xq26	Gu et al., J Med Genet 33:52, 1996	
MRX36	ARX	Xp21.3	Frints et al., Am J Med Genet 112:427, 2002	Frints et al., Am J Med Genet 112:427, 2002
MRX37		Xp22.31-Xp22.32	Bar-David et al., Am J Med Genet 64:83, 1996	
MRX38	ARX	Xp21.3	Schutz et al., Am J Med Genet 64:89, 1996	Stepp et al., BMC Med Genet 6:16, 2005
MRX39		Xp11	Teboul et al., J Genet Hum 37:179, 1989	
MRX40		Xq28	May et al., Hum Mol Genet 4:1465, 1995	
MRX41	GDI1	Xq28		D'Adamo et al., Nat Genet 19:134, 1998; Bienvenu et al., Hum Mol Genet 7:1311, 1998
MRX42		Xq24-Xq25	Holinski-Feder et al., Eighth International Workshop on Fragile X and X-Linked Mental Retardation, Picton, Canada, 1997	

(continued)

Designation	Gene	Locus	Original Report	Gene Identification
MRX43	*ARX*	Xp21.3	Hamel et al., Am J Med Genet 85:290, 1999; Hamel et al., Eighth International Workshop on Fragile X and X-Linked Mental Retardation, Picton, Canada, 1997	Bienvenu et al., Hum Mol Genet 11:981, 2002
MRX44	*FTSJ1*	Xp11.23	Hamel et al., Am J Med Genet 85:290, 1999; Hamel et al., Eighth International Workshop on Fragile X and X-Linked Mental Retardation, Picton, Canada, 1997	Freude et al., Am J Hum Genet 75:305, 2004
MRX45	*ZNF81*	Xp22.1-Xp11	Hamel et al., Am J Med Genet 85:290, 1999; Hamel et al., Eighth International Workshop on Fragile X and X-Linked Mental Retardation, Picton, Canada, 1997	Kleefstra et al., J Med Genet 41:394, 2004
MRX46	*ARHGEF6*	Xq26	Hamel et al., Eighth International Workshop on Fragile X and X-Linked Mental Retardation, Picton, Canada, 1997; Yntema et al., J Med Genet 35:801, 1998	Kutsche et al., Nat Genet 26:247, 2000
MRX47	*PAK3*	Xq21.3-Xq24	des Portes et al., Am J Med Genet 72:324, 1997	Bienvenu et al., Am J Med Genet 93:294, 2000
MRX48	*GDI1*	Xq28	des Portes et al., Am J Hum Genet 60:903, 1997	D'Adamo et al., Nat Genet 19:134, 1998; Bienvenu et al, Hum Mol Genet 7:1311, 1998
MRX49	*CLCN4*	Xp22.2	Claes et al., Am J Med Genet 73:474, 1997	Kalscheuer et al. 15th International Workshop on Fragile X and Other Early-Onset Cognitive Disorders, Berlin, Sept. 4–7, 2011
MRX50		Xp11.4-Xp11.21	Claes et al., Am J Med Genet 73:474, 1997	
MRX51		Xp11.4-Xp11.3	Claes et al., Am J Med Genet 85:283, 1997	
MRX52		Xp11.21-Xq21.32	Hamel et al., Am J Med Genet 85:290, 1999	
MRX53		Xq22.2-Xq26	Ahmad et al., Am J Med Genet 100:62, 2001	
MRX54	*ARX*	Xp21.3	Ben Jemaa et al., Am J Med Genet 85:276, 1999	Bienvenu et al., Hum Mol Genet 11:981, 2002
MRX55	*PQBP1*	Xp11.23	Deqaqi et al., Ann Genet 41:11, 1998	Kalscheuer et al., Nat Genet 35:313, 2003
MRX56		Xp21.1-Xp11.21	Holinski-Feder et al., Eighth International Workshop on Fragile X and X-Linked Mental Retardation, Picton, Canada, 1997	
MRX57		Xq24-Xq25	Holinski-Feder et al., Eighth International Workshop on Fragile X and X-Linked Mental Retardation, Picton, Canada, 1997	
MRX58	*TM4SF2*	Xq11	Holinski-Feder et al., Am J Med Genet 86:102, 1999	Zemni et al., Nat Genet 24:167, 2000
MRX59	*AP1S2*	Xp22.2	Carpenter et al., Am J Med Genet 85:266, 1999	Tarpey et al., Am J Hum Genet 79:1119, 2006
MRX60	*OPHN-1*	Xq12	Billuart et al., Nature 392:923, 1998	Billuart et al., Nature 392:923, 1998
MRX61		Xq13.1-Xq25		

(continued)

Designation	Gene	Locus	Original Report	Gene Identification
MRX62	*UPF3B*	Xq25-Xq26	Graham et al., Am J Med Genet 80:145, 1998	Laumonnier et al., Mol Psychiatry 15:767, 2010
MRX63	*ACSL4 (FACL4)*	Xq22.3	Raynaud et al., Eur J Hum Genet 8:253, 2000	Meloni et al., Nat Genet 30:436, 2002
MRX64	*dup MECP2*	Xq28	Pai et al., J Med Genet 34:529, 1997	Friez et al., Pediatrics 118:1687, 2006
MRX65		Xp11.4-Xq21.33	Yntema et al., Am J Med Genet 85:305, 1999	
MRX66		Xq21.33-Xq234		
MRX67				
MRX68	*ACSL4 (FACL4)*	Xq22.3	Longo et al., J Med Genet 40:11, 2003	Longo et al., J Med Genet 40:11, 2003
MRX69		Xp11.21-Xq22.1		
MRX70		Xq23-Xq25		
MRX71		Xq24-Xq27.1		
MRX72	*RAB39B*	Xq28	Russo et al., Am J Med Genet 94:376, 2000	Giannandrea et al., Am J Hum Genet 86:185, 2010
MRX73		Xp22-Xp21	Martinez et al., Am J Med Genet 102:200, 2001	
MRX74		Xp11.3-Xp11.4		
MRX75		Xq24-Xq26	Caspari et al., Am J Med Genet 93:290, 2000	
MRX76	*ARX*	Xp21.3		Bienvenu et al., Hum Mol Genet 11:981, 2002
MRX77		Xq12-Xq21.33	Sismani et al., Am J Med Genet 122A:46, 2003	
MRX78		Xp11.4-Xp11.23	DeVries et al., Am J Med Genet 111:443, 2002	
MRX79	*MECP2*	Xq28		Winnepenninckx et al., Hum Mutat 20:249, 2002
MRX80		Xq22-Xq24	Verot et al., Am J Med Genet 122A:37, 2003	
MRX81		Xp11.2-Xq12	Annunziata et al., Am J Med Genet 1189A:217, 2003	
MRX82		Xq24-Xq25	Martinez et al., Am J Med Genet 131A:174, 2004	
MRX83				
MRX84		Xp11.3-Xq22.3	Zhang et al., Am J Med Genet 129A:286, 2004	
MRX85		Xp21.3-Xp21.1		DeBrouwer et al., Hum Mutat 28:207, 2007
MRX86				
MRX87	*ARX*	Xp21.3		LaPeruta et al., BMC Med Genet 8:25, 2007
MRX88	*AGTR2*	Xq22-Xq23	Vervoort et al., Science 296:20401, 2002	Vervoort et al., Science 296:20401, 2002
MRX89	*ZNF41*	Xp22.1-cen	Shoichet et al., Am J Hum Genet 73:1341, 2003	Shoichet et al., Am J Hum Genet 73:1341, 2003

(continued)

Designation	Gene	Locus	Original Report	Gene Identification
MRX90	*DLG3*	17q12-q21	Makino et al., Oncogene 14:2425, 1997	Tarpey et al., Am J Hum Genet 75:318, 2004
MRX91	*ZDHHC15*	Xq13.3	Gustavson et al., Clin Genet 26:245, 1984	Mansouri et al., Eur J Hum Genet 13:970, 2005
MRX92*	*ZNF674*	Xp11	Lugtenberg et al., Am J Hum Genet 78:265, 2006	Lugtenberg et al., Am J Hum Genet 78:265, 2006
MRX93				
MRX94				
MRX95	*MAGT1/ OSTb*	Xq13.1-Xq13.2	Molinari et al., Am J Hum Genet 82:1150, 2008	Molinari et al., Am J Hum Genet 82:1150, 2008

Other genes that cause Nonsyndromal XLID:

*Association of ZNF674 and XLID considered uncertain
AFF2 (FMR2)
FGD1
NLGN4
SLC6A8
ATRX (XNP)
KDM5C (JARID1C)
CDKL5 (STK9)
SLC16A2 (MCT8)

INDEX